Orthopedic Assessment
in Massage Therapy

Dedication

To my parents, Audrey and Wade Lowe.

Orthopedic Assessment in Massage Therapy

Whitney Lowe, LMT

Director
Orthopedic Massage Education &
Research Institute www.omeri.com

Forewords by

Benny Vaughn, LMT, ATC, CSCS

Director
Texas Athletic Therapy Center
Fort Worth, TX

Judith DeLany, LMT

Director
NeuroMuscular Therapy Center
St. Petersburg, FL

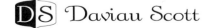

Daviau Scott Publishers
PO Box 3500, PMB 409
Sisters, OR 97759

Printed in the United States of America

ISBN 0-9661196-3-0

Library of Congress Control Number: 2005908840
Catalogue information is available from the Library of Congress

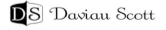 Daviau Scott

To order additional texts please contact the
distributor at www.omeri.com or 888-340-1614.

Whitney Lowe has done it again! He has written another exceptional text that improves on his previous book of assessment skills for the massage therapist. In his new textbook, Lowe presents the most updated and referenced information on orthopedic assessment as it applies to massage therapy. The role of orthopedic assessment skills is critical and absolutely necessary to determine the best massage therapy strategy for optimum results. Assessment is one of the key factors to moving massage therapy into the health care delivery system as a treatment option for soft-tissue conditions. Lowe's book will improve the practitioner's treatment effectiveness and aid in their ability to provide therapeutic care.

Lowe does an excellent job of organizing the text materials for easy referencing of specific subject areas, making this textbook a great, user-friendly manual for either the working therapist or student. His detailed description of assessment techniques and the symptoms often associated with soft-tissue conditions, allows the massage therapist to recognize when a certain orthopedic presentation requires further attention from other medical, health, and fitness professionals.

The sign of a true professional is not only knowing *when to* but knowing *when not to* provide treatment. Knowing *when to* is dependent on how well the professional massage therapist can assess the client's complaint. This, in turn, allows the massage therapist to improve their effectiveness and ensure that the client's primary complaint is addressed.

Lowe's writing is exceptional and takes complex, science-based, outcome-generated orthopedic assessment information and makes it relative to the professional massage therapist. Yet, his writing style is easy to understand. He covers key elements of orthopedic assessment including a review of function, movement, and the contributing factors that interfere with biomechanics and function.

All the right things have been done in this text to present and teach the techniques of assessment and the biomechanical considerations for soft tissue complaints. A generous number of charts and diagrams are provided to assist in understanding. Lowe's assessment approach can advance the practitioners' massage therapy skills to a new level, allowing them to produce effective results and outcomes. Massage therapists, regardless of their chosen style of work, should invest in their orthopedic assessment skills knowledge by adding Whitney Lowe's books to their libraries.

Benny Vaughn LMT, ATC, CSCS
Fort Worth, TX USA
May 2006

Complementary (integrative) medicine emerged gradually over the last decade to become a part of primary healthcare throughout the world. The gap between traditional medicine and other modalities previously thought of as alternative has now been bridged by the effort of those who have attempted to explain them, to conduct research to support their efficacy and to provide comprehensive, well designed trainings to ensure competency in practice. The success of multidisciplinary approaches in patient care has prompted the development of numerous clinics worldwide, each seeking to interface multiple practitioners' efforts in order to achieve a more positive outcome and more long lasting result.

The field of massage therapy has only recently been received into the more traditional medical settings, despite the fact that it has been incorporated in wellness approaches for hundreds of years in some cultures. Massage-related research now shows (and will continue to clarify) evidence of the effects of massage on the various systems of the body, including lymph, endocrine, nervous, and, of course, musculoskeletal. As this research becomes more focused, we will see clearer pictures of how, when and why massage therapy gains results and begin to discern its effectiveness with particular conditions, such as numerous orthopedic disorders, migraine headaches, fibromyalgia, referred pain and other chronic (often debilitating) conditions. New precautions and contraindications may emerge as we begin to understand more about the application of massage for serious diseases - cancer patients, chemotherapy patients, and those with AIDS and other dangerously harmful pathologies. It is important that all those who are practicing massage therapy base their work on current knowledge – the depth of which is growing at an alarming rate.

In order to practice competently within this medically oriented arena, a firm foundation in anatomy, physiology and functional biomechanics, as well as exceptional manual therapy training and practical experience, are required. The acquisition of skills and the development of the ability to comprehend complex conditions should initially come from massage school training. Unfortunately, there is no worldwide or even national standardization of training that will insure that practitioners are capable of assessing a region or a condition to determine if they should proceed or if they should refer the patient to another practitioner. To which type of physician they should refer is yet another unresolved problem. This is not the fault of the practitioners nor perhaps even of the schools that trained them. The base training in the field of massage therapy has simply not yet caught up with the practical application of massage therapy in medical settings.

This may seem like the cart is before the horse; however, it is apparent that both the horse (massage education) and the cart (the emergence of medically-oriented massage) have been on a fast-paced, bumpy ride of long duration. Massage therapy education has experienced a huge evolution in the last decade. What was once an industry of individual, privately owned schools, each with its own focus of preferred modalities and styles, now also includes large corporations with ownership of multiple schools as well as colleges with degree programs. Associate (USA), bachelor (England) and master (under development in Ireland) programs have been implemented or are rapidly being developed to include massage therapy and to carry the field into new realms of professional status. As these programs have emerged, standards of education, requirements toward state licensure and a push toward national certification have also occurred out of necessity, bringing with them all the benefits as well as the perils of professional progress.

During this time, Whitney Lowe has been an integral part of massage therapy's growth and development. Lowe completed his massage therapy basic education in 1988, in an era in which the massage field was still quite immature in the US and practically non-existent within medical settings. After enhancing his massage therapy education, including obtaining certifications in neuromuscular therapy and sports massage, he began working in the orthopedic field at Emory Clinic Sports Medicine Center in Atlanta, Georgia. Lowe has taught for 17 years in the massage school setting and in his own continuing education seminars, as well as presented at state and national conventions and conferences throughout the US. As a leader who helped integrate massage into medical settings he also served as a member of American Massage Therapy Association Sports Massage Education Council (1995-96), a member of the Health Care Professionals Advisory Committee, American Medical Association CPT Panel, and director for three years and chairperson for

one year for National Certification Board for Therapeutic Massage & Bodywork. In each of these positions he was able to both propel and steer the massage therapy field's professional maturation.

Since its inception in 1996, Lowe has served as a member of the editorial advisory board of peer-reviewed Journal of Bodywork & Movement Therapies as well as being a contributing author to that journal and to magazines and other journals. He has strived through these efforts to bring the standards of published materials on manual therapies into a more academic model. With these goals in mind Lowe has now given us a yet another valuable text as a contribution that can both validate medically oriented massage therapy as well as significantly alter massage therapy education.

Lowe's first assessment text was a culmination of Lowe's extensive experience in education and service. It was a valiant effort to provide massage therapy with more than just an overview of orthopedic assessment – it offered massage therapists in medical settings comprehensive guidelines for practice. How could one improve on such a fine text? Teach with the book and see what happens! In doing so, what happened for Lowe was the eruption of a passion, almost obsession, for assisting practitioners in developing clinical reasoning. He realized that no recipe, no routine could help the practitioner know how to treat common orthopedic conditions. Specifically, how and why particular techniques are useful, what symptoms mean and when a particular approach is needed. With Lowe's sheer determination that is evident in these pages, this text integrates traditional orthopedic methodology (HOPRS) into massage therapy, offers clear steps in clinical reasoning and differential evaluations, and, coupled with better explanations of biomechanics, helps to clarify what assessment can evidence for the practitioner. The chapters move region by region through the body, with each chapter offering discussions of common injuries, pathologies and syndromes that might be encountered within the region. It now stands as an equal assessment companion to the more treatment oriented Orthopedic Massage: Theory and Technique.

This text makes a significant contribution to the integration of massage therapy into medical and athletic settings. It fills a big gap in foundational knowledge and is a valuable tool for massage educators, both in massage school and in continuing education. For practitioners who seek to understand the functions and dysfunctions of the musculoskeletal frame, this book is a gem – not in the rough – but smoothly polished to greatly enhance skill and understanding.

Judith DeLany
St. Petersburg, Florida
2006

Massage therapy has seen phenomenal growth over the last twenty years and is now poised to become a part of mainstream Western medicine, although it has been used as a medical treatment in many cultures around the world for hundreds of years. Repetitive motion disorders, chronic stress, and sports-related injuries have become a fertile ground for innovative approaches of soft-tissue manipulation. Massage therapy has tremendous potential for treating numerous soft-tissue orthopedic problems and can help address the epidemic of soft-tissue pain and injury problems that currently overwhelm our health care system.

Massage is in a unique position to fill a gap in our medical system regarding musculoskeletal disorder treatment. Currently there is an emphasis on drugs and surgery as treatment approaches for many orthopedic disorders. While those treatments certainly have their place, the majority of musculoskeletal disorders are in many cases better treated with conservative approaches, such as massage. Although oriented toward massage practitioners, this text is designed to be a resource for anyone using soft-tissue treatments to treat orthopedic problems, regardless of specialty.

Massage therapy is frequently mentioned in the popular media and in discussions of complementary and alternative medicine. As a result, most people today consider massage a viable option for addressing the numerous aches and pains of soft-tissue disorders. Massage is included in basic wellness programs, hospital care, and used for stress reduction and treatment of a wide variety of conditions. While pain and injury treatment with massage started with an emphasis in athletics, it has expanded to include dysfunction arising from a variety of occupational, recreational, and daily activities.

As massage emerges as a viable treatment option, the client's expectations also increase. The client who reads about the positive aspects of massage treatment in the popular magazines will want that experience when he or she goes to see a massage therapist. The modern day massage practitioner must be armed with greater diversity and depth of knowledge, skills, and abilities to meet society's new demands. There are no recipes or formulas for this treatment; effective care requires addressing client complaints with adequate training and clinical skills.

As the professional landscape expands into greater responsibilities for massage therapists as health care providers, the educational preparation of practitioners must also improve. Massage therapy training programs must prepare students for these new challenges. While not every massage student will want to pursue clinical or medically-oriented massage approaches, familiarity with basic concepts of assessment is a fundamental skill that is valuable for all practitioners.

Even those clients who come for relaxation or wellness massage may describe a soft-tissue disorder they would like to have addressed. Without some form of assessment it is difficult, if not impossible, for the practitioner to make a sound decision about how, or if, a client should be treated. This is one of the most important reasons why assessment skills should be taught in entry-level massage training programs.

Until recently, orthopedic assessment has not been adequately addressed in training programs in part because educators and practitioners misunderstand the concept of assessment. Unfortunately some confuse assessment with diagnosis, and in an attempt not to violate massage's scope of practice, they shy away from any form of clinical information gathering that is essential for safe and effective practice. While it is out of the legal scope of practice for massage therapists to diagnose conditions, assessment is not diagnosis. A physician's diagnosis integrates assessment to make a final conclusion about a patient's pathology or condition. Massage assessment attempts to identify the tissues involved and their potential dysfunction in order to properly treat the client's pain or impairment.

There are a number of exceptional textbooks on orthopedic assessment. However, most orthopedic assessment texts are far too detailed and complicated for the needs of the massage practitioner. The depth and cost of these texts makes them fairly inaccessible to the entry-level massage student. In addition, the field of massage therapy is unique enough that an orthopedic assessment text written specifically for the massage therapist is beneficial. *Orthopedic Assessment in Massage Therapy* is based on established assessment protocols, but is focused on the information and skills that will be most used by the massage practitioner.

The OAMT is uniquely organized and has a significantly different format from other orthopedic assessment texts. Most assessment textbooks provide general information about evaluation of a joint region and then follow up with a series of special orthopedic tests. An approach like this can be helpful as a comprehensive atlas of orthopedic testing procedures. However, it can also cause the individual to run through a virtual laundry list of tests in an attempt to find the nature of the client's pathology without cultivating a broader clinical picture. Developing the complex critical thinking necessary for skillful orthopedic assessment requires that many aspects of the evaluation process be considered in unison.

To provide a larger framework that encourages clinical reasoning development, this book is structured with a unique format. The text is organized regionally, and then by the conditions commonly seen in the massage setting. The conditions are then organized into the HOPRS format. This organization provides for easier learning and allows the reader to better understand how HOPRS concepts might actually be applied. Students and practitioners gain greater clinical reasoning and critical thinking skills as a result of this 'applied' type of learning.

While a great deal of information about evaluating orthopedic conditions is presented in this text, the reader is encouraged to remember that not every soft-tissue pain is an orthopedic disorder. Specialized study or interest in the field of orthopedics may cause us to think of orthopedic problems first. However, it is essential to remember that the client's pain complaint may be something other than a common orthopedic disorder, such as a tumor, systemic disease, viscerosomatic reflex, or other pathology. It is standard of professional practice to refer a client when it is possible that a more serious condition is involved or when treatment may be contraindicated.

The human body is an amazing marvel of structure, biomechanics, and neurophysiological integration. Unfortunately, the demands of the modern world often put us at odds with the tissues of our movement system. It is my sincere hope that practitioners will use the information contained within this text to sharpen their clinical skills and in the process help ease some of the physical pain that plagues so many people today.

Whitney Lowe
Sisters, OR

Acknowledgments

Putting together a book is a monumental task that by necessity involves many individuals. While the author gets the primary credit, the finished product is highly dependent on the crucial contributions of many individuals. I am indebted to Alexandra Hamer and others who spent countless hours proofreading the text and graphics for accuracy and clarity.

Having been in this profession for a number of years I have developed friendships with colleagues whose work I greatly respect and who have influenced this project as well. While there are too many to name in this small space, in particular I would like to offer special thanks to Judith Delany and Benny Vaughn for their contributions of the forewords. Also thanks to Bob King, David Kent, Leon Chaitow, and Erik Dalton for a number of good ideas along the way. A well designed reference text must also be influenced by the perspective of the educator. Special thanks to Rick Garbowski for his constant input and guidance on how to make this book an effective teaching tool.

The graphic design of this text is greatly aided by the outstanding anatomical images provided by Primal Pictures in London as well as those from Lippincott Williams & Wilkins. Thanks to all those that participated in these various photo shoots. Finally I owe a particular debt of gratitude to the thousands of students, educators, and professional massage practitioners I have had the opportunity to work with throughout my career. It is from all of your contributions, questions, and discussions that my insights about massage have developed and grown.

Contents

1 Introduction to Assessment

Clients increasingly turn to soft-tissue treatment for musculoskeletal pain and injuries as an alternative to mainstream interventions because of value and effectiveness. Consequently, massage treatment of soft-tissue pain and injury conditions increased dramatically in the last decade and has become one of the most frequently used methods of complementary and alternative medicine in the United States. Massage is used not only by the massage practitioner, but also nurses, chiropractors, physical therapists, athletic trainers, occupational therapists, and osteopathic physicians.

The majority of these problems are minor musculoskeletal disorders or pain conditions that do not require surgery. Massage therapy is a valuable complement to traditional treatment methods that focus on rest, exercise, rehabilitation, and activity modification. From everyday aches and pains to soft-tissue disorders and injuries, massage is an effective method of treatment.

For massage to provide these beneficial effects, the practitioner must be adequately trained. To move beyond relaxation massage to more advanced applications, the practitioner's skill base, knowledge, and experience must increase accordingly. Practitioners choosing spa or relaxation oriented practices are also encouraged to adopt assessment protocols to provide improved treatment. Learning assessment is a prerequisite for providing safe, effective, and targeted advanced massage therapy.

Orthopedic Assessment in Massage Therapy (OAMT) provides the first half of the training required to treat minor musculoskeletal pain and injuries – assessment. This aspect of the massage approach is a mandatory step, without which treatment would be a guessing game. The second half of training, advanced massage techniques and their application and effects, is presented in the companion text, *Orthopedic Massage: Theory and Technique.*

While a great deal of information about evaluating orthopedic conditions is presented in the OAMT text, the reader is encouraged to remember that not every soft-tissue pain is an orthopedic disorder. It is essential to remember that the client's pain complaint may be something other than a common orthopedic disorder, such as a tumor, systemic disease, viscerosomatic reflex, or other pathology. It is standard professional practice to refer the client when it is possible that a more serious condition is involved or when treatment may be contraindicated.

What is Orthopedic Assessment?

Why Do I Need This?

Assessment is an evaluation process - a systematic process of gathering information. Without knowing this information, treatment would be based on assumptions, not clinical reasoning. Assessment performs the following important functions:

- Indicates which tissues are most likely involved.
- Indicates the status of the involved tissues.
- Directs the choice of most appropriate treatment.
- Helps determine progress toward treatment goals.
- Determines if a client's condition falls within your scope of practice and expertise.
- Helps distinguish between conditions that present with similar symptoms.

Even with a physician's diagnosis, the practitioner is wise to perform their own evaluation in order to inform their treatment. Additionally, treatment should not be considered predetermined recipes. Rather, the individual characteristics of the client's condition should be explored for nuances that may alter the treatment protocol.

Orthopedic Assessment

Orthopedic assessment is the evaluation of soft-tissue pain and injury conditions which fall into the classification of *orthopedic conditions*. The field of orthopedics is the medical specialty that deals with the primary tissues that create or limit movement in the body (locomotor tissues). Rather than being only about the skeleton, as sometimes thought, *orthopedics involves the entire musculoskeletal system, which includes muscle, nerves, fascia, tendon, ligaments, joints, and cartilage.* Orthopedic conditions result from any number of activities and range from mild pain to cumulated trauma disorders (repetitive stress) to acute injury and/or chronic pain conditions.

Assessment VS. Diagnosis

There is a distinct difference between assessment and diagnosis. A medical diagnosis is the *identification of a disease, illness, or condition made by a licensed medical professional.* A physician uses information gathered during assessment--along with other test results--to make a diagnosis. But the process of assessment, in and of itself, is not a diagnosis. Instead, whether performed by a physician or a massage therapist, assessment is simply a process of information-gathering which the practitioner uses to develop a treatment plan.

Massage practitioners do not have the scope of practice to make diagnoses. It is important for the practitioner to avoid telling the client they have a particular condition when no medical diagnosis has been performed. However, identifying the tissues involved and assessing their dysfunction is within the scope of practice for massage and a necessary function for proper treatment.

Learning to speak to the client in terms of tissues, function, and location is best. (For example: 'possible median nerve impingement in the carpal tunnel' vs. 'carpal tunnel syndrome'). This may feel awkward at first, but learning to articulate conditions in this manner actually trains one to think about tissues and their complexity, rather than boiling down a client's condition to code words and recipes.

Benefits and Function of Assessment

Assessment is a process of gathering information, from which the data is then used to make clinical decisions about treatment. It is an ongoing process that continues throughout the duration of the treatment(s). The basic rule of assessment is to 'rule out, not in'. Because one cannot know the true nature of a client's complaint until evaluation occurs, one starts with a broad perspective. As the assessment (HOPRS, Box 1.2) proceeds, tissues and pathologies that don't fit the evaluation results or symptoms are ruled out. Evaluation narrows the possibilities and reveals the tissues involved or dysfunctional.

Several functions are provided in an assessment:

1.   The most important reason for the massage practitioner to perform assessment is *to determine if massage therapy is appropriate.* Massage is not benign; it can produce significant tissue changes, which is why it functions as a form of soft-tissue treatment. Ordinarily, these changes are positive. However, massage can be contraindicated and the practitioner must be able to apply clinical reasoning to determine what results will likely come from massage, and if these are desired.

2.   Initial evaluation *assesses the severity of a condition.* Practitioners should refer clients whose pain or injuries need evaluation by another healthcare professional. Practitioners should also refer if their skill base or knowledge is not sufficient for a particular client's treatment. It is the responsibility of the practitioner to know his or her therapeutic limitations and capabilities.

BOX 1.1   BENEFITS OF ORTHOPEDIC MASSAGE

Information derived from assessment is used to develop an appropriate treatment plan and provides a baseline in which to gauge treatment results and their effectiveness.

General & initial questions answered by assessment

   Is massage appropriate?

   Could massage treatment be contraindicated?

   How severe or serious does the problem appear?

   Should the client be referred?

   Can the practitioner help the client?

Information gained from assessment

   What are the clients symptoms?

   What is the client's history?

   What is the client's pain experience and level?

   What tissues are involved in the problem?

   How are the tissues involved?

   What biomechanical forces are in play?

   What are the structural aspects of the problem?

   What type of tissue damage has occurred, if any?

Questions regarding the treatment plan

   What type of treatment does the condition call for?

   What treatment goals are reasonable to expect?

   How is the treatment progressing?

   Is the approach effective, is it resolving symptoms?

   Is the condition stabalizing? Is this the goal?

   Are there any negative results from treatment?

   What new findings has the practitioner found?

   Is treatment still appropriate?

   Does the client need referring?

   Does the treatment plan need adapting?

   Can treatment be improved?

---

3.   Assessment is primarily used to *determine the tissues or structures involved and estimate their status.* Massage treatment aims at reducing symptoms by addressing the causes. In the least, the practitioner determines whether the tissues involved are muscle, fascia, tendon, ligament, capsular, etc. In addition, the practitioner will evaluate the type of dysfunction in the tissue (tear, hypertonicity, myofascial trigger point, nerve conduction impairment, etc.). Along these lines, the biomechanical forces that produce these tissue effects are estimated, for example compressive load, excess tensile load, repetitive stress, and so forth. Without the diagnostic tools used by physicians, massage practitioners can never be fully sure about

the nature of the client's condition. However, a basic idea can be formed that allows the practitioner to create a clinically reasoned treatment plan.

4.   Assessment also *gauges the client's pain levels and symptoms*. Evaluation allows the practitioner to get to know the client's symptoms: pain levels and locations, movement restrictions, and other symptoms. This information drives treatment choices such as what techniques to use and how, when, and what intensity level. It also allows the practitioner to gauge treatment progress.

5.   The assessment process *builds the client/therapist relationship* and in-treatment questions help the practitioner keep track of the client's experience. In addition, the practitioner will develop a better understanding of the client's pain levels, threshold, and locations. A practitioner who spends a little time creating a therapeutic and communicatively open environment with the client will have better results.

6.   Initial evaluation *provides a baseline against which progress can be measured*. Throughout the duration of treatment - both within a single session and among multiple sessions - ongoing assessment monitors the client's responses to the treatment. It allows the practitioner to establish whether the treatment needs adapting or is proving to be beneficial. If the client has been referred, ongoing assessment can produce new findings or results which can then be shared with the referring physician.

Caveats to Assessment

An important caveat with assessment is that it is *not an exact science*. There are no specific evaluation techniques that can provide a 100% positive result in establishing the tissues and dysfunction involved. In some cases the nature of the client's pain is fairly straightforward. In other cases, assessment becomes an ongoing investigation that can result in changes in treatment. For example, with neck and arm pain it might be fairly easy to establish that the client has hypertonicity in the upper back and neck from doing a repetitive task. But if the client has irregular arm symptoms of paresthesia and numbness, treatment will require more thought and evaluation.

It is extremely *important that immediate assumptions are not made*. Numerous conditions have symptoms that mimic each other. Distinguishing between conditions with similar symptoms and presentations is paramount for effective treatment.

In some cases a reason for the client's complaint simply cannot be established. Regardless of experience or knowledge, the practitioner may not always be able to find a reason for their client's symptoms. In this case, continual exploration and monitoring, and thinking outside of the box are the best approaches. If treatment is not working and the primary symptoms continue, referral to a more experienced healthcare professional may be advised.

Orthopedic assessment skills are developed and require practice. Recent massage therapy graduates or

---

> ### Box 1.2 Components of Orthopedic Assessment
>
> The established orthopedic assessment approach referred to as HOPRS provides the structure for massage assessment in this text (see Chapter 3).
>
> H - History
> O - Observation
> P - Palpation
> R - Range-of-motion & Resistive Tests
> S - Special Orthopedic Tests

---

those with less experience will need to learn these new skills just as they did their entry level training skills. With practice, practitioners will become more at ease in applying these procedures. Practitioners with more healthcare or massage experience will find the learning process and integrating these techniques into their practice easier.

Students and practitioners will learn to combine their knowledge about tissues, pathology and conditions, with appropriate treatment approaches and critical thinking skills in their clinical practice. This text provides the practitioner a path toward those goals.

Integrating Assessment

Integrating assessment into massage practice can feel awkward at first. But like any new skill, practice will improve efficiency and comfort. Practitioners often find that their client's are greatly appreciative and impressed by the care shown to them through assessment.

Assessment has a wide range of applications, from the simplest and quick inquiry to full-length testing. The practitioner will determine the extent of the assessment needed through the initial interview and history. Use these tips to help determine how and when to use these new skills:

1.   *Why is the client seeking massage?* The client may have a predetermined goal. Is that goal simple relaxation or treatment for a specific complaint? The initial interview, palpation, and history will reveal the level to which an assessment is advised. If none is, or if the request is for relaxation therapy, then put testing aside and focus on evaluating the client's tissues as you perform treatment.

2.   If the client is seeking more specified treatment or their history reveals the potential for a pain and injury pathology, then *it is the role of the professional practitioner to advise the client on the benefits of further evaluation*.

3.   *Follow the HOPRS protocol and system* laid out in this text. Begin with interview and history, but then move on to palpation and basic tests. Use special tests only if they are truly warranted. Don't skip range-of-motion testing in favor of special tests! The work horses of assessment

are these basic tests. They often provide more information than the special tests.

4.   *Assessment often does not require a lengthy testing process.* In many cases a full blown assessment may not be necessary. Experience will allow one to quickly jump to the appropriate assessment protocols. Take more time with the challenging conditions. Efficiency is the goal.

5.   Remember that *assessment is a skill*. Using the skills improves one's understanding of musculoskeletal conditions overall. With continued use and practice, assessments become more efficient and smooth.

6.   In time, connections will be noted between various signs and symptoms and the investigation will almost lead itself in many cases. At the beginning it will be difficult to know which clues are most relevant and which ones are not. This is where experience will come in to play. *After seeing similar conditions a number of times, the practitioner has an experiential background against which to see similar patterns* and know that a particular case has similarities to another. As knowledge is combined with experience the nature of the client's complaint is more accurately and quickly discovered.

Clinical Reasoning

The evaluation process is not about absolutes. There may be alternate interpretations of any clinical case and a number of different ways to proceed with treatment for most conditions. Having an open mind and being able to reflect and question oneself when faced with more complex conditions is an important part of advanced work.

The practitioner's eventual success relies strongly on their development of clinical reasoning skills. *Clinical reasoning is the ability to reflect upon and analyze gained information and make reasonable conclusions or decisions.* In assessment, it is the ability to answer the critical questions about the client's condition and treatment.

Clinical reasoning questions would include:
- What happened?
- What tissues are likely involved?
- How or what forces were involved in the injury?
- How are the tissues involved?
- What is the physiological nature of the condition?
- What is the rehabilitation process for the injury?
- What role would soft-tissue treatment play?
- What is the physiological nature of the treatment?
- Why would the chosen treatment work? How?

To answer these questions, familiarity with common conditions and their presentation along with a working knowledge of anatomy, physiology, and kinesiology is fundamental. In addition, equal knowledge of treatment techniques, how they work and *why*, is necessary.

Remember that any client may have a combination of different factors or conditions present. Because various conditions can occur simultaneously or mimic each other, the clinical reasoning process in assessment is a crucial skill for safe and effective treatment.

Poorly evaluated conditions can result in inaccurate or inappropriate treatment. At the least the treatment may be ineffective; at the worst it could harm the client. The result of not engaging assessment or clinical reasoning skills may also lead a practitioner to miss the need for referral to another health professional. This error could have serious consequences for the client's health.

How to use this book

This book streamlines the process of interpreting the large quantity of information that comes from assessment. Follow these basic guidelines to best use this text..

To understand soft-tissue injuries it is essential to understand how the tissues function in a healthy state as well as when they are injured, this is found in Chapter 2. The information in this chapter forms the groundwork for understanding the entire process of assessment.

Chapter 3 presents the HOPRS system, which is used as the framework for soft-tissue assessment in this text.

The remaining chapters cover the major regions of the body. The wealth of information on soft-tissue disorders is organized into discrete conditions in order to provide a structure to aid learning and understanding. Each soft-tissue pathology is structured in the HOPRS format so the user can learn about it in the same process as it is evaluated in the clinic.

Each regional chapter includes these elements:
- Primary single plane movements of that body region.
- Condition overview and characteristics.
- HOPRS aspects of the conditions.
- Suggestions for treatment.

In addition, reference charts are provided to make looking up information easy while in the clinic:
- Primary muscle actions in single plane movements. Knowing the basic muscle actions is essential for evaluating pain with particular movements.
- Charts of major nerve trunks of the region and the muscles innervated by them.
- Charts of manual resistive tests most effective for emphasizing a particular muscle, the associated nerve root, and related primary motor nerve trunk. Knowing these greatly aids in interpreting neurological dysfunction as well as muscle and tendon injury.

There is much information to digest regarding the numerous orthopedic soft-tissue pain and injury conditions. By no means should one expect to remember it all. Keep the text handy and use it as a reference tool to help guide clinical treatment decisions.

Soft-tissue evaluation forms the basis of any successful clinical massage treatment. Like a carpenter who must know how to use his or her tools appropriately, successful application of assessment principles sets the stage for the practitioner to be far more successful in treating both common conditions and advanced injuries or pain.

2 The Soft Tissues

Effective treatment of orthopedic disorders requires a working knowledge of the primary soft tissues of the body. Understanding how these tissues function under normal circumstances is essential for evaluating soft-tissue dysfunction. With an understanding of normal function one can advance to evaluating tissues that are in a pathological state.

This chapter provides a brief discussion of the anatomy and physiology of the major soft tissues involved in locomotion as they function under normal circumstances. The anatomy and physiology sections are followed by descriptions of primary tissue dysfunctions. Dysfunction is discussed below in general terms and further exploration of these conditions is found in Chapter 4. The initial anatomy, physiology, and pathology information provided here is necessary for understanding the soft-tissue conditions discussed in Chapters 5-11.

Understanding Soft-Tissue Pathology

Pain or discomfort is the primary reason that clients seek treatment from a massage therapist. Pain, whether significant or mild, is an indicator of pathology or disturbance to normal function in the painful area. Pain can also be referred from a site of dysfunction in another area. Pain and injury conditions can be acute or chronic. An **acute** problem occurs immediately after an offending or traumatizing action. The link between the event and pain onset is direct. An example is stepping off a curb and twisting the ankle. The cause of an acute injury is easier to identify because the person usually remembers significant details about the event. These details are crucial for determining appropriate care.

With **chronic** dysfunction, there is a repetitive or prolonged stress of structures that eventually leads to degeneration or dysfunction. This stress can happen over a short or long period of time (for example, several years in postural dysfunction). The primary characteristic is that a single movement does not produce the disorder, but a cumulative effect of many movements or long periods of stress overtax the structures involved. An example is low back pain that results from long periods of muscle tightness in the lumbar muscles. Chronic injuries or pain conditions can be challenging to assess because it is harder to pinpoint their exact cause.

FORMS OF TISSUE DISRUPTION

Soft-tissue orthopedic pathologies are produced by either **mechanical disruption of tissue, neurological dysfunction,** or a combination of both. Soft-tissue disorders often have components of both mechanical and neurological impairment and treatment decisions must address both. **Conditions that involve neurological dysfunction are characterized by errors in signal processing within the central nervous system (CNS) and peripheral nervous system (PNS)**. In simple terms, the neurological system is a central information processing station (the CNS) with relay lines sending signals to and from the distant parts of the body (the PNS). Signals that go away from the CNS, known as efferent signals, produce muscle contraction. Signals that report from the PNS back to the CNS, known as afferent signals, provide feedback information to the brain about pressure, temperature, pain, or position in space.

Dysfunctional signal transmission in either the CNS or PNS can create altered neuromuscular function even in the absence of adverse mechanical forces. If there are excessive neurological motor signals, hypertonic muscles or myofascial trigger points can develop. When there is motor signal deficiency, muscle atrophy results. In either case, the involved tissues may not sustain any mechanical damage. Alterations in signal transmission can also elicit sensory symptoms. Causative factors that produce neurological dysfunction without mechanical involvement include systemic disorders, nutritional imbalance, stimulant intake (such as caffeine), or postural adaptation.

Soft-tissue injuries result from mechanical forces that overwhelm the strength and resilience of the tissue(s). As a result there is disruption to the continuity of the tissue as it compresses, stretches, tears, breaks, or chips. The human body is affected by five mechanical forces: compression, tension, torsion, bending, and shear. Almost all soft-tissue injuries occur from compression or tension (or a combination). Nerve tissue is also susceptible to mechanical force injuries. Although the symptoms may be neurological, the source of the disorder can be mechanical in nature.

Due to their pliability soft tissues are not damaged by most of the forces to which they are exposed. Mechanical disruption injury results only when soft tissues are exposed to high force loads or a force load that is applied repetitively. For repetitive motion to produce soft-tissue injury the force load does not have to be large. For example, a small tensile load on the common wrist extensor tendons might not cause any damage, but the same small force load applied dozens of times every day during an occupational activity can easily cause a breakdown in the collagen matrix of the tendon and lead to tendinosis. This repetitive breakdown process is what happens in cumulative trauma disorders (CTDs) and repetitive stress injuries (RSIs), such as lateral epicondylitis or rotator cuff tendinosis.

Types of Mechanical Forces
Compression
When structures are pressed together they exert a force against each other. When that force is greater than the integrity of the tissue(s) involved, structural breakdown occurs. Compression injuries develop from sudden, direct impacts or chronic pressure over long periods. Examples of acute compression injury include contusions, meniscal damage, and acute ulnar neuropathy. Chronic compression disorders include shoulder impingement syndrome, olecranon bursitis, a chronic herniated nucleus pulposus, and nerve compression syndromes.

Tension
Tension, also called tensile stress, is a pulling force applied to one or more tissues. A tensile stress injury develops when a force pulls two ends of a tissue away from each other. In tensile stress injuries most tissues stretch to some degree before they tear. Muscle strains, tendinosis, and ligament sprains are examples of tensile stress disorders. Tarsal tunnel syndrome or adverse sciatic nerve tension are nerve dysfunctions produced by excessive tensile stress to the nerve.

Shear
Shear is a sliding force between two tissues and produces excess friction. A condition of the distal extremity tendons called tenosynovitis is an example of shear stress. Due to excess friction the tendon and surrounding synovial sheath become inflamed and irritated, and adhesions may develop between the tendon and its sheath. Spondylolisthesis is another example.

Torsion
Torsion is force applied in a rotary or twisting fashion. Due to the body's anatomy, individual soft-tissues are rarely exposed to enough torsion stress to damage the tissue. However, torsion forces applied to joints can produce excessive tensile or compressive forces and produce soft-tissue injury. For example twisting the knee produces torsion stress to the knee joint, causing tensile stress to the cruciate ligaments inside the joint that resist the rotary movement of the knee.

Bending
Soft tissues rarely develop injuries from bending because they are pliable, whereas bones are susceptible to bending stress because they are rigid. Bending is a combination of compression and tension as one side of a tissue is compressed while the other side is stretched. Most bone fractures occur from bending stress.

Tissue Roles & Dysfunctions

For the sake of evaluation, soft tissues are divided into two categories: contractile and inert.[1] **Contractile** tissues are those that are actively engaged to create movement and include muscles and tendons. Although a tendon does not generate a contraction within its own fibers, it is considered a contractile tissue because it transmits the contraction force of a muscle to the bone.

Inert tissues lack the capacity to directly produce movement of bones. These tissues include the joint capsule, ligament, bursa, cartilage, fascia, dura mater, and nerves. Other soft tissues, such as vascular structures and organs, are not included in this classification because they do not have a fundamental role in locomotion.

MUSCLE

As the primary contractile tissue, **muscles' principle roles are to maintain posture, create movement, slow or stop movement, and provide sensory feedback about the body's position in space and contact with the outside world.**[2] By shortening and elongating, muscles stabilize, accelerate, and decelerate bone movement. Individual fibers in the muscle contract when stimulated by nerve impulses; when nerve impulses cease, contraction stops.

Movement is created through concentric or eccentric activation, and through gravity or momentum (without muscular effort). When gravity or momentum creates the motion, no muscle contraction occurs and elongation or shortening is passive. There are three types of muscle contraction used in orthopedic assessment: concentric, eccentric, and isometric.

Muscle injuries are prevalent, making up 30% of the injuries seen in physicians' offices.[5] The frequency of muscle injury is due to the fact that muscle is such a predominant tissue in the body. Muscles are used in every action that humans perform. Factors that lead to muscle injury include overuse, lack of proper conditioning, fatigue, chronic tension, and numerous other stressors. These factors can lead to a number of pathological processes in muscle tissue. The primary muscle tissue

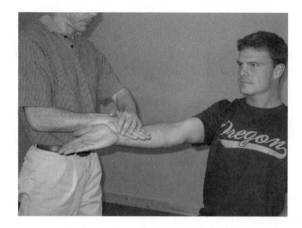

Figure 2.2 Manual resistive tests use isometric contractions to evaluate symptoms.

pathologies are muscular hypertonicity, myofascial trigger points, atrophy, strain, and contusion.

Muscle Contractions
Concentric
During active contraction the muscle's two ends move closer together to overcome resistance and the muscle shortens. **Concentric contractions** are acceleration movements because they increase action against resistance. For example, with a person in the standing position, the biceps brachii muscle engages in a concentric contraction when the forearm is flexed at the elbow and the wrist is brought toward the shoulder (Figure 2.1).

When the practitioner is familiar with the actions of specific muscles, concentric contractions are relatively easy to identify. It is the concentric contractions of muscles that are referred to as the muscles' actions in many anatomy and physiology texts.

Eccentric
Although it sounds like a contradiction in terms, the muscle actually elongates in an **eccentric contraction**. Eccentric activation might be a more appropriate term to describe this muscle action. Nerve impulses excite the muscle's fibers stimulating it to contract, but the contraction is overcome by the resistance force. During eccentric contraction, the muscle gradually releases its contraction.

Eccentric contractions are most often used when decelerating movement or resisting gravity (a form of deceleration). Using the example given above, an eccentric contraction takes place when the forearm raised during the concentric phase is slowly lowered to the beginning position (extension) (Figure 2.1). Identification of eccentric contractions is important, as they are the most common cause of muscular injury.[3, 4]

Isometric
An **isometric contraction** is one in which no movement is produced at the joint despite the active contraction of

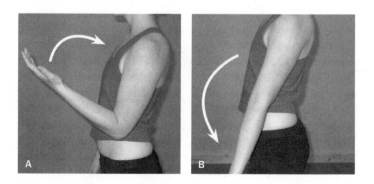

Figure 2.1 Elbow flexion using concentric contraction (A), elbow extension using eccentric contraction when slowly lowering the arm (B) .

the muscle. If an outside resistance equals the amount of contraction stimulus in the muscle, then no movement results. Isometric contractions are used to hold the body in a static position and resist gravity (Figure 2.2). Muscles use isometric contraction in their role as stabilizers.

Elongation

While focus is given to muscle contractions, an equally important part of muscle function is its ability to **elongate**. Muscle tissue has the property of *extensibility*, which means it can stretch as well as contract. A limiting factor to how effectively a muscle generates force is its level of extensibility. A muscle that remains in a shortened position for a long period of time is likely to become dysfunctional. Weakness or fibrous tissue can develop, limiting its ability to fully elongate. *Contracture* is a state in which fibrous tissue binds a muscle in a shortened position. If a muscle is unable to properly elongate due to excessive neurological stimulation, it is considered *hypertonic*.

Muscular Hypertonicity

Excess muscle tension is the most common muscular dysfunction. Despite its frequency of occurrence, this problem rarely receives the level of attention it deserves. Perhaps the idea of tight muscles is too simple to be considered an orthopedic condition. However, biomechanical disturbances around various joints are routinely described by researchers and clinicians as *muscle imbalance* and *tightness*.

Muscle tightness results from an increased rate of contraction stimulus causing the muscle to hold a higher degree of resting *tonus* than it normally would. Some form of stress generally creates this degree of increased tone. Types of stress primarily responsible include mechanical (e.g. postural distortions), chemical (e.g. excessive caffeine intake), or psychological.[6] The body's response is to increase neuromuscular tone in reaction to the stressor. Box 2.1 includes indications of excessive muscular tension.

Myofascial Trigger Points

Another dysfunctional process that occurs in muscle tissue is the *myofascial trigger point (MTrP)*. These are found in hypertonic muscles, but can be present in other tissues as well. Although awareness of this pathology is still limited, MTrPs are gaining attention in the health care community. Janet Travell describes a myofascial trigger point as:

> …**a hyperirritable spot in skeletal muscle that is associated with a hypersensitive palpable nodule in a taut band**. The spot is painful on compression and can give rise to characteristic referred pain, referred tenderness, motor dysfunction, and autonomic phenomena.[6]

The exact pathophysiology of MTrPs is still not well-understood. However, interesting findings have surfaced in recent years. Researchers have found altered cellular muscle metabolism at the site of MTrPs, but it has not been determined whether this is a cause or an effect.[7] In other research, electromyographic activity at the site of the MTrP also seems altered.[8] Also notable is that pain referral patterns appear to be related to perception errors by the brain.[6, 9] Further research is necessary to fully understand the physiological causes of trigger points.

MTrP identification is primarily based on clinical examination and not on reproducible diagnostic testing. Consequently, greater clinical examination skills are necessary for verifying the presence of MTrPs.[10, 11] The ability to identify MTrPs is a crucial skill for health care professionals addressing soft-tissue disorders. Furthermore, correct evaluation requires practitioners to have adequate palpation skills. With their emphasis in hands-on therapy, massage practitioners are uniquely positioned to contribute to the evaluation and treatment of myofascial trigger point pain.

Knowing the **characteristic referral patterns** for MTrPs is important. There are numerous charts and maps of MTrP pain referral patterns that are useful references. However, practitioners are encouraged to use these diagrams only as a starting reference point because pain referral patterns can differ between individuals. Interestingly, studies have found the sites of MTrPs to be similar to the acupuncture points in traditional Chinese medicine.[12] A characteristic MTrP pain referral pattern is shown in Figure 2.3.

Muscles develop trigger points in reaction to stress. These stresses often involve biomechanical overload on the muscle, but could also result from chemical stimulants such as caffeine, excess heat or cold, nutritional deficiencies, or psychological stress.[6, 13] Referred pain created by an MTrP increases muscle tension either in the muscles housing the MTrP and/or in the pain referral zone. Muscles that perform the same action as an injured muscle can also develop MTrPs while compensating for the dysfunction.

While there is no official list of diagnostic criteria, several characteristics of MTrPs differentiate them from pain produced by other soft-tissue sources. The key charac-

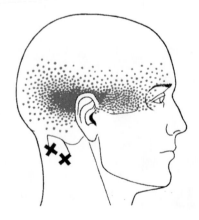

Figure 2.3 Myofascial trigger point referral pattern for the suboccipital muscles.

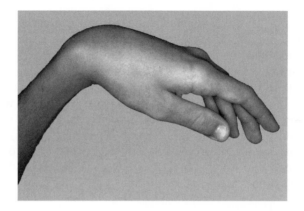

Figure 2.4 Atrophy of the wrist extensors produces characteristic wrist drop. (3-D image courtesy of Primal Pictures Ltd. www.primalpictures. com.)

teristics offered by Huguenin and Simons for MTrPs are listed in Box 2.2.[9, 14]

Atrophy

Muscular atrophy is a **decrease or wasting of muscle size** and is usually caused by denervation or disuse. *Denervation* is a **loss or impairment of nerve supply** to the muscle and results from nerve compression syndromes, systemic disease, or traumatic damage to the nerve or neuromuscular interface. The lack of proper neurological stimulation leads to loss of size and contractile strength, as well as to abnormal biomechanics.[15]

Disuse atrophy is relatively common and can cause problems with proper biomechanical function. Atrophy can result when a limb must be immobilized for a long period after a traumatic injury. Atrophy can also develop when movement is restricted due to pain. Disuse atrophy advances quickly, with the muscle losing strength and size in a short period of time (Figure 2.4).[15]

Disuse atrophy develops in the primary anti-gravity muscles more rapidly than other muscles, although the reason for this is not established.[16] Anti-gravity muscles are those that are responsible for resisting the downward pull of gravity while in the normal upright position. For example, disuse atrophy affects the quadriceps more than the hamstring muscles because the quadriceps are anti-gravity muscles. The affects are more pronounced if the muscle is immobilized in a shortened position.[15] Immobilization for knee injuries frequently requires the knee to be set in an extended position where the quadriceps are shortened and the hamstrings are lengthened. Immobilizing the quadriceps in their shortened position accelerates their atrophy.

Strain

A *strain*, sometimes referred to as a *pulled* muscle, is a muscle injury **that causes fibers to tear within the tissue**. Muscle strains are produced by **excessive tensile stress.** A muscle strain generally does not result from excess stretch alone, but from a combination of tension and contraction. Due to muscle mechanics, strains are more likely when the muscle is in eccentric contraction rather than concentric or isometric.[17, 18]

There are three grades of muscle strain: **first degree** or mild, **second degree** or moderate, and **third degree** or severe. In a first-degree strain, few muscle fibers are torn. There may be some post-injury soreness, but the individual usually returns to normal activity levels quickly. With second-degree strains more fibers are involved. There is a greater level of pain and a clear region of maximum tenderness in the muscle tissue.

A complete rupture of the muscle-tendon unit occurs with a grade three strain. Because of extensive damage, strains are sometimes classified as third degree even though the muscle still has a few fibers intact. Significant pain is likely at the time of injury. Pain can be minimal afterwards, because the ends of the muscle are separated and limb movement does not cause additional tensile stress.

Third-degree strains generally require surgical repair. In some instances, surgery is not performed because the muscle does not play a crucial role and the potential dangers of surgery outweigh the benefits. Ruptures to the rectus femoris are an example because the other three quadriceps muscles make up for the strength deficit caused by the strain. Further characteristics of muscle strains are included in Chapter 4.

The muscles most susceptible to strain injuries are **multiarticulate muscles**, which are those that cross more than one joint. The more joints crossed by a muscle, the greater their vulnerability for strain injury. All involved joints cannot achieve full range of motion at the same time due to limited extensibility of the muscle-tendon unit. If the muscle is stretched across multiple joints, it is susceptible to tearing from excess tensile stress.

Strains can develop in any part of the muscle, but ordinarily occur at the **musculotendinous junction**.[19] The junction of muscle and tendon places one tissue with higher pliability (muscle) directly adjacent to another with limited pliability and more tensile strength (tendon). As a consequence, the point of interface between the two tissues becomes a site of mechanical weakness; this is where strains often occur.

Contusion

A *contusion* results from a direct blow to the muscle that causes **disruption in the fibers and/or their neurovascular supply**. *Ecchymosis* (bruising) forms as the blood from damaged capillaries leaks into the muscle tissue and interstitial space. Muscle contusion healing depends on the severity of the impact trauma and the level of disruption of muscle fibers and neurovascular structures.

In some cases, a severe contusion develops into a condition is known as *myositis ossificans*. During the healing process, **ossification** (bone tissue development) takes place within the muscle injured by the contusion. Awareness of this condition is important. Deep pressure on an area with myositis ossificans can cause further muscle damage and can be detrimental to the healing process.[20] The anterior muscles of the body vulnerable to direct blows such as the quadriceps group, biceps brachii, brachialis, and deltoid muscles are most at risk for myositis ossificans.

TENDON

The primary function of a tendon is to transmit the contraction force of its associated muscle to the bone. Consequently, the tendon needs to have sufficient tensile strength. Tendons have various shapes, such as the sheet-like aponeurosis of the latissimus dorsi or the long, pencil-like structure of the biceps brachii. They are constructed with parallel collagen fibers running the length of the tendon. The longitudinal arrangement of the collagen fibers gives the tendon its tensile strength.

Tendons are a fundamental part of the contractile unit. The tensile strength in a tendon can be more than twice that of its associated muscle.[21] As a result, they are rarely torn. Even in muscles where complete ruptures occur, such as the biceps brachii or triceps surae group, the rupture is usually at the musculotendinous junction or in the muscle fibers.

In some cases the muscle fibers remain intact and the tendon tears or pulls away from its attachment site on the bone. This is known as an *avulsion*. More often tendons are damaged with internal structural pathologies such as *tendinosis* and *tenosynovitis*. These conditions generally result from repetitive overuse as opposed to an acute injury.

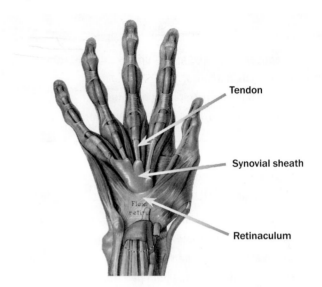

Figure 2.5 In the wrist and palm, the synovial sheath protects the tendons from friction by the binding retinaculum. (Mediclip image copyright, 1998 Williams & Wilkins. All rights reserved.)

Tendinosis/Tendinitis

The most common pathological problem involving tendons used to be referred to as tendinitis but is now more correctly known as *tendinosis*, which means **abnormal condition of the tendon**. Tendinitis implies an inflammatory condition and it was previously believed that chronic overuse lead to tendon fiber tearing and inflammation. *True tendinitis*, which is tendon fiber tearing with inflammation, does occur but it is a rare condition.[22]

Recent investigation of tendon overuse dysfunction shows that most overuse tendon pathologies are devoid of inflammatory cells and instead **involve a breakdown in the collagen matrix**.[23-26] Because of the lack of inflammatory activity in these conditions, the term *tendinosis* is encouraged. The term tendinosis does not specify the pathological process, only that the tendon is dysfunctional. High levels or prolonged periods of tensile stress on the tendon can lead to collagen breakdown. While any tendon can develop tendinosis, tendons in the extremities are more susceptible. Another result of chronic load on the tendon is **alteration in the tendon's vascularity** (blood flow). An increase in vascularity is indicated in some studies, while other research shows decreased vascularity.[22, 27-29] Either problem contributes to chronic tendon pathology.

Even though there is significant research and evidence showing that it is the pathology of tendinosis occurring, physician diagnosis and rehabilitation practitioners often call this injury tendinitis. Rehabilitation in many cases continues to focus on anti-inflammatory treatment strategies, rather than collagen rebuilding. In some cases use of anti-inflammatory medication can be detrimental for healing collagen degeneration.[28] Overuse tendon disorders can take a long time to heal due to the slow rebuilding

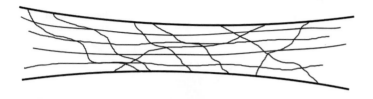

Figure 2.6 Ligament fibers run longitudinally as well as in transverse and diagonal directions to increase strength and pliability.

of collagen. If tendon fiber tearing (tendinitis) were the primary problem, the tissue would heal rather quickly as it moves through the various stages of the inflammation and tissue repair process. Collagen rebuilding is a slow process and tendinosis can become chronic or recurrent.

Tenosynovitis

Another chronic overuse tendon problem is *tenosynovitis*, which is an **inflammation and/or irritation between a tendon and its surrounding synovial sheath**. This condition affects only those tendons enclosed within a synovial sheath, also called the **epitenon**. The synovial sheath surrounds tendons in the distal extremities and a few other locations, such as the biceps brachii long head tendon as it travels through the bicipital groove. The sheath reduces friction between the tendon and the retinaculum (or, infrequently, a ligament) that binds the tendon close to the joint (Figure 2.5). The tendon must be able to glide freely within the sheath.

Chronic overloading or excess friction leads to adhesion between the tendon and its sheath. The adhesions cause a roughening of the surface between the tendon and its sheath and a subsequent inflammatory reaction results. The rough tendon surface routinely produces **crepitus** (grating sensations) when the muscle-tendon unit and affected joint are moved through their range of motion.

The symptoms of tendinosis and tenosynovitis are similar, but one can distinguish between the two by determining if the tendon has a synovial sheath. If it does, tenosynovitis is possible. If there is no sheath, tendinosis is probably the cause.

Avulsion

An *avulsion* is an acute tendon injury resulting from high tensile loads, in which **a tendon is forcibly torn away from its attachment site on the bone**. In a majority of tensile stress injuries of the musculotendinous unit fiber tearing occurs at the musculotendinous junction, but in some cases these fibers remains intact and the tendon pulls away from its bony attachment site.

Avulsion injuries occur in regions where a large muscle attaches at a relatively small site on the bone, such as the hamstring attachment at the ischial tuberosity. The tensile force on the attachment site is greater than the tendon's tensile strength, causing it to pull free from the bone. In some cases the tendon pulls a bone fragment with it and the injury is called an *avulsion fracture*. If serious enough, the damage requires surgical repair.

Enthesitis is a tendon pathology that is similar to an avulsion and is **an inflammatory irritation of the attachment site of the tendon into the bone**.[6] Prior to the tendon tearing away from its attachment site, it can pull excessively on the **periosteum**. The periosteum is a pain sensitive tissue, which causes the irritation to be out of proportion to the damage.

LIGAMENT

The primary function of ligament tissue is to connect adjacent bones and establish stability in the skeletal structure. Ligament fibers are oriented primarily in a longitudinal direction in order to provide the greatest resistance to tensile stress.[29] However, forces acting on joints can come from multiple directions and, as a result, some fibers are oriented in a transverse or diagonal direction increasing the ligament's pliability and strength (Figure 2.6). Ligamentous tissue makes up a significant amount of the fibrous capsule around synovial joints.

Ligament Sprain

Ligaments are usually injured from an acute overload of tensile stress on the fibers, causing a *sprain*. Increasing tensile forces cause the ligament to stretch. The severity of a tensile stress injury depends on the level of force the ligament must withstand. Ligament fibers have a small degree of pliability and resistance to stretch, due to a greater amount of elastin as compared with tendon fibers. If the tensile stress is minor, the ligament can absorb the force with minor stretching of the fibers.

If the force is significant, the **ligament fibers can stretch past the tissue's initial level of pliability** and undergo what is called *plastic deformation*.[29] This means that **the tissue stretches but does not recoil to its original length**, and a permanent degree of tissue elongation can occur. There are three phases in ligament tensile stress injuries based on the relative load-to-length ratio (Figure 2.7). In the initial **elastic phase** the ligament increases in length as additional tensile load is applied. As the load increases, the ligament enters the **plastic deformation** phase where more load is applied, but length is not significantly increased. In this phase the ligament will not return to its original length when the load is released. Further increasing load causes tissue failure and the ligament is torn.

Ligament sprains are categorized as **first**, **second**, or **third degree** sprains. In first degree sprains there is elastic phase damage to the ligament. The type of damage in second degree sprains runs from end of elastic to the beginning of plastic deformation phases. Third degree damage can fall into the end of the plastic deformation phase to complete rupture. The characteristics of the degrees of ligament sprain are discussed in Chapter 4.

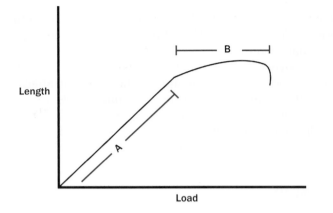

Figure 2.7 The graph indicates the relative load-to-length curve for ligament tissue damage. During the elastic phase (A), length increases equally with load. In plastic deformation (B), load exceeds the ligament's springback ability and the ligament becomes permanently stretched. Finally, the ligament tears (C).

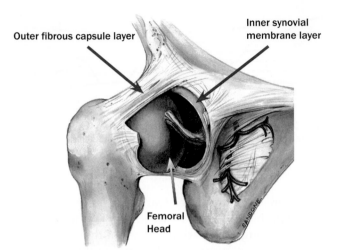

Figure 2.8 Opened hip joint showing the layers of joint capsule. (Mediclip image copyright, 1998 Williams & Wilkins. All rights reserved.)

JOINT CAPSULE

The joint capsule has two layers. The outermost layer is called the **fibrous capsule** and the inner layer is called the **synovial membrane** (Figure 2.8). The fibrous capsule makes up a large portion of the joint capsule around synovial joints. **The capsule acts like a ligament to maintain stability and support. It also houses synovial fluid and protects the synovial membrane.** The fibrous capsule is richly innervated and even minor damage can cause significant pain and discomfort. The synovial membrane secretes **synovial fluid**, which lubricates the joint, supplies nutrients, and removes metabolic waste products.

Capsular tear
The joint capsule is damaged similarly to ligament tissue in an acute injury. A *capsular tear* is a tensile stress injury of the joint capsule. These injuries occur when a joint is dislocated or exposed to stress that **tears the supporting ligamentous structure.** Capsular tears are evaluated in the same manner as ligament sprains.

Capsular adhesion
The capsule is also susceptible to fibrotic changes. **Fibrous adhesion of the capsule to itself or to adjacent tissues** is called *capsular adhesion*. For example, the common injury of adhesive capsulitis of the shoulder, often confused with bursitis, results from adhesion in the glenohumeral joint capsule to itself or other adjacent fibers.

Capsular adhesion is sometimes evaluated with a movement restriction called a *capsular pattern*. The capsular pattern is **a pattern of movement restriction that is characteristic to each individual joint**. It is represented by a sequential listing of the movements that are most likely to be limited to those that are least likely to be limited. Not all joints have capsular patterns. For example, those joints that are not directly controlled by muscles, such as

the sacroiliac joint, do not have capsular patterns.[30]

If the joint's pattern of motion restriction does not evidence the characteristic capsular pattern for that joint, the restriction is referred to as a **non-capsular pattern**. For example, in the shoulder the capsular pattern dictates that restrictions due to capsular problems occur first in lateral rotation, then abduction, and eventually medial rotation. Therefore, in the early stages of capsular restriction limitations are seen only in lateral rotation. As the pathology progresses, further limitations are found in abduction and eventually medial rotation. If there is pain and limited motion in abduction, but no pain or restriction with lateral rotation, it is considered a non-capsular pattern and the joint capsule is likely not involved.

FASCIA

Fascia is an exceptionally abundant tissue in the body. Its consistency ranges broadly from thin membranes to relatively thick bands. The primary function of fascial tissue is to **provide support, shape, and suspension for the soft tissues** of the body. From an orthopedic perspective, the fascia associated with muscle tissue is of primary concern because dysfunction within the fascial system can produce significant movement system problems.[31, 32]

Fascial tearing
The majority of fascia is highly elastic, but extreme tensile stress can cause *fascial tearing* or *perforation*. A tensile stress injury to fascia can cause **scar tissue** to develop, leading to movement restrictions. Fascial tearing is likely to be painful because fascia is richly innervated.

Fascial shortening
A significant pathological problem involving fascia occurs when it remains in a shortened position for prolonged periods. While fascial tissue has a great deal of elasticity, it **tends to adapt to shortened or elongated positions**

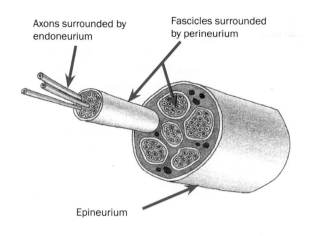

Axons surrounded by endoneurium

Fascicles surrounded by perineurium

Epineurium

Figure 2.9 Layers of the peripheral nerve. (Illustration courtesy of Alexandra Hamer.)

and adhesions can link adjacent fascial fibers.[32, 33] This **fibrous cross-linking** within fascial tissue leads to shortening of the fascia, creating resistance to elongation. Fascia has a **viscoelastic** property so that when it is over-stretched it can recoil to some degree, but not to its original length.[33]

Recent investigation into the fascia's physiological properties indicate that it may have contractile cells similar to those found in smooth muscle fibers.[34] Presence of contractile cells within fascia would explain its apparent ability to shorten. This also provides a valuable working theory for the effectiveness of fascial treatment methods such as myofascial release. Schleip's research suggests that the low level tangential forces of myofascial treatment techniques actually cause the contractile units in the fascia to decrease their contractions, creating the characteristic tissue release felt by practitioners. With either chronic shortening or over-lengthening some degree of deformation in fascial tissue can become permanent, which can contribute to postural distortions.[40]

NERVE

Peripheral **nerves** have a dorsal root that carries sensory information and a ventral root that carries motor signals. The nerve roots blend together shortly after leaving the spinal cord, converging to create the major trunks of the peripheral nerves. The peripheral nerves then extend through the upper and lower extremities and other areas of the body.

The majority of nerve is made up of axons. **Axons** are often surrounded by a **myelin sheath**, which functions to speed signal transmission. Around each axon and its sheath are several connective tissue layers. The first layer is the **endoneurium**, which surrounds the individual axons. The axons are collected into bundles called **fascicles** and surrounded by another connective tissue layer called the **perineurium**. The fascicles are bundled together within a layer called the **epineurium**. Bundled fascicles make up

the entire peripheral nerve (Figure 2.9). These connective tissue layers function primarily to provide support and protection for the nerve. Consequently, these layers play important roles in nerve tissue pathology.

In addition to connective tissue layers and nerve fibers, there is a complex web of tiny circulatory vessels within the peripheral nerve. An adequate **vascular supply** is needed for the nerve to function properly. Consequently, *ischemia* from compression is likely to cause neurological symptoms, such as the sensation of pins and needles (paresthesia). The nerve also carries its own nutrient proteins necessary for proper function. These substances move through the nerve fiber in a flowing cytoplasm called **axoplasm**. The movement of axoplasm within the nerve is called the **axoplasmic flow**. Disturbances to this flow affect the nerve not only locally but along its entire length. Axoplasmic flow disturbance is discussed further in the description of the double crush phenomenon below.

Because the major peripheral nerve trunks have motor and sensory fibers, nerve damage can produce sensory or motor dysfunction. Understanding nerve injury symptoms requires familiarity with dermatomes, cutaneous innervation, and myotomes. **Dermatomes are areas of skin supplied by fibers from a single nerve root**. The fibers from that one nerve root make up several peripheral nerves and innervate a specific area of the body. For example, the C8 nerve root has branches that make up portions of several upper extremity nerves, such as the median and ulnar nerves. Sensory symptoms from C8 nerve root irritation are felt in the ulnar side of the hand and medial side of the forearm and arm (Figure 2.10a).

Each peripheral nerve is made up of fibers deriving from the different nerve roots. **A skin region supplied by a peripheral nerve is called the cutaneous innervation** of that nerve (Figure 2.10b). Note that there is some overlap between the dermatome and the area of cutaneous innervation. For example, the ulnar nerve in the arm has fibers from C7, C8, and T1, yet its sensory fibers only supply the ulnar aspect of the hand and the last two fingers, whereas the C8 dermatome covers the ulnar aspect of the hand, as well as the entire medial forearm and arm.

Information about dermatomes and regions of cutaneous innervation is valuable in the clinical evaluation process. Using the example above, if sensory symptoms are felt throughout the C8 dermatome, one would suspect nerve root involvement rather than a problem with the ulnar nerve. This is because the symptoms extend outside the ulnar nerve's cutaneous innervation area in the ulnar side of the hand. If symptoms are only in the ulnar side of the hand, ulnar nerve pathology is more likely. Keep in mind that symptoms may appear in only a part of the dermatome. Whenever sensory symptoms are reported in an extremity one should consider the possibility of the nerve root being the source of the problem.

Myotomes are somewhat similar to dermatomes. A myotome is **a group of muscles that are innervated by the same nerve root**. However, a single muscle can have

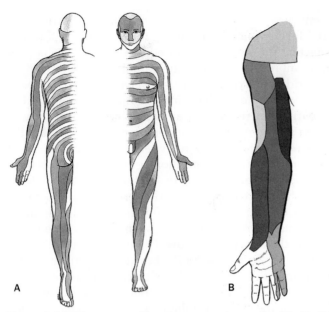

Figure 2.10   Dermatomes (A) and cutaneous innervation (B). (Mediclip image copyright, 1998 Williams & Wilkins. All rights reserved.)

fibers that come from several different nerve roots. Each peripheral nerve also has a number of muscles that it innervates. If there is weakness apparent in a group of muscles innervated by the same nerve root, i.e. the same myotome, then the problem is most likely at the nerve root level. Muscle weakness in a myotome is not always easy to detect because the muscle may only have a small number of fibers that come from the affected nerve root.

Nerve Compression or Tension

Nerve compression or tension **is pressure or stretch on the nerve that eventually causes a pathological reaction or complete rupture**. Nerve injuries generally develop from compressive loads, such as a direct blow to the nerve or a chronic low level of compression. With excess tensile stress the overall diameter of the nerve decreases compressing the fibers within the nerve; this condition is called adverse neural tension.

There are two terms that are used to describe nerve injuries and which indicate the location of the pathology in the nerve. A *radiculopathy* is a **nerve pathology that occurs at the nerve root**. A common radiculopathy is the herniated nucleus pulposus (HNP) or herniated disc, in which the disc presses on the nerve root. **Pathology farther along the length of the nerve** is called a *neuropathy*. It is also called a *peripheral neuropathy* indicating that the injury is in the peripheral nerves, distant from the nerve roots and spinal cord. Many nerve compression syndromes, such as thoracic outlet and carpal tunnel syndromes, are examples of peripheral neuropathies.

Pathological changes also develop in the nerve if there is a *double or multiple crush phenomenon*, which causes an axoplasmic flow limitation.[35] In this situation there is **more than one region of compression on a nerve trunk**.

Sections of the nerve distal to the first site of compression become nutritionally deficient because of axoplasmic flow blockage. Consequently, these distal regions are more susceptible to irritation from even a minor degree of compression (becoming the second site of crush). For example, with a proximal compression on the brachial plexus everything distal to that site is more susceptible to pathology. Even a minor degree of compression on the median nerve in the distal forearm or hand could then become symptomatic. The double (or multiple) crush phenomenon explains why clients might have simultaneous symptoms of thoracic outlet syndrome and carpal tunnel syndrome.

The symptoms of compression and tension pathologies can be similar because the degenerative process in the nerve is similar. Nerve damage from these forces is characterized in the same three levels of severity described below in the section on nerve degeneration. There are several signs or symptoms characteristic of nerve compression or tension pathologies listed in Box 2.3. Compressive or tensile forces occur in numerous locations along the nerve. The areas most at risk for increased neural tension or compression are listed in Box 2.4.[36]

Nerve Degeneration

In *nerve degeneration*, the axons and myelin sheath degenerate first. As damage progresses, the connective tissue layers surrounding the nerve trunk and its individual fibers are eventually destroyed. **Degeneration of the axon and myelin sheath** is defined as *wallerian degeneration*.[37] Because a few of the connective tissue layers remain intact after the nerve's central components are damaged, some supporting structure of the nerve is left intact. This remaining structure can provide a template for regeneration of axons if the damage is not severe.

Nerve degeneration results from mechanical forces or from systemic disorders that attack the nerve, such as multiple sclerosis. Nerve injuries are classified by severity into three levels: neurapraxia, axonotmesis, and neurotmesis.[38, 39] The characteristics of each are described below. Note that either compression or tension injuries can produce these levels of nerve injury.

Neurapraxia is the least severe nerve injury and involves the blocking of axon conduction (Figure 2.11a). The nerve continues to conduct some signals above and below the primary area of compression or injury, but conduction velocity slows. Common symptoms include mild sensory and motor deficits, which are usually alleviated when pressure is removed from the nerve. There is no wallerian degeneration apparent with neurapraxia.

The next level of nerve damage is called *axonotmesis* in which wallerian degeneration of the fiber has begun (Figure 2.11b). There is a loss in continuity of the axon, but the surrounding endoneurium may still be intact. The outer layers of connective tissue are still intact as well. Typical symptoms include sensory and motor dysfunction, as well as significant pain. If the connective tissue

Box 2.3 Nerve Compression, Tension Pathology Symptoms

Reduced sensory input

Reduced motor impulses

Sensory symptoms in a specific dermatome if at nerve root

Motor weakness in muscles in the involved myotome

Sensory symptoms in region supplied by the involved
    peripheral nerve if at peripheral nerve level

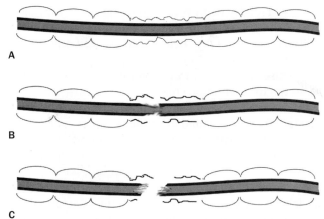

Figure 2.11 Neurapraxia, axon conduction blocked (A); axonotmesis, degeneration of the axon and myelin sheath (B); and neurotmesis, nerve is axons and connective tissue layers severly damaged..

layers are intact the nerve axon is likely to regenerate, although slowly. The rate of regeneration of nerve axons is estimated to be 1 mm per day or 1 inch per month and slower in many cases.[36]

A severe nerve injury is *neurotmesis*. At this level, damage affects not only the axons, but also their connective tissue layers (Figure 2.11c). Because these layers are damaged, recovery from neurotmesis may not be possible. Neurotmesis occurs in severe crush injuries or situations where the nerve is severed. Axons can regenerate once severed, but because the connective tissue template is disrupted the axons may not grow back in their original locations. This is one reason some surgical repairs produce altered sensation or function in the region when the individual regains use.

CARTILAGE

There are three types of **cartilage**. The two affected by orthopedic disorders are hyaline and fibrocartilage. A third type, elastic cartilage, is found in areas such as the external portion of the ear and the epiglottis and is not involved in orthopedic disorders.

Hyaline cartilage acts as a necessary **protective cushion** on the ends of long bones and is also called **articular** cartilage. It provides a smooth gliding surface for move-

ment at the joints, producing flexibility and support. **Fibrocartilage**, the strongest type of cartilage, is designed to provide **rigidity and support** as well as guiding proper joint movement. Fibrocartilage is located in areas of high compressive force between bones, such as the intervertebral discs and the menisci of the knee.

Cartilage degeneration

A common pathology affecting hyaline cartilage is compressive stress that causes **breakdown in the integrity of the cartilage matrix**, eventually causing degenerative changes in the joint. Osteoarthritis is a type of *hyaline cartilage degeneration*. Because cartilage is mostly devoid of nerve fibers there may be no pain from the cartilage degeneration, but instead from the richly innervated subchondral bone, the layer of bone just below the cartilage. With cartilage degeneration, friction develops on the surface of the bone thereby producing pain.

Similar to hyaline cartilage, **injury to fibrocartilage is**

Box 2.4 Areas Most at Risk for Increased Neural Tension or Compression

In tunnels created by soft tissues, bony tissues, or a combination; for example the hand's carpal tunnel, the elbow's cubital tunnel, the foot's tarsal tunnel.

Where the nervous system branches to other areas; for example the region where the posterior interosseous nerve branches from the main radial nerve near the elbow.

Where the nervous system is fixed to adjacent structures for stability; for example where the deep peroneal nerve attaches to the upper region of the fibula.

At the point of contact where the nerve passes closely to unyielding surfaces such as bone, cartilage, ligament, or retinacula; for example where the brachial plexus passes over the first rib.

At tension points, which are the locations where opposing forces meet midway when a nerve is pulled in opposite directions; for example where superior and inferior tensile forces on the sciatic nerve meet midway down the lower extremity.

usually caused by compressive damage from overuse or sudden injury. The compressive forces causing problems are often those involving heavy loads placed on the cartilage over a long period of time. Poor posture, for example, can increase the compressive load on the intervertebral discs in the lumbar spine creating disc pathology.

While cartilage is often injured from compressive loads, tensile forces can also produce injury. The tearing of the glenoid labrum, a cartilage rim around the glenoid fossa in the shoulder, is an example. The biceps brachii long head tendon attaches to the supraglenoid tubercle of the scapula and has fibers that merge through the glenoid labrum. Excessive pulling on the attachment site produces tensile loads on the cartilage strong enough to tear the upper glenoid labrum.

Because of limited innervation to hyaline and fibrocartilage, identifying cartilage damage is difficult. Assessing cartilage problems relies on client history and certain signs and symptoms the individual demonstrates or describes that are indicative of cartilage injury. Pain is a relevant factor in regions where the hyaline cartilage has worn away and the subchondral bone is irritated.

BURSA

The bursae are small fluid-filled sacs that provide cushioning to reduce friction between adjacent tissues. Contrary to images in anatomical texts, the majority of bursae are thin and flat. As friction reducers, bursae are most vulnerable to chronic or acute compressive force injuries.

Bursitis

By far the most common type of bursa pathology is compressive damage that results in inflammation, called bursitis. This is generally an overuse pathology, but can result from acute compressive injury. The shoulder bursitis experienced by swimmers, for instance, develops from repetitive overhead motions of the arm. A number of bursae, such as the olecranon bursa and the prepatellar bursa, are superficial which allows their inflammatory reactions to be more easily identified. Knowledge of anatomy and biomechanics will assist in the identification of bursa injuries. Bursae inflammation is sometimes caused by systemic illness, not mechanical compression.

References

Some information in this chapter is adapted from: Lowe W. *Orthopedic Massage: Theory and Technique*. Edinburgh: Mosby; 2003. Used by permission.

1. Cyriax J. *Textbook of Orthopaedic Medicine Volume One: Diagnosis of Soft Tissue Lesions*. Vol 1. 8th ed. London: Bailliere Tindall; 1982.
2. Neumann DA. *Kinesiology of the Musculoskeletal System*. St. Louis: Mosby; 2002.
3. AAOS. *Athletic Training and Sports Medicine*. 2nd ed. Park Ridge: American Academy of Orthopaedic Surgeons; 1991.
4. Garrett WE. Muscle strain injuries. *Am J Sports Med*. 1996;24(6 Suppl):S2-8.
5. Kirkendall DT, Garrett WE, Jr. Clinical perspectives regarding eccentric muscle injury. *Clin Orthop Relat Res*. Oct 2002(403 Suppl):S81-89.
6. Simons D, Travell J, Simons L. *Myofascial Pain and Dysfunction: The Trigger Point Manual*. Vol 1. 2nd ed. Baltimore: Williams & Wilkins; 1999.
7. McPartland JM. Travell trigger points--molecular and osteopathic perspectives. *J Am Osteopath Assoc*. Jun 2004;104(6):244-249.
8. Baldry PE. *Myofascial Pain and Fibromyalgia Syndromes*. Edinburgh: Churchill Livingstone; 2001.
9. Huguenin L. Myofascial trigger points: the current evidence. *Physical Therapy in Sport*. 2004;5:2-12.
10. Al-Shenqiti AM, Oldham JA. Test-retest reliability of myofascial trigger point detection in patients with rotator cuff tendonitis. *Clin Rehabil*. Aug 2005;19(5):482-487.
11. Gerwin RD, Shannon S, Hong CZ, Hubbard D, Gevirtz R. Interrater reliability in myofascial trigger point examination. *Pain*. Jan 1997;69(1-2):65-73.
12. Melzack R. Myofascial trigger points: relation to acupuncture and mechanisms of pain. *Arch Phys Med Rehabil*. Mar 1981;62(3):114-117.
13. Treaster D, Marras WS, Burr D, Sheedy JE, Hart D. Myofascial trigger point development from visual and postural stressors during computer work. *J Electromyogr Kinesiol*. Apr 2006;16(2):115-124.
14. Simons DG. Review of enigmatic MTrPs as a common cause of enigmatic musculoskeletal pain and dysfunction. *J Electromyogr Kinesiol*. 2004;14(1):95-107.
15. McComas A. *Skeletal Muscle: Form and Function*. Champaign: Human Kinetics; 1996.
16. Liebenson Ce. *Rehabilitation of the Spine*. Baltimore: Williams & Wilkins; 1996.
17. Faulkner JA, Brooks SV, Opiteck JA. Injury to skeletal muscle fibers during contractions: conditions of occurrence and prevention. *Phys Ther*. 1993;73(12):911-921.
18. Hoskins W, Pollard H. The management of hamstring injury--Part 1: Issues in diagnosis. *Man Ther*. May 2005;10(2):96-107.

TABLE 1 COMMON SOFT TISSUE INJURIES

Muscle	Tendon	Joint Capsule
Hypertonicity	Tendinosis	Capsular Tear
Myofascial Trigger Points	Tenosynovitis	Capsular Adhesion
Atrophy	Avulsion	
Strain		Fascia
Contusion	Ligament	Fascial Tearing
	Sprain	Fascial Shortening
Nerve		
Nerve Compression	Cartilage	Bursa
Neural Tension	Compressive Degeneration	Bursitis

19. Garrett WE, Jr., Safran MR, Seaber AV, Glisson RR, Ribbeck BM. Biomechanical comparison of stimulated and nonstimulated skeletal muscle pulled to failure. *Am J Sports Med.* 1987;15(5):448-454.
20. Ernst E. The safety of massage therapy. *Rheumatology (Oxford).* 2003;42(9):1101-1106.
21. Nordin M, Frankel V. *Basic Biomechanics of the Musculoskeletal System.* 2nd ed. Malvern: Lea & Febiger; 1989.
22. Khan KM, Cook JL, Taunton JE, Bonar F. Overuse tendinosis, not tendinitis - Part 1: A new paradigm for a difficult clinical problem. *Physician Sportsmed.* 2000;28(5):38+.
23. Almekinders LC, Temple JD. Etiology, Diagnosis, and Treatment of Tendinitis - An Analysis of the Literature. *Med Sci Sport Exercise.* 1998;30(8):1183-1190.
24. Cook JL, Khan KM. What is the most appropriate treatment for patellar tendinopathy? *Br J Sports Med.* 2001;35(5):291-294.
25. Kraushaar BS, Nirschl RP. Tendinosis of the elbow (tennis elbow). Clinical features and findings of histological, immunohistochemical, and electron microscopy studies. *J Bone Joint Surg Am.* 1999;81(2):259-278.
26. Whiteside JA, Andrews JR, Conner JA. Tendinopathies of the Elbow. *Sport Med Arthroscopy.* 1995;3(3):195-203.
27. Astrom M, Westlin N. Blood flow in chronic Achilles tendinopathy. *Clin Orthop.* Nov 1994(308):166-172.
28. Fadale PD, Wiggins ME. Corticosteroid Injections: Their Use and Abuse. *J Am Acad Orthop Surg.* 1994;2(3):133-140.
29. Nordin Ma, Frankel V. *Basic Biomechanics of the Musculoskeletal System.* 3rd ed. Baltimore: Lippincott Williams & Wilkins; 2001.
30. Magee D. *Orthopedic Physical Assessment.* 3rd ed. Philadelphia: W.B. Saunders; 1997.
31. Myers TW. *Anatomy Trains.* Edinburgh: Churchill Livingstone; 2001.
32. Schultz RL, Feitis R. *The Endless Web.* Berkeley: North Atlantic Books; 1996.
33. Cantu R, Grodin A. *Myofascial Manipulation: Theory and Clinical Application.* Gaithersburg: Aspen; 1992.
34. Schleip R. Fascial plasticity - a new neurobiological explanation. *Journal of Bodywork and Movement Therapies.* 2003;7(1):11-19.
35. Upton AR, McComas AJ. The double crush in nerve entrapment syndromes. *Lancet.* Aug 18 1973;2(7825):359-362.
36. Butler D. *Mobilisation of the Nervous System.* London: Churchill Livingstone; 1991.
37. Tortora G, Grabowski S. *Principles of Anatomy and Physiology.* 8th ed. New York: Harper Collins; 1996.
38. Seddon HJ. Three types of nerve injury. *Brain.* 1943;66:237.
39. Sunderland S. *Nerves and Nerve Injuries.* 2nd ed. Edinburgh: Churchill Livingstone; 1978.
40. Schleip R. Fascial plasticity - a new neurobiological explanation. Journal of Bodywork and Movement Therapies. 2003;7(1):11-19.

3 The HOPRS Method

The HOPRS format outlined in this chapter provides an effective method for gathering and interpreting clinical assessment information. This process allows the clinician to proceed logically from the most general information presented in the initial case history through evaluation of tissue pathology to specialized physical examination procedures.

There are several reasons for using a systematic method for gathering information. Accurate assessment relies on the practitioner's ability to interpret results from investigative questions and procedures. Detailed orthopedic assessment produces a large amount of information about the client's condition. Without a systematic method of organization, the information could become a scattered accumulation of facts and observations and leave the practitioner at a loss for how to proceed in clinical treatment.

In addition, the practitioner must have an accurate method for measuring and documenting results within a treatment session and between multiple sessions. Comparative analysis is how clinical improvement is measured. The practitioner is also able to share this information with other health professionals and third party payers. Assessment results might also be required as evidence in a legal case associated with the client's injury.

Finally, in many cases, a practitioner has a limited amount of time to conduct assessment procedures and complete a treatment session. Streamlining the evaluation process with a systematic method makes assessment more efficient.

HOPRS Method

OVERVIEW

There are a number of structured methods of orthopedic assessment. One of the most effective is a system easily remembered by the acronym **HOPRS**, standing for **History, Observation, Palpation, Range-of-Motion and Resistance Testing**, and **Special Tests**. In some texts, range-of-motion and resistance testing are included in the special tests section and the acronym used is **HOPS**.

However, these tests are more appropriately treated as individual procedures separate from special tests.

The HOPRS procedure is arranged in an order that eases assimilation and interpretation of the information gathered. The first part, history, is the subjective report from the client about his or her condition. In the history, the client shares important information about their condition, such as when and how the problem started, symptoms, previous or related conditions, and how the condition has impacted daily life. There is no substitute for a well-taken history, as the skilled interviewer can extract a wealth of information in this part of the evaluation.

Observation and palpation occur at the beginning of the assessment and continue throughout the process. Observation includes anything the practitioner sees that gives clues to the presenting complaint. Palpation involves information the practitioner gathers from physical contact with the client from initial palpatory assessment and throughout massage treatment.

Range-of-motion and resistance testing, the fourth part of HOPRS, evaluates active and passive motion and resisted isometric muscle contractions. Active range of motion is performed first, followed by passive range of motion if needed, and then manual resistive tests. The reason for this order is discussed in more detail later in the chapter. The final section, special tests, includes orthopedic testing procedures that are used to evaluate tissue involvement and pathology. These tests have unique names, usually derived from the individual who developed the test. Each test is designed to elicit a particular response to determine the likelihood of a particular condition.

SOAP Notes

Documenting the results of the assessment is important for the reasons discussed earlier. There are different methods of documentation, but in health care professions the **SOAP** note is primarily used. **SOAP** is an acronym for the four part process of the documentation note: **Subjective, Objective, Assessment**, and **Plan**. The texts by Thompson and Kettenbach are valuable resources for employing the use of SOAP notes in massage therapy.[1, 2]

The HOPRS evaluation procedure fits well into the SOAP note format (Figure 3.1). History information is put into the Subjective section. Responses from the OPRS sections belong in the Objective portion. Once the HOPRS evaluation process is finished, the first two sections of the SOAP note are completed. By interpreting the information from the HOPRS evaluation in the first two sections of the SOAP note, the practitioner gains an impression of the client's condition and the tissues involved. These impressions are documented in the third section of the SOAP note, Assessment. Following Assessment, a beneficial treatment approach or Plan is constructed. Each component of the HOPRS protocol is discussed below along with guidelines on how to perform the procedures.

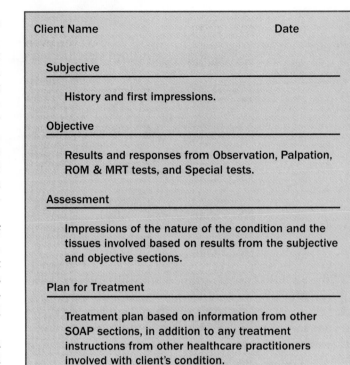

Client Name	Date

Subjective

   History and first impressions.

Objective

   Results and responses from Observation, Palpation, ROM & MRT tests, and Special tests.

Assessment

   Impressions of the nature of the condition and the tissues involved based on results from the subjective and objective sections.

Plan for Treatment

   Treatment plan based on information from other SOAP sections, in addition to any treatment instructions from other healthcare practitioners involved with client's condition.

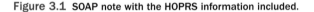

Figure 3.1 SOAP note with the HOPRS information included.

HISTORY

The first part of the HOPRS assessment is the **history**. The practitioner conducts a relaxed interview with the client dressed. A medical questionnaire, of which there are several types, is useful. Setting these out in a waiting room allows the client to fill the form out without taking up treatment time. As discussed in Chapter 1, a thorough history is more detailed than the standard set of questions about indications and contraindications for treatment. A detailed client history is crucial in determining the nature of soft-tissue conditions.

Clients with chronic dysfunction, pain, or injury conditions should be asked detailed questions to identify their complaint. Though subjective, the importance of client history should not be underestimated; the information acquired is some of the most valuable and affects treatment progression. Identifying pertinent information in the history can prevent contraindicated therapeutic approaches. It can also help the practitioner gauge progress and effectiveness of the therapy.

The history must pursue a logical line of inquiry, which requires skill on the part of the practitioner. The practitioner's ability to ask pertinent questions is guided by knowledge and understanding of various pathological problems. The better understanding a practitioner has of common orthopedic conditions, the better equipped they are to select questions that effectively isolate the client's problem. It is important to know why certain questions are asked and what the answers indicate. However, even without a comprehensive knowledge of the pathologies in this text, a productive interview can still be conducted.

Interview Style and Facilitation

Much of the success in history-taking results from the individual's interview style. First impressions are powerful. The communication dynamics established during the initial interview set the stage for communication patterns throughout the therapeutic relationship. Inadequate interpersonal skills play a dominant role in poor or failed therapeutic outcomes in many health care professions.[3] Therefore it is essential to create a communication experience for both client and practitioner that is open, clear, and engenders trust.

An important aspect of an effective interview style is the practitioner's ability to listen.[4,5] Listening skills include the ability not to rudely interrupt, while also facilitating the gathering of quality information from the client.[6] Effective listening requires that the practitioner concentrate on what the client is saying versus allowing his/her thoughts to dominate. This is sometimes difficult and takes practice. Listening is also about paying attention to both the obvious information and the finer details that may prove important later. More than anything, good listening skills demonstrate genuine, empathic interest.

Facilitation is also relevant in the history. Control over the interview process allows the practitioner to use time efficiently. It can be a delicate balance between offering proper listening skills and keeping the interview on track. Gentle interruption and redirecting the client responses are important facilitation techniques. With practice the practitioner becomes better at facilitating the interview and keeping the client on topic.

Interview Questions

The order and way in which questions are asked is important. Several guidelines should be observed in the interview. The interviewer should ask only one question at a time. Too many questions at once may cause the client to leave out significant details and prevent an important line of inquiry. Open-ended and closed-ended questions are used to produce different types of information.

The interview should progress from general questions to the more specific. General questions cover issues such as the client's age, previous medical history, current medications, work and recreational activities, sleep habits, stress levels, and the primary reason for the visit. It is best to start the history with basic open-ended questions such as, "Why are you seeking massage therapy?" Closed-ended questions limit the client's response. For example, yes-no questions give the client only two choices. Open-ended questions elicit more information than close-ended, as they allow the client more freedom to relate what is relevant to them.

After gathering basic information, the client is asked questions that probe further into the primary reason for treatment. While there is no exact list of questions, some guidelines are helpful. In the regional chapters, the history sections provide information on the client's experience with the condition. From these sections, practitioners can create specific questions about the client's pain and functioning.

General Questions

The following questions provide a basic framework for conducting the interview.

WHAT IS THE NATURE OF YOUR COMPLAINT?

The client should describe the primary complaint, whether the condition is acute or chronic, and how it affects their functional abilities. There may be more than one aspect to the complaint, so allow the client an opportunity to fully explore their symptoms of pain, discomfort, or impairment.

HOW WOULD YOU DESCRIBE YOUR PAIN OR DISCOMFORT?

It is often only mild discomfort that leads some clients to massage; however, many seek orthopedic or clinical massage care due to pain. The quality of pain gives clues as to the type of tissue injured. Sharp, burning pain is indicative of neurological disorders. Dull, aching pain usually results from muscular disorders such as myofascial trigger points. While it is not possible to make an exact determination of the tissue injured from the description of the pain, the quality of pain is a helpful indicator. It is important to identify the severity of the client's pain, keeping in mind that each person has a different pain threshold. A frequently used pain scale is the visual analog scale (Figure 3.2).[7] It is easy for the client to understand and gives a reference point for the subjective experience of the client's pain. The scale can be used in successive treatments to measure the client's perception of pain over the course of time.

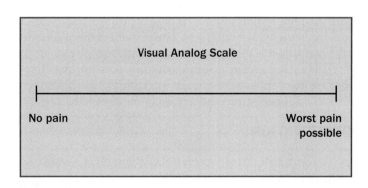

Figure 3.2 The Visual Analog Scale can be used in the initial and subsequent sessions to gauge changes in the client's pain.

WHERE DO YOU FEEL PAIN?

Some disorders cause pain locally while others produce pain in distant locations. Identifying exactly where the client feels pain helps determine if the present complaint is from local or referred pain and which tissues may be involved. It is helpful to ask the client to place her/his finger directly on the area that reproduces the pain. If the client is able to reproduce the primary pain by pressing directly on an area, anatomical knowledge helps identify what structures under the palpating finger could cause the pain. If the client is unable to press on something that reproduces the primary pain, the injured tissue may be either deep and inaccessible, or in another location and referring pain.

WHEN DID THE PAIN ARISE?

How long the condition has been present affects the choice of treatment. Whether the onset is gradual or sudden gives clues about pathology. Additional questions along this line elicit specifics about biomechanical factors associated with the onset of the complaint.

ARE THERE SPECIFIC ACTIVITIES THAT AGGRAVATE THE PAIN OR DISCOMFORT? WHAT RELIEVES THE PAIN?

These questions explore additional biomechanical explanations for the complaint. Identifying positions or movements that aggravate or alleviate the pain helps identify the involved tissues. In addition, the client may describe factors such as ice, hot baths, or medications that improve or exacerbate the problem.

HAVE YOU HAD THIS OR A SIMILAR CONDITION BEFORE? IF SO, HOW WAS IT RESOLVED?

Some pain complaints are recurrent, caused by, or related to, a previous injury or illness. If the complaint was successfully resolved before, beneficial treatment approaches may be easier to identify. If previous attempts at treatment were unsuccessful, helpful clues are also provided about which tissues are injured or treatment methods that might not be productive.

HAVE YOU CONSULTED OTHER HEALTH PROFESSIONALS FOR THIS PROBLEM? IF SO, WHAT WAS THE RESULT?

It is beneficial to know if the client has seen another health care provider, particularly if the condition could be a serious acute injury or illness. The present complaint may be a condition that should be evaluated by a physician. It is also helpful at this point to identify whether previous therapeutic approaches were successful as this gives additional insight into the nature of the problem.

OBSERVATION

The next portion of the HOPRS procedure, **observation**, takes note of visual cues that help identify the presenting complaint. Significant information is gained through observation. Visual analysis begins at first sight of the

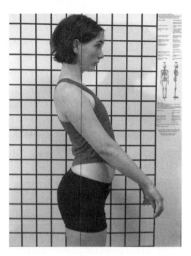

Figure 3.3 A postural grid chart and plumb line are used for accurately assessing postural distortions.

client and continues through the duration of the treatment program or session. It is beneficial for the practitioner to be observant in the initial meeting as movement patterns may be notable. Patterns of compensation or substitution may be evident as the client attempts to avoid pain or discomfort. In these naturally occurring opportunities, the practitioner has a chance to observe the client in an unobtrusive manner.

Postural distortion is a particularly important characteristic evaluated during observation. It is important to note that the ideal postural alignment shown in medical texts is only a reference point. Unique structural differences exist among individuals and are to be expected. However, posture can play a significant role in dysfunction and should be evaluated. An accurate postural evaluation requires a frame of reference, such as a plumb line and a wall chart grid (Figure 3.3).

Patterns of body symmetry reveal information about muscular tension, congenital disorders, previous injury, or tissue dysfunction. However, asymmetry is not always pathological. It is common to have some degree of difference between sides. An observed deviation should be considered in the assessment to determine if it produces dysfunction. If dysfunctional, consider whether it is significant enough to be a primary cause for, or contributes in some way, to the pathology.

There are several other visual indicators to watch for during the remainder of the assessment process. Skin texture and appearance may point to certain orthopedic problems or systemic disorders. Muscle contours should be evaluated to see if they are smooth and indicative of appropriate muscle tone. Atrophy of muscle tissue is an indicator of neurological impairment. Take note of visual signs of inflammation, such as redness or swelling, particularly if the condition is a recent injury. Previous injuries that may be contributing to the complaint might be seen.

Movement observation requires a frame of reference.

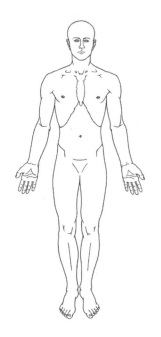

Figure 3.4 Anatomical position. (Mediclip image copyright, 1998 Williams & Wilkins. All rights reserved.)

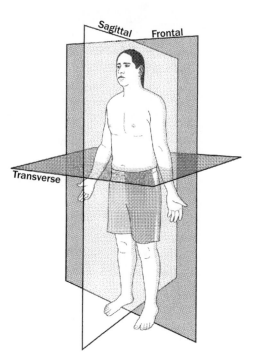

Figure 3.5 Cardinal planes. (Mediclip image copyright, 1998 Williams & Wilkins. All rights reserved. Adapted.)

Anatomical position is the static position of reference for visual assessment (Figure 3.4). Movements, postural distortions, and body position are described in relation to anatomical position. The three cardinal planes, frontal, sagittal, and horizontal, are used as a visual template to describe motion (Figure 3.5). For every plane there is an associated axis of rotation perpendicular to the plane itself.

The **frontal** (also called **coronal**) plane divides the body into two sections (front and back). Joint movements in the frontal plane occur around an antero-posterior axis. Common movements in this plane include abduction, adduction and lateral flexion. In the **sagittal** plane, the body is divided into a left and right section. Joint movements in the sagittal plane are around a medio-lateral axis of rotation. Common movements in this plane include flexion and extension. The **transverse** plane divides the body into upper and lower segments. The axis of rotation for movements in the transverse plane is a superior-inferior axis. Common movements in this plane include

medial and lateral rotation as well as left and right rotation of the spine.

There are a number of anatomical terms used for documenting positions during the assessment. A brief review of these terms is included in Box 3.1. Anatomical position is the reference point for all motion evaluation. Box 3.2 lists the primary single-plane movements that occur in the cardinal planes. Because these movements only occur in one plane, they are the simplest movements to reproduce accurately and are used extensively in range-of-motion and resistance testing.

PALPATION

Assessment through **palpation** is an essential skill for the soft-tissue practitioner. The human hand is a sensitive tool that can produce valuable information about soft-tissue disorders. A benefit of massage therapy is that palpation occurs not only during the initial evaluation, but throughout the treatment process. Consequently, changes in tissue response can be continually evaluated.

Investigative palpation is a complex psychomotor skill that involves far more than poking or prodding someone while searching for pain. It includes not only the muscular activity of performing the palpatory movement, but also the processes of perception and cognition. While performing palpation, the practitioner perceives a multitude of sensations with the hand. Perceiving often subtle information requires practice and palpatory skills are developed.

Box **3.1** Anatomical Direction Terms	
Anterior	Toward the front of the body
Posterior	Toward the back of the body
Superior (cephalad)	Toward the head
Inferior (caudal)	Toward the feet
Medial	Toward the midline of the body
Lateral	Away from the midline of the body

Box 3.2 Single-Plane Movements

Flexion	involves a decrease in the joint's angle. In most cases flexion brings the anterior surfaces of the involved bones closer together.
Extension	involves an increase in the joint's angle. When the angle reaches 180^0 the joint is in full extension. Many joints are in full extension in anatomical position. Movement past full extension (180^0) is called either extension or hyperextension; this text uses hyperextension.
Abduction	is movement of a limb away from the midline of the body.
Adduction	is movement of a limb toward the midline of the body.
Medial Rotation	is rotary movement of a segment where the anterior surface rotates toward the midline of the body.
Lateral Rotation	is a rotary movement of a segment where the anterior surface rotates away from the midline of the body.

There are several primary characteristics of an effective palpatory examination. Investigative palpation is the first therapeutic physical contact between the practitioner and the client. As such, it sets the tone for much of the interaction between the client and practitioner. It is essential to convey compassion during the palpatory exam and throughout the treatment.

Another skill essential in palpation is visualizing the structures underneath the fingers. Visualization strengthens knowledge and comprehension of anatomy in three dimensions, as opposed to the two dimensional images in anatomy texts. It also aids in identifying the structures requiring treatment.

Types of Palpatory Information

Different types of information are acquired during palpatory evaluation. Rattray & Ludwig suggest the **Four Ts** of palpation - *temperature, texture, tenderness,* and *tone* - as a framework for evaluating findings during palpation.[8] In addition to these four categories a fifth, *referred sensation*, has been added.

Temperature

Variations in tissue temperature may indicate a number of problems. Inflamed tissues may feel warm, whereas those with impaired vascular flow may feel cool.

Texture

Sensations of texture difference are felt in the skin as well as in deeper structures. In the skin, systemic disorders may be evident with symptoms such as dryness, lack of pliability, excess moisture, cracking, splitting, sores, excess pliability, rashes, or a host of other irritations. Texture difference in structures below the skin yields valuable information as well. The practitioner may identify any number of the following variations in sub-cutaneous tissues: edema; scar tissue or fibrosis; lack of proper mobility; structures that should not be present in healthy tissue such as neoplasms, cysts, bone spurs, or tumors; anatomical alterations such as joint misalignment, muscle tightness, crepitus, or fiber direction; muscle atrophy or other changes due to metabolic or systemic disorders.

Tenderness

Pain and discomfort are primary signs of tissue disorder. Typically, pain is not evident until additional pressure is applied to the injured tissue. The practitioner should pay particular attention to the type of pain produced, for example: sharp, shooting, dull, aching, diffuse, localized, or other kinds of sensation. Types of pain correlate with the types of tissues affected.

Tone

Tone correlates to muscle tissue and provides information as to the health, habitual usage, and state of the tissue. The practitioner is primarily attempting to identify whether a muscle is hypertonic, indicating excessive neurological excitement, or hypotonic, which indicates impairment of neurological function. Note that muscles can feel hypertonic (tight) when in fact they are being overstretched and pulled taut due to postural distortion.

Referred Sensation

Palpation can produce sensations in other regions or areas. An example is pressure on a peripheral nerve that produces paresthesia distally along the length of an extremity. While the practitioner may not feel the nerve tissue, the client's response to the pressure provides information about the structure being palpated. It is important to encourage the client to give thorough information about any sensations (not just pain) experienced in response to palpation. Myofascial trigger points are another example of a pathological phenomenon that can produce referred pain or neurological sensations.

Appropriate Pressure

Appropriate pressure should be used during palpatory evaluation. One of the biggest mistakes inexperienced clinicians make when learning to feel structures during palpation is to use too much pressure. In some cases it is necessary to use significant pressure, especially if the structure being accessed is relatively deep. However, even deep pressure should only be used after slowly and gently working through the more superficial tissues. The clinician may miss subtle sensations in the superficial tissue in the zeal to press into the deeper tissues and feel something significant.

More specific information can be derived from palpation with an increased load applied to the target tissue. If there is a structural problem in a muscle-tendon unit there will be more tenderness if the site of injury is palpated while the muscle is being stretched or contracted, such as during a manual resistive test. Likewise, a sprained ligament can be palpated while it is under tensile stress during a ligamentous stress test and is likely to be more tender. The increased degree of tenderness in these tissues will help localize and identify the primary source of pain if there is structural damage to the soft tissues.

RANGE-OF-MOTION AND RESISTANCE TESTING

In the R portion of the HOPRS procedure the practitioner evaluates the client's ability to move actively, passively, and against manual resistance. Different information is derived from **active range-of-motion (AROM), passive range-of-motion (PROM),** and **manual resistive tests (MRT).** These tests produce some of the most valuable data in the assessment process. By cross-referencing information between AROM, PROM, and MRTs, a more accurate picture of the pain or dysfunction is created.

The system presented here for organizing the information acquired in motion and resistance testing is based on the concepts of **selective tissue tension** developed by James Cyriax.[9] Listing motions in their single-plane movements categorizes the range-of-motion tests and allows the tests to be accurately reproduced in later assessments by the practitioner or other healthcare practitioners.

Active motion is performed first to determine the motion possible within the client's pain tolerance prior to further stressing the involved tissues. In addition, results from AROM make certain PROM evaluations unnecessary. For example, it is unlikely that a client will be pain-free during active motion and have pain on the same motion when performed passively. Therefore, if active motion is pain-free, it is often unnecessary to do passive ROM. If the practitioner suspects certain motions might be painful, these motions should be tested near the end of the evaluation to decrease aggravation of the injured tissues and reduce client discomfort. MRTs are performed after AROM and PROM evaluations because MRTs put more stress on the muscle-tendon unit.

Contractile and Inert Tissues

In order to use this data effectively, the practitioner must understand which tissues are being used in each of these different procedures. Active movements use both **contractile** and **inert tissues.** Contractile tissues (muscle and tendon) produce movement, while inert tissues (nerves, bursa, and fascia) are moved in the process. If there is pain during active movement, it can result from a problem in any of these tissues. Because both contractile and inert tissues are involved in AROM, it is the most general of these testing procedures.

Passive movement emphasizes the inert tissues, but may reveal problems when certain contractile tissues are stretched. Because the client uses no muscular activity to perform passive motion, the contractile units are not engaged. Passive motion moves inert tissues and pain during passive movement indicates a good likelihood that an inert tissue is involved. Muscles whose **concentric** action is opposite the passive motion being engaged are stretched at the end range of passive movement. For example, medial rotators are stretched in passive lateral rotation. If pain arises only near the end range, dysfunction may exist in the tissues that are being stretched.

MRTs only use contractile tissues because no motion occurs during the test, only muscle contraction. Therefore, if there is pain during an MRT, it is likely the result of a problem in the muscle-tendon unit.

It is important to remember that the procedures listed here are not absolute or definitive tests. These tests should be considered as one aspect of the broader assessment process. Test results should be compared with findings from other portions of the assessment in order to gain further understanding of the client's pathology.

Active Range-of-Motion Tests

A variety of information is gained from observing active movements, including the client's willingness to move, their available range of motion, muscle strength, pain, and coordination. An adequate understanding of kinesiology and biomechanics is necessary to perform AROM evaluations correctly. In addition, the practitioner must evaluate whether the motion is performed by **concentric** or **eccentric** muscle activity in order to determine which tissues are responsible for that particular movement (see Chapter 2).

How To Perform AROM Tests

The following are basic steps for performing active range-of-motion testing.

DETERMINE THE MOTIONS POSSIBLE AT THE BODY REGION OR JOINT BEING EVALUATED.

For range-of-motion evaluation, the practitioner must know what motions the body region or joint being assessed is capable of performing. Chapters 5–11 include a description of the primary single-plane movements related to the joints of that region.

SELECT THE MOTION TO BE EVALUATED.
All single-plane movements of the joint should be evaluated one at a time in order to perform a comprehensive assessment. If there are movements suspected to be painful, have the client perform these last to minimize tissue irritation and discomfort.

In some situations select motions are eliminated from the AROM evaluation. One reason to eliminate a specific motion from the AROM evaluation is severe pain. If during the initial history, the client reports severe pain with a particular motion, that motion is sometimes omitted from the evaluation process because the practitioner has already learned it is painful. If the motion is performed, exaggerated sensitivity in the region could result and adversely affect results in the remainder of the assessment.

Some motions can be eliminated from the AROM evaluation due to time restraints in the evaluation. The client may have stated in the history that certain motions were pain free and caused no limited movement. In the interest of brevity those motions could be eliminated because it has already been determined that there is no pain or restriction when they are performed.

DETERMINE THE TISSUES INVOLVED IN THE ACTIVE MOTION.
AROM tests involve both contractile and inert tissues. Clarifying which contractile and inert tissues are involved in AROM evaluations is critical to gaining valuable information from these procedures. The inert tissues involved are the same regardless of the body's position. However, the contractile tissues recruited during an AROM evaluation could differ depending on the position of the body and the resistance offered by gravity.

AROM evaluations primarily focus on the contractile tissues whose concentric action is the same as the motion being performed. Mistaking eccentric action for concentric is a common mistake when beginning AROM testing. For example, the shoulder flexors are engaged when performing active shoulder flexion from a standing or seated position. However, when the arm is returned to the starting position, extension is the motion being performed. It is not the shoulder extensors performing this action, but the shoulder flexors which contract both concentrically during the initial motion and eccentrically on the return to neutral. Careful consideration and thought about the tissues performing the action is important.

INSTRUCT THE CLIENT HOW TO PERFORM THE CHOSEN MOVEMENT.
In some cases demonstrating the movement first ensures the client fully understands what they are being asked to do. In other cases, it is enough to provide a basic instruction such as, "turn your head to the right."

HAVE THE CLIENT PERFORM THE MOTION.
With a unilateral complaint, test the uninvolved side first. Testing the uninvolved side first establishes a baseline for what normal motion should be. Any complaint involving

the axial skeleton should be tested on both sides. Have the client perform the full range of motion for the action being tested.

NOTE REPORTED PAIN, DISCOMFORT, OR MOVEMENT LIMITATION.
Treatment notes should document the client's pain or discomfort. Estimate as closely as possible the point during the motion at which pain occurs. Accuracy in measuring pain location is increased if a goniometer is used. The practitioner might observe a lack of smoothness in movement, but the client may not report pain or discomfort. Lack of smoothness could indicate a neuromuscular coordination problem and should be documented in the treatment notes. Valuable information is gained when all of the results are evaluated.

Pain with AROM
Pain with active movement indicates a problem in either contractile or inert structures engaged during that movement. It can be difficult to isolate whether the pain is from contractile or inert tissues, so further assessment is necessary. Common causes of pain during AROM include muscle strain, binding fibrous scar tissue, impingement of soft tissue, tendinosis or tendinitis, tenosynovitis, excessive neural compression or tension, joint capsule damage, degenerative changes, or internal structural pathologies within the joint.

No pain with AROM
If there is no pain with AROM it is likely there is minimal or no damage to a structure, contractile or inert, involved in the active movement. However, there may be damage that is not immediately evident. For example, a mild muscle strain may not be painful because not enough muscle fibers are recruited to produce pain. When the muscle is tested with an MRT, pain can result because a greater amount of muscle activation is required, which loads the muscle enough to produce pain. Additional testing will be needed to identify the source of pain and it is essential to cross-reference findings with other evaluation procedures.

Other information from AROM evaluation
Faulty biomechanical patterns such as compensation, guarding, or splinting may indicate an attempt to avoid pain. These reactions may be indicative of soft-tissue damage or dysfunction and need to be evaluated with other portions of the assessment process.

Passive Range-of-Motion Tests
Passive range-of-motion testing focuses primarily on inert tissues because contractile tissues are not employed during passive movement. However, at the end of passive movement some contractile tissues are stretched and can be evaluated in PROM. For example, at the end of passive elbow flexion, the elbow extensor muscles are stretched. While the action being performed is elbow flexion, it is

the extensors, not the flexors that are stressed during this movement.

In addition to evaluating pain, the practitioner should pay attention to the quality of movement throughout the passive range of motion. Consequently palpation plays an important role here, although it is palpation of movement versus specific tissues. As the practitioner moves a client's limb passively through a range of motion, sensations that indicate binding, restriction, or crepitus in the movement might be felt. There may or may not be pain associated with these restrictions. The practitioner must be sensitive to the subtle feelings in the quality of movement in order to identify these problems.

End Feel

Identifying joint involvement requires evaluating the quality of movement at the end range of passive movement. The practitioner evaluates both normal motion and what is called **accessory motion.** Accessory motion is the amount of movement at the end range that goes beyond the end of the client's active movement, but remains within normal anatomical limits.[10] For example, when a client actively hyperextends the wrist, a certain range of motion is achieved. By applying pressure to the palm of the hand in the direction of further hyperextension, the practitioner can achieve slightly more motion without going past the natural anatomical boundary. The additional motion is accessory joint motion. When performing PROM the limb is moved all the way through normal and accessory motion.

The end of accessory motion is an important indicator of joint or soft-tissue pathology. The sensation felt at the end of accessory motion is called the **end feel**.[9] Whether or not an end feel is pathological or normal depends on the joint. For example, the end feel described below as bone-to-bone is normal for elbow extension, but pathological at the end of lateral shoulder rotation. In some cases, the terms used to describe end feel are general qualitative terms such as firm or soft. Although there is some variation in terms used to describe end feel, the following are generally used.

BONE-TO-BONE
Results from two bony surfaces contacting each other at the end of the movement range. An example is the olecranon process contacting the olecranon fossa at the end of elbow extension. Elbow extension is one of the few motions in the body where a bone-to-bone end feel is normal. Usually, soft tissues limit motion before the bones contact each other.

SOFT-TISSUE APPROXIMATION
When motion is stopped by the compression of muscle tissue between opposing limb segments it produces soft-tissue approximation. An example is full flexion of the elbow where motion stops as the biceps brachii and brachialis contact the wrist flexors.

TISSUE STRETCH
This is the most common normal end feel and results from stretching the soft tissues surrounding the joint. The stretch of soft tissue limits movement and is further described as **leathery, firm,** or **soft**. Medial rotation of the shoulder, which stretches the lateral rotator muscles and glenohumeral joint capsule, is a good example of a tissue stretch end feel that is soft.

In other situations, the tissue stretch is rapid due to sudden ligament tension, giving a **firm** end to the motion that feels similar to a bone-to-bone end feel. It is sometimes called a firm end feel. Extension of the knee, where the cruciate ligaments suddenly become taut, is an example.

MUSCLE SPASM
Muscle spasm involves limitation to movement that feels abrupt and occurs prior to where the end range of motion should be. Pain is usually associated with this end feel. Muscle spasm is a pathological end feel because there is no joint that has muscle spasm as its normal end feel.

SPRINGY BLOCK
This end feel is pathological and is caused by a loose body within the joint space. The loose body alters the normal end point of motion in the joint. However, it may not alter the motion in the same way each time it is performed. For example, when a torn meniscus is present in the knee, the loose body may wedge between the tibia and femur and prevent normal joint mechanics. When flexion or extension is attempted, the limb can spring back a little due to the loose body of cartilage being pinched in the joint. In many cases, when the motion is repeated, the joint does not spring back in the same way because the loose body has moved slightly in the joint.

EMPTY
An empty end feel is one in which no apparent mechanical obstruction exists to movement, but the client suddenly halts or stops movement because of pain. For example, extreme neural tension in the extremities produces this end feel.

How To Perform PROM Tests
The following are the basic steps for performing passive range-of-motion tests.

DETERMINE THE MOTIONS POSSIBLE AT THE JOINT BEING EVALUATED
For range-of-motion evaluation, the practitioner must know what motions the joint being assessed is capable of performing. Chapters 5–11 include a description of the primary single-plane movements related to the joints of that region.

SELECT THE MOTION TO BE EVALUATED
Any movement that is painful with active motion should be evaluated with passive movement. The single-plane

movements are evaluated one at a time, just as with active motion. If there are movements suspected to be painful, evaluate these last so not to increase tissue irritation or sensitivity. If there is no pain with active movement, it is unlikely pain will be found with passive movement. Therefore, the passive movement can be eliminated, especially if there is limited time and efficiency of the assessment is important. However, end feel is not evaluated with active movement, so performance of some PROM evaluations that are pain free during active movement could be necessary so the end feel of that motion can be properly assessed for joint pathology.

DETERMINE WHICH TISSUES ARE INVOLVED IN THE PASSIVE MOTION

Passive movements focus predominantly on the inert tissues around the joint being moved. However, a muscle whose concentric contraction is in the opposite direction of the passive movement is stretched during the movement. Hypertonicity in these muscles may prematurely limit passive movement.

DETERMINE THE NORMAL END FEEL FOR THE MOTION BEING TESTED

The end feel for the joint is evaluated at the end of the PROM evaluation. Chapter's 5–11 include a chart listing the normal end feel for the primary joints of that region.

HAVE THE CLIENT RELAX AS MUCH AS POSSIBLE

Because the focus of a PROM test is on inert tissues, active muscle contraction should be removed from the testing process as much as possible.

PERFORM THE PASSIVE MOVEMENT

With a unilateral complaint, test the uninvolved side first. Testing the uninvolved side first establishes a baseline for what normal motion should be. As with active motion, any complaint involving the axial skeleton should be tested on both sides.

Gently hold the body part being tested and move it slowly through the desired range of motion. Do not force movements at any point. Pay careful attention to the end feel at the end of the available range. Also pay attention to any sensations of crepitus, restriction, or binding that are felt while holding and moving the limb. If severe pain is elicited, it is not necessary to continue movement through the remainder of the range of motion.

NOTE ANY REPORTED PAIN, DISCOMFORT, OR MOVEMENT LIMITATION

Treatment notes should document any pain or discomfort felt by the client during the passive movement. Also note any pathological end feel. As with active motion, estimate as closely as possible the point during the motion at which pain occurs. A goniometer can be used for greater accuracy. Valuable information is gained when all of the results are evaluated.

Because PROM tests are performed after AROM, the results from both procedures are considered together to help identify potential tissues at fault. If pain occurs

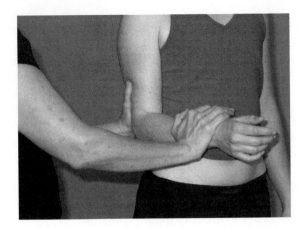

Figure 3.6 In MRT, resistence is often performed when the muscle is close to the middle of its range of motion.

during AROM but not PROM, contractile tissues are suspected. If there is pain during AROM and PROM, inert tissues are likely the cause. Remember that it is unusual to have no pain with AROM and pain with PROM because the same tissues are moved in both tests.

Pain with PROM

If passive movement reproduces the client's pain prior to reaching the end range, inert tissues are indicated. However, which inert tissue is causing the pain may not be immediately clear. Common causes of pain with passive motion are fibrous scar tissue restrictions, ligamentous injury, joint capsule injury, impingement of soft tissues such as bursa or nerves, osteoarthritis, or other joint pathologies.

If passive movement reproduces the client's complaint near the end range of motion, nerves or muscles that are stretched might be at fault. A pathological end feel may produce pain at the end of passive motion.

No pain with PROM

If there is no pain with passive movement it is unlikely the injury involves inert tissue. However, keep in mind that the PROM evaluation may have been performed in a plane that did not precisely stress the involved tissue. Additional testing will be needed to identify the source of pain and it is essential to cross-reference findings with other evaluation procedures.

Manual Resistive Tests

Manual resistive tests are also called resisted isometric movements because they require an isometric muscle contraction. The purpose of an MRT is to evaluate proper function of the contractile tissues (muscle and tendon) during movement. The MRT is designed to confirm and elaborate on findings from AROM and PROM tests. In the MRT, information is acquired by selectively applying tension to the muscle-tendon unit during an isometric contraction without moving inert tissues. Because there is

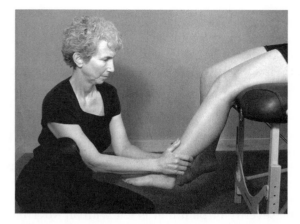

Figure 3.7 For best results, the practitioner places the client's body segment in the start position. The client then holds the position and resists the practitioner's force.

no movement occurring at the joint during the isometric contraction, inert tissues are not involved. (MRTs should not be confused with the muscle testing that is a technique of applied kinesiology).

An MRT can yield information about the function of motor nerves. Weakness during an MRT may indicate loss of muscular strength due to a nerve compression syndrome. To determine which muscles might be weak when specific nerves are affected, see the tables at the end of Chapters 5—11 which list muscles and the nerves that supply them.

How To Perform MRTs

The following are the basic steps for performing muscle resistive tests.

DETERMINE THE MOTIONS POSSIBLE AT THE JOINT OR BODY SEGMENT BEING EVALUATED.

For resistance testing, the practitioner must know what motions the joint being assessed is capable of performing as well as the principle muscles responsible for creating those motions. Chapters 5–11 include a description of the primary single-plane movements related to the joints of that region.

SELECT THE MOTION TO BE EVALUATED.

All single-plane movements of the joint should be evaluated one at a time for a comprehensive assessment. It is especially important to evaluate any resisted motion that causes pain or discomfort with active movement. In some cases certain resisted motions can be eliminated from the MRT evaluation. If there is severe pain with active motion, performing a resisted action of the same motion may be too painful for the client.

If a client reports no pain with active motion, an MRT may still be necessary. In some cases the number of muscle fibers recruited to perform active motion is too small to reproduce the client's symptoms. An MRT may be needed to recruit enough fibers to reproduce symptoms.

DETERMINE THE TISSUES INVOLVED IN THE RESISTED MOTION.

MRTs evaluate contractile tissues so it is important to identify which muscles are recruited. Chapters 5–11 include a list of the primary muscles involved with each single-plane movement. It is rare for any action to involve only one muscle so chances are that several muscles will be recruited during any MRT. However, certain positions minimize the contribution of accessory muscles or those that don't have a strong contribution to the resisted action.

FIND A POSITION THAT EFFECTIVELY ENGAGES THE DESIRED MUSCLE(S).

Different positions can be used to recruit the desired muscle(s) during the MRT. A typical position is to resist the muscle's action when it is close to the middle of its range of motion (Figure 3.6). Another method is to use a position that is more mechanically taxing on the muscle, such as with the muscle fully shortened or fully lengthened. Greater mechanical effort is required when the muscle is in either its fully shortened or fully lengthened position. However, it is not advisable to put muscles that span more than one joint, such as the hamstrings, in a fully shortened position when performing an MRT because a sudden muscle cramp may result. Chapters 5–11 show the most common positions used to perform MRTs for each of the single-plane motions.

HAVE THE CLIENT PERFORM A CONTRACTION AGAINST RESISTANCE.

If there is a unilateral complaint, testing the uninvolved side first helps establish a baseline for what normal strength should be. When evaluating muscle strength, comparison with the unaffected side is particularly important.

The best way to achieve an accurate test result is to place the client's body segment in the appropriate start position and instruct the client to hold the position and not allow the practitioner to move it. The practitioner then attempts to move the limb in the direction opposite the target muscle's concentric action while the client resists the movement (Figure 3.7). The client's resistance contracts the target muscle. The contraction does not have to be a maximal contraction, but a strong effort is required. The contraction is held only long enough to determine if there is pain or weakness from the resisted movement.

There are several advantages of this method. First, the practitioner can more accurately target the desired muscle action by placing the client in the correct position, versus the client initiating the movement. Second, it is the practitioner who determines the amount of resistance that is used during the test. Sometimes very strong clients will perceive the MRT as a strength contest and use an unnecessary amount of force. Third, fewer instructions to the client are needed to perform multiple MRTs because the instruction in each test is simply, "Hold this position and don't let me move it." With fewer instructions, more tests can be accomplished in a shorter period of time.

Another MRT method instructs the client to engage the desired motion with a certain amount of strength. The practitioner then resists the client's effort. Some practitioners use a quantifiable amount of effort by saying something like, "When I say push, I want you to push your arm away from your body using about 40% of your strength." However, it is difficult for anyone to accurately gauge what 40% of their strength is. Using a qualitative modifier is generally better. For example, the practitioner might say, "When I say push, I want you to push your arm away from your body using a moderate amount of effort." In some cases, especially with strong individuals, the client's effort is greater than needed. Usually, the first method described above is preferable.

NOTE ANY REPORTED PAIN, WEAKNESS, OR DISCOMFORT.
Treatment notes should document any pain or discomfort felt by the client. In addition, weakness perceived by the practitioner during the test should be noted. Muscle weakness is graded on a scale from five to zero with five being the strongest contraction and zero the weakest (Box 3.3).[7, 13] Resisted movements that are strong, equal to the unaffected side, and pain free indicate that the problem is not in the muscle-tendon unit. Valuable information is gained when all of the results are evaluated.

BOX 3.3 GRADES OF MUSCLE WEAKNESS

Grade 0	No muscle contraction apparent, indicating no neurological activity in the muscle.
Grade 1	Trace neurological activity found in the muscle. Slight contractile activity, joint motion absent.
Grade 2	Poor strength with complete range only possible when gravity is minimized. Significant dysfunction found in the muscle.
Grade 3	Only fair strength with complete range against gravity, but not more resistance.
Grade 4	Good strength, but strength deficit evident with muscle not as strong as should be.
Grade 5	Normal muscle strength with maximal resistance available.

Muscle Weakness Scale

```
0       1       2       3       4       5
|-------|-------|-------|-------|-------|
Weakest                          Strongest
Contraction                      Contraction
```

Pain with an MRT

If a resisted movement is strong or relatively strong and causes pain, it indicates some type of injury to the muscle-tendon unit. Pain may indicate a problem with the muscle, tendon, or the insertion site of the tendon into the bone. Common causes include muscle strain, tendinosis, or tenosynovitis. Problems of neuromuscular activity that induce chronic muscle spasm may also produce pain. Coordinate this information with other portions of the assessment process. Resisted movements that are weak and painful indicate problems such as a strain or other tissue damage that cause a reflex muscular inhibition.

The severity of pain that is felt with an MRT usually reflects the severity of injury. In some cases, palpating a site of local injury in a muscle during an MRT is painful, when the MRT alone is not. Here the tissue damage is identified because additional stress (in the form of palpation) is applied during manual resistance.

No pain with MRT

If there is no pain with an MRT, the problem may not involve the contractile structure being isolated. However, muscular involvement can not be ruled out completely. In some cases the problem does not produce pain because not enough fibers are recruited in the MRT to reproduce symptoms. Also, myofascial trigger points, which may be painful during static postures or during various movements, may not be painful during an MRT, especially in the larger extremity muscles. Therefore, lack of pain with an MRT should not rule out trigger point activity as a cause of soft-tissue pain.

Weakness with MRT

If weakness is evident when performing a manual resistive test, a neurological deficit may exist. Possible causes include peripheral neuropathy, radiculopathy, upper motor neuron lesion, or systemic disease. Serious muscle weakness is a good reason to refer the client for further neurological evaluation. Resisted movements that are weak and painless may be indicators of a ruptured muscle-tendon unit or neurological dysfunction (see grading scale for muscle weakness in Box 3.3). The art of muscle testing for neurological deficit is complex and the client may benefit from seeing a healthcare practitioner trained in this skill. The reader who is interested in learning more about using muscle testing for evaluating neurological pathology is encouraged to consult the texts by Kendall and Hislop.[11, 12]

SPECIAL ORTHOPEDIC TESTS

Special tests are performed after completion of the history, observation, palpation, and AROM, PROM and MRT evaluations. **Special orthopedic tests** are designed to evaluate the likelihood of a specific problem, such as carpal tunnel syndrome or a sprained medial collateral ligament at the knee. These tests were created through biomechanical analysis of each injury condition. Test results are either positive, suggesting possible presence of the condition, or negative, implying the condition is likely absent. Remember that no test is completely accurate and that these procedures only provide a likelihood that a condition is either present or not. Also note that these are assessment procedures NOT diagnostic tests. Regional orthopedic tests for individual conditions are presented in Chapters 5-11.

The information gained from the other sections of the HOPRS format directs the choice of special tests to perform. Once familiar with several tests in a region, it may be tempting to run through an entire list of tests to find the problem, but this approach is inefficient and leaves out valuable components of the assessment process. The selection of special tests should be based on critical thinking and reasoning that leads one to believe that a particular test will yield beneficial information.

Many special orthopedic tests are designed to provoke or reproduce an existing pain complaint. It is important to be able to reproduce the primary pain to determine if the dysfunctional or injured tissue is correctly identified. However, the practitioner should express the sense of compassion and care that is essential in the therapeutic relationship when performing tests that might produce pain or discomfort for the client.

The practitioner should not focus disproportionate attention on the special tests and neglect other parts of the assessment process. In many clinical cases, the most useful and valuable information is derived from the history, observation, palpation, and ROM sections.

Sensitivity and specificity

Some special tests are more accurate than others. It is helpful to know when a test has a high degree of accuracy and is more reliable. The two factors that determine a test's accuracy are sensitivity and specificity. **Sensitivity** is a measure of how accurate the test is at identifying everyone that has the condition being evaluated. **Specificity** is a measure of how accurate the test is at producing a negative result and ruling out those that don't have the condition. In order for a test to be accurate it must have a high degree of sensitivity as well as specificity.

High-tech Diagnostic Procedures

Although soft-tissue practitioners will not order or perform any of the following tests, they should be familiar with these assessment methods. Optimum evaluation of a client's condition sometimes requires a combination of several testing methods and the client may need to be referred for more advanced testing procedures and diagnosis. A client might also be referred for massage after having had these evaluation procedures. Understanding these procedures contributes to the practitioner's assessment and to effective communication with other health care professionals.

COMMON HIGH-TECH TESTS

Included below are some of the usual high-tech diagnostic procedures used in the orthopedic environment.

X-Ray

The oldest of the current high-tech diagnostic studies, x-ray has been in use since the early part of the last century. A simple x-ray study is also called a **plain radiograph**. This procedure identifies fractures, dislocations, or obvious pathologic structural changes in certain tissues. In some cases a procedure called a **stress radiograph** is used to evaluate the integrity of a soft tissue, such as a ligament, by placing the target tissue under tensile stress during the radiograph. For example, valgus stress might be applied at the knee during the x-ray to investigate whether or not the MCL is intact. If there is more space between the tibia and femur than there should be, there is an indirect indication of ligament stretching or disruption.

While plain radiographs are used widely, there are problems with their accuracy in evaluating certain conditions. For example, small stress fractures, early infection, and other conditions not affecting bone are rarely visible on a plain radiograph. For this reason a number of other specialized x-ray procedures are used, including discography, fluoroscopy, arthrography, myelography, CAT scan, and bone scan.

Discography

This is a procedure used specifically for evaluating the integrity of discs in the spine, which do not show up well on a plain radiograph. It involves visualization of the cervical and lumbar discs after direct injection of a radiopaque (impenetrable to x-ray) dye into the disc. With the dye injected into the disc, the radiologist can achieve a more accurate picture of the intervertebral disc structure to evaluate problems.

Fluoroscopy

Recorded as a videotape or a series of still images, fluoroscopy is a technique used for obtaining a live or moving x-ray image. The x-rays go through the patient and strike a fluorescent plate that is coupled with a device to intensify and sharpen the image. That device is then connected to a television camera and the images may be watched on a TV monitor. Fluoroscopy is particularly helpful when it is important to see movement of various structures. It is also frequently used to visualize abdominal blockages when a radioactive substance like barium is swallowed.

Arthrography

An x-ray procedure showing the outline of a joint after a radiopaque medium and/or air has been injected into the joint. The injection of the material allows an outline of the soft-tissue or joint structures to be constructed. Tendon, ligament, or meniscal tears are more accurately seen with this procedure than with a plain radiograph.

Arthrography is generally used for detecting tears in knee ligaments or pathology in the shoulder such as rotator cuff tears or damage from a dislocation. The results of arthrography procedures are called **arthrograms**.

Myelography

This test is similar to arthrography except it is specific to the spinal column. It is an x-ray examination taken with air or a contrast medium injected into the spinal column to examine the spinal cord and canal for disc protrusions or lesions. It is used with fluoroscopy so that protrusions of a disk on or near a nerve root can be evaluated with different motions of the spine. Myelography is more helpful than plain radiographs in evaluating disc pathology. The results of myelography procedures are called **myelograms.**

CAT Scan

CAT Scan (also called **CT scan**) is an abbreviation for **Computerized Axial Tomography**. In this procedure, a computer is used to compose a picture that results from numerous x-ray images. A series of images is constructed by rotating one degree at a time and then composing a computerized picture based on the density of various tissues.

The CAT's advantage is that it distinguishes between adjacent tissues of similar composition, which may be indistinguishable on x-ray. For example, a plain radiograph will only show shadows of various soft tissues, but a CAT scan can show details of these structures and also include blood vessels, nerves, etc. This procedure is particularly effective for pinpointing tumors because of their density in contrast to adjacent structures.

Bone Scan

The bone scan is one of the regularly used nuclear medicine studies. A radioactive isotope is injected into the body and it migrates to areas where bone is being re-built. The metabolic activity is exaggerated where there is bone pathology, such as a stress fracture, and therefore more of the radioactive isotope is drawn to the area. The radioactive isotope is essentially a tracer that can be followed during x-ray viewing. This procedure is not as clear as an x-ray, but its advantage is the ability to see areas where bone is being constructed.

MRI

MRI is an abbreviation for **Magnetic Resonance Imaging** and is also a computer-generated image. MRI provides an unprecedented degree of detail. Forces from very strong magnets excite the atoms of structures being studied, which in turn emit radio waves that are translated by the computer into a picture. It produces a detailed picture of specific parts, spaces, and tissues.

MRI is used in diagnosis of central nervous system disorders such as multiple sclerosis because of the accurate image it can produce of the gray and white matter in the brain and spinal cord. It is helpful for identifying infections, degenerative disorders, tumors, and various other soft-tissue pathologies. MRI is the procedure of choice to detect injuries involving ligament and tendon damage because of the accuracy of the image it can produce. However, the high cost of this procedure makes it less likely to be used for many non-surgical musculoskeletal disorders like tendinosis, minor sprains, or muscle strains.

Ultrasound

Ultrasound involves high frequency sound waves used to outline soft tissues. Ultrasound evaluation is used to outline intra-pelvic or intra-abdominal masses. An advantage of ultrasound is that it gives real-time images and movement of tissues may be observed during the procedure. Another advantage is that no radiation is used. However, ultrasound waves don't reflect clearly from bone or air, so this procedure is not accurate for looking at bony tissue.

EMG and Nerve Conduction Studies

EMG and nerve conduction studies are measurements of electrical activity in the neuromuscular system. An EMG (electromyogram) is the graphical measurement of muscle contraction resulting from electrical stimulation, ordinarily from a motor nerve impulse. The EMG is helpful in determining if there is a problem involving motor nerves or the neuromuscular junction. Diseases that damage muscle tissue or impair transmission of motor signals such as amyotrophic lateral sclerosis (ALS) or myasthenia gravis are evaluated with EMG studies.

Nerve conduction studies (NCS) are beneficial for examining impulses, both sensory and motor. Electrodes are placed on the surface of the skin or just underneath the skin to measure the rate at which nerve impulses are transmitted along the length of the nerve. If there is a nerve compression syndrome or pathology, the NCS will identify slowing of impulse transmission in the region.

Isokinetic Evaluation

Isokinetic Evaluation uses a computer-assisted strength resistance device that offers accommodating resistance. Accommodating resistance means the machine senses how much effort a muscle is exerting through its range of motion and immediately adjusts its resistance so that the limb maintains a constant velocity. The areas of appropriate strength and areas with weakness are revealed in the test. This test is frequently used in rehabilitation clinics to evaluate improvement in muscle strength and joint function following injuries and surgery. Isokinetic evaluation is used to test and improve muscular strength and endurance, especially after injury.

References

1. Kettenbach G. *Writing SOAP Notes*. 3rd ed. Philadelphia: F.A. Davis Company; 2004.
2. Thompson D. *Hands Heal: Communication, Documentation, and Insurance Billing for Manual Therapists*. Baltimore: Lippincott Williams & Wilkins; 2005.
3. Swain J, Clark J, Parry K, French S, Reynolds F. *Enabling Relationships in Health and Social Care*. Oxford: Butterworth Heinemann; 2004.
4. Roter D, Lipkin M, Jr., Korsgaard A. Sex differences in patients' and physicians' communication during primary care medical visits. *Med Care*. Nov 1991;29(11):1083-1093.
5. Beck RS, Daughtridge R, Sloane PD. Physician-patient communication in the primary care office: a systematic review. *J Am Board Fam Pract*. Jan-Feb 2002;15(1):25-38.
6. Rhoades DR, McFarland KF, Finch WH, Johnson AO. Speaking and interruptions during primary care office visits. *Fam Med*. Jul-Aug 2001;33(7):528-532.
7. Magee D. *Orthopedic Physical Assessment*. 3rd ed. Philadelphia: W.B. Saunders; 1997.
8. Rattray F, Ludwig L. *Clinical Massage Therapy: Understanding, Assessing and Treating over 70 Conditions*. Toronto: Talus Incorporated; 2000.
9. Cyriax J. *Textbook of Orthopaedic Medicine Volume One: Diagnosis of Soft Tissue Lesions*. Vol 1. 8th ed. London: Bailliere Tindall; 1982.
10. Hengeveld E, Banks K, eds. *Maitland's Peripheral Manipulation*. 4th ed. Edinburgh: Elsevier; 2005.
11. Hislop H, Montgomery J. *Daniels and Worthingham's Muscle Testing*. Philadelphia: W.B. Saunders; 2002.
12. Kendall F, Kendall-McCreary E, Geise-Provance P. *Muscles: Testing and Function*. 4th ed. Baltimore: Williams & Wilkins; 1993.
13. Hislop H, Montgomery J. Daniels and Worthingham's Muscle Testing. Philadelphia: W.B. Saunders; 2002.

4 General Soft-Tissue Disorders

Soft-tissue disorders develop in all regions of the body. In some cases, a condition is given a specific medical reference because of its specialized characteristics. Carpal tunnel syndrome for example is essentially a general soft-tissue disorder, in this case nerve compression. In Chapters 5—11 several general soft-tissue disorders are treated as discrete conditions due to their frequency of occurrence and specific characteristics.

Although some general soft-tissue disorders do not have specific condition names, their presence should not be underestimated. Unfortunately, many of these disorders are overlooked in favor of other high-profile conditions or joint dysfunctions.[1] For example, soft-tissue shoulder pain from myofascial trigger points or muscle tightness can be erroneously identified as shoulder arthritis, even though arthritis in the glenohumeral joint is not common. In addition, public and medical overemphasis of a condition can lead to misinterpretation of a client's symptoms.

Carpal tunnel syndrome and fibromyalgia are good examples. When symptoms, such as wrist pain or the combination of fatigue and back pain, are assumed to be caused by high-profile conditions, other causes may be overlooked. Wrist pain and neurological symptoms in the hand can be caused by nerve compression in other areas of the upper extremity, not just in the carpal tunnel. Fibromyalgia is an over-diagnosed condition. Hypertonicity, poor ergonomics, and repetitive stress can cause chronic back pain and sleep problems, leading to fatigue and exhaustion which mimic the symptoms of fibromyalgia. Relatively simple musculoskeletal problems, such as hypertonic muscles, are frequently the cause of a client's musculoskeletal condition.

Proper assessment is crucial for understanding a client's symptoms and the nature of their complaint. In some cases, a client needs referral to a physician who can more thoroughly evaluate and diagnose the condition. In this chapter hypertonicity, myofascial trigger points, strains, nerve compression and tension pathologies, ligament sprains, tendinosis, tendinitis, tenosynovitis, and osteoarthritis are discussed in broad terms as they apply to all regions of the body.

Common Tissue Dysfunction

MUSCULAR HYPERTONICITY & MYOFASCIAL TRIGGER POINTS

Muscular hypertonicity and *myofascial trigger points* are two of the most common orthopedic problems. Despite the fact that these problems are pervasive, they are under-diagnosed in the traditional healthcare environment.[2] Massage is a highly beneficial treatment for these conditions, so it is valuable for the practitioner to appropriately identify them.

Characteristics

Hypertonic (tight) muscles result from various problems such as *biomechanical stress, reflex spasm* due to injury, *postural distortion, metabolic disorders, neurological dysfunction, systemic disorders,* and *psychological stress*.[3-7] As a response to these stressors, there is **an increased level of neurological activity in the motor fibers that supply the affected muscle**. The increased activity raises the level of resting **tonus** (contractile activity while at rest) causing tightness in the muscle.

As a result of the neuromuscular dysfunction, myofascial trigger points may also develop.[3] Myofascial trigger points may be present in muscles that do not appear hypertonic but house **taut bands** within them.[8] Research shows that metabolic, chemical, and psychological stressors can also cause trigger points, but additional research is required for understanding these causes.[8]

Pain can result from hypertonic muscles or trigger points. Myofascial trigger point pain can also affect not only the muscle housing the trigger point, but also muscles in the pain referral zone. See the discussion of muscular hypertonicity and myofascial trigger points in Chapter 2 for more detail about their pathophysiology.

Muscular hypertonicity has acute and chronic onsets. In an acute onset, muscular tightness develops immediately after an injury and is called a spasm. Postures or activities that keep the body in a static position for prolonged periods are particularly problematic for causing muscular hypertonicity and trigger points.[9, 10]

Chronic muscular tightness can lead to alterations in the biomechanical patterns of movement. In some cases the client can become so accustomed to the compensation patterns that the altered position of tightness feels normal.[11] In other cases, there is chronic pain or dysfunction directly evident from the muscular dysfunction. For example, neck pain could directly result from muscular tightness or myofascial trigger points without significantly altering the biomechanical patterns in the area.

In many cases, pain is not the primary detrimental effect of hypertonicity or trigger points. Biomechanical alterations or postural distortions produced by tightness or trigger points can lead to other conditions. For example, muscle tightness or trigger points in the shoulder muscles can alter glenohumeral mechanics and contribute to *subacromial impingement*. Biomechanical problems can be misdiagnosed by other healthcare professionals in favor of more familiar conditions while the underlying muscular dysfunction goes unaddressed.[13]

History

With hypertonicity, clients typically report pain or tightness. Pain is diffuse and exists throughout the muscle as opposed to appearing in a small, localized area. If myofascial trigger points exist, there may be exaggerated tenderness in a specific location and referred pain or other neurological sensations in another area.[12] Myofascial trigger points refer pain or neurological sensations to other regions in characteristic patterns. (Figure 4.1).[8] Diagrams of common myofascial trigger point pain referral patterns specific to the regions are provided in Chapters 5–11. Knowledge of pain referral patterns is important, as active trigger points are often mistaken for other pathologies.

Myofascial trigger points can sometimes cause paresthesia (pins and needles sensations). Evaluate paresthesia thoroughly because either nerve damage or trigger point

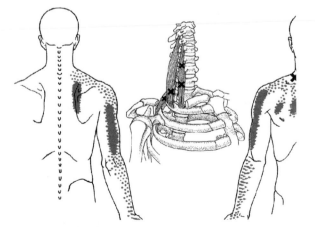

Figure 4.1 Myofascial trigger points of the scalene muscles. (Mediclip image copyright, 1998 Williams & Wilkins. All rights reserved.)

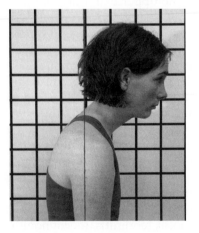

Figure 4.2 The upper-crossed syndrome is a common postural distortion produced by hyptertonicity. See Chapter 9.

GRADES OF MUSCLE STRAIN

First Degree	Second Degree	Third Degree
Few fibers torn	About half of fibers torn	All fibers torn
Minor weakness	Moderate to major weakness	Moderate to major weakness
Minor spasm	Moderate to major spasm	Moderate spasm
Minimal loss of function	Moderate to major function loss	Major loss of function
Minor swelling	Moderate to major swelling	Moderate to major swelling
Minor pain on MRT	Moderate to major pain on MRT	Minor or no pain on MRT
Pain on stretch	Pain on stretch	No pain on stretch (if muscle is only tissue injured)
No palpable defect	No palpable defect (usually)	Palpable defect present
Decreased ROM	Decreased ROM	Increased or decreased ROM

referral could produce these symptoms. Ask about recent trauma to the area. A resulting pattern of muscular tightness may linger long after an acute injury. Ask about occupational or recreational postures and mechanical stresses, as chronic hypertonicity and trigger points usually develop in response to improper biomechanical patterns or postural overload. In many cases the client is not aware of the muscular dysfunction because the tightness arose gradually as an adapted pattern.

Observation

No visual characteristics positively identify trigger points or hypertonicity. However, postural distortion resulting from hypertonicity is common (Figure 4.2). For example, forward slumped and medially rotated shoulders involve tightness in the anterior shoulder girdle muscles. It is important not to mistake well-defined muscles in someone with low body fat for hypertonicity. A well-toned muscle may be visible, but not necessarily hypertonic. During range-of-motion evaluations there may be visible movement restrictions. Trigger points are invisible, but the local twitch response (LTR) may be visible with palpation.

Palpation

The affected muscle feels tight in relation to adjacent muscles. With myofascial trigger points, palpation may refer pain or other neurological sensations to a characteristic target region and could also produce a local twitch response when palpated.[14] See the diagrams at the end of Chapters 5–11 for illustrations of the common target regions for trigger point referrals.

Range-of-Motion and Resistance Tests

AROM: With moderate or significant hypertonicity, pain may be felt during active motion that contracts the affected muscle. Discomfort is also possible as the hypertonic muscle is stretched in the direction opposite its concentric action. Myofascial trigger points usually do not produce pain or discomfort during active (concentric) movement if the body segment is moved without additional resistance. If there is increased resistance during active movement, such as standing up from a squatting position, some pain could be felt. Trigger points can produce pain or characteristic referrals when the muscle in which they lie is actively stretched.

PROM: With significant hypertonicity, there may be pain or discomfort near the end range of passive motion as the hypertonic muscle is stretched. The same is true for myofascial trigger points.

MRT: Manual resistive tests sometimes cause pain with muscular hypertonicity, but not often. If there are active myofascial trigger points in the hypertonic muscle, pain or characteristic neurological phenomena may be referred during the MRT. Hypertonicity or myofascial trigger points could cause weakness during the MRT.

Suggestions for Treatment

Muscular hypertonicity is effectively treated with various massage and stretching techniques. Longitudinal strokes which are performed parallel to the affected muscle's fiber direction are most important, as they encourage tissue lengthening. Static compression techniques are particularly effective for reducing irritation of myofascial trigger points. Stretching methods are also important for reducing trigger point activity and restoring proper neuromuscular tone.[3, 15]

MUSCLE STRAINS

A *muscle strain* involves **tearing of muscle-tendon unit fibers**. Strains can occur to the tendon, but are more prevalent in muscle tissue, especially near the musculotendinous junction. The junction is vulnerable because it is an interface of different tissue types and therefore a structural weak point.[16]

Characteristics

Strains result from *muscular fatigue*, lack of proper conditioning, loss of flexibility, poor recovery after exercise, inadequate warm-up prior to vigorous activity, high force loads, and *repetitive overuse*.[17] Any muscle can experience a strain, but certain muscles are more susceptible. Those exposed to high force loads such as the hamstrings or shoulder muscles are commonly strained.[18, 19] Small muscles, such as the intrinsic spinal muscles, are also susceptible to strains due to their small size and the repetitive postural loads that can cause the fibers to fatigue.[20]

Strains develop during excess tensile stress and most often with eccentric muscle activity.[17] The injury is likely to occur when the muscle contracts against strong resistance with excessive force. When a muscle strain occurs, fibers of the muscle or tendon are torn along with the connective tissue, capillary beds, and nerve endings in the area. As a result, blood from the broken capillaries can leak into the interstitial space causing a *bruise*. Pain is felt from *edema* and damage to the free nerve endings.

Muscle strains are generally caused by acute injuries. However, repetitive tensile forces on the muscle can cause small degrees of fiber tearing and produce a chronic strain. Strains, both acute and chronic, frequently develop in muscles that have previously experienced a strain. Scar tissue that repaired the original strain is a weak point in the muscle's continuity and therefore a location vulnerable to re-injury.

There are three grades of muscle strain: **first degree** or mild, **second degree** or moderate, and **third degree** or severe. The characteristics associated with muscle strain grades are listed in Box 4.1. The muscles most susceptible to strain are those that cross more than one joint (multiarticulate muscles). The more joints the muscle crosses, the more the muscle must be able to stretch, making it more susceptible to strain.

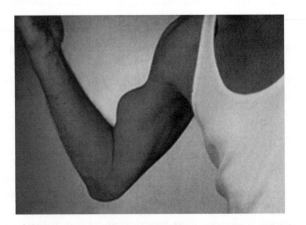

Figure 4.3 Biceps brachii Popeye deformity produced by a third degree strain. (3-D image courtesy of Primal Pictures Ltd. www.primalpictures.com.)

History

In acute strains, the client reports a sudden pain in the muscle associated with an activity that used that muscle. Swelling might be reported in the area immediately after the injury, but is likely to subside after the initial inflammatory phase (an estimated 72 hours). In larger muscles of the body, such as the hamstrings, the client periodically reports a loud popping sound at the time of injury. In a chronic strain, it is less likely that the client will be able to describe a single event as the cause of the injury. The client reports pain that is aggravated when the muscle is used and which subsides with rest. It is important to find out whether the client has suffered a previous injury to the area.

Observation

The most visible indicator of a strain is *ecchymosis* (bruising), but it is not always present. If the strain is severe, a defect in the continuity of the muscle fiber may be apparent. When visible, the defect looks like a divot or dent in the muscle. Some redness, which is indicative of an inflammatory reaction, may be visible. In some third-degree strains the severed muscle-tendon unit pulls completely toward one end producing a large bundle of muscle. This defect when it develops with a biceps brachii rupture is sometimes called a *Popeye deformity* (Figure 4.3).[21]

The client's movements will appear guarded, even before engaging in ROM evaluations. The client may demonstrate visible apprehension when performing these movements, due to pain or restriction. Restrictions in range of motion are observable.

Palpation

There is localized tenderness in the muscle where the fiber tearing has occurred. If the strain is more severe (2nd or 3rd degree), there may be a palpable defect in the muscle as well. If there is a 3rd degree strain (complete rupture) the muscle may not be tender to palpation, although a palpable defect is likely. There is a lack of tenderness because the two ends of the muscle are completely separated.

Edema may be palpable, particularly if the damaged muscle or tendon is superficial. Muscles in the surrounding area are generally hypertonic due to reflex muscle splinting and feel tight or dense.

Range-of-Motion and Resistance Testing

AROM: Active motion in the direction of the muscle's primary concentric action may produce pain if there is sufficient resistance and the strain is severe enough. If the strain is minor, there may not be enough muscle fibers recruited during the motion to produce pain. For example, a mild hamstring strain might not produce pain during active knee flexion if only the weight of the leg is being lifted. However, if the same motion (knee flexion) were performed with resistance, such as with an ankle weight or in an MRT, pain would be far more likely.

Pain or discomfort is likely near the end range of AROM

when the action stretches the damaged muscle. Refer to the list of primary actions of the muscles in Chapters 5–11 to determine which actions would stretch or contract a particular muscle.

PROM: Passive motion is not painful when the affected muscle is shortened, but lengthening causes pain.

MRT: Pain occurs with an MRT when the primary action of the involved muscle is engaged. The degree of pain is relative to the severity of the injury and the amount of contraction required. If there is a complete rupture of the muscle, it may not appear painful at all, but there will be dramatic weakness because the two ends are separated and cannot produce a contraction force.

When performing an MRT for a muscle strain, use the primary action of the involved muscle. The primary resisted actions to test the major muscles of the body are listed in tables at the end of Chapters 5–11. Keep in mind that when a resisted action is used, it does not necessarily mean that only the target muscle is recruited. It is important to minimize the contribution of accessory muscles as much as possible.

Suggestions for Treatment

Following a strain, resting from offending activities for several weeks provides the body time to heal damaged tissue. Another primary goal of treatment is to reduce tension in the affected muscle with massage techniques such as effleurage, stripping, broad cross-fiber sweeping, etc. Massage is also highly useful for helping to develop a functional scar at the site of tearing and prevent scar tissue from adversely binding adjacent fibers. Deep transverse friction massage is used for this purpose.

NERVE COMPRESSION & TENSION PATHOLOGIES

Nerves may be damaged by compression or tension forces. These pathologies can occur in many locations along the nerve or at the nerve root level. A **compression or tension injury to a nerve root** is called a *radiculopathy*. A **compression or tension injury to a peripheral nerve** is called a *neuropathy*. For detailed information about the physiology of nerve damage from compression or tension, see the section on nerve injury in Chapter 2.

Characteristics

Nerve compression or tension injuries usually occur in regions where a nerve travels through a narrow pathway, such as a **fibro-osseous tunnel** (Figure 4.4).[22] These injuries can also occur in areas where there is moderately free movement of the nerve, such as the posterior thigh, but the nerve is fibrously tethered to adjacent tissue.[23] At the end of Chapters 5–11 there is a list of common nerve entrapment sites for each body region.

In a nerve compression injury, bone, muscle, ligament, or other adjacent tissue presses on the nerve and causes an interruption of its signal transmission producing sen-

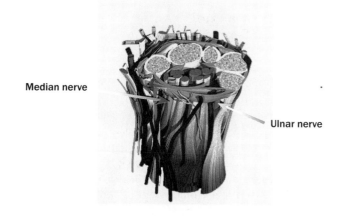

Figure 4.4 Cross-section of the left wrist showing fibro-osseous tunnels of the median and ulnar nerves. (3-D anatomy image courtesy of Primal Pictures Ltd. www.primalpictures.com.)

sory or motor impairment. In neural tension injuries, the overall diameter of the nerve decreases as the nerve is stretched, which produces the same symptoms as nerve compression.[22] The degree of nerve damage from compression or tension is described in three stages ranging from mild to severe: **neurapraxia, axonotmesis,** or **neurotmesis,** respectively. The pathophysiology of each stage is described in the section on nerve injuries in Chapter 2.

Neural compression and tension pathologies are acute or chronic. Acute compression injuries occur with direct blows to a superficial nerve, such as the ulnar nerve near the olecranon process of the elbow (the region known as the funny bone). Acute tension injuries result from sudden stretch of a nerve, such as the brachial plexus with lateral whiplash during a side-impact automobile collision.

Chronic compression injuries develop with low levels of pressure that is left on the nerve for a long time. Nerve damage can occur even with very little pressure if it is applied over a period of time.[24] Low levels of pressure make some nerve compression injuries difficult to detect. Chronic tensile injuries can also develop even with low to moderate levels of tension on a nerve if they are held for long periods.[25, 26]

Acute compression or tension injuries can occur from any number of activities. Chronic injuries are more likely to develop from repetitive occupational or recreational motions, postural distortion, or prolonged periods of mechanical stress on the nerve. Identify the mechanical demands of the occupation or recreational activity to determine if adverse compression or tension is placed on any particular nerve or nerve root. For example, repetitive pronation of the forearm during occupational activities could cause the pronator teres muscle to compress the median nerve.

In either acute or chronic injury it is important to determine whether sensations are increased with compression or stretching. In some cases, compression and stretching occur simultaneously. For example if there is compression

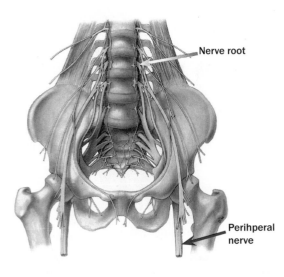

Figure 4.5 Nerve roots and peripheral nerves of the lumbar and sacral plexuses. Damage affects the dermatomes; injury to peripheral nerves affects their cutaneous innervation. (Mediclip image copyright, 1998 Williams & Wilkins. All rights reserved.)

Nerve root

Perihperal nerve

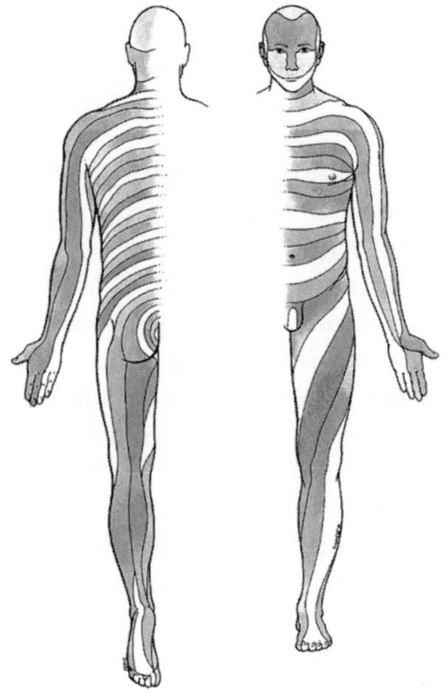

Figure 4.6 Each band indicates the dermatome of a particular nerve root. Dermatomes of the regions are provided in Chapters 5-11. (Mediclip image copyright, 1998 Williams & Wilkins. All rights reserved.)

of the tibial nerve in the tarsal tunnel, neurological sensations may increase with ankle dorsiflexion as the nerve is stretched taut against adjacent structures. Knowledge of anatomy and the paths of peripheral nerves throughout the body is essential for this analysis.

Primary sensory symptoms from nerve compression or tension pathologies include searing or electrical pain, numbness, burning sensations, and paresthesia. Ask questions about the location of these sensations to see if they occur in the cutaneous innervation of a particular nerve or whether they are spread throughout one or more involved dermatomes. If damage is to the nerve root (Figure 4.5), sensory symptoms can occur anywhere within that nerve's dermatome (Figure 4.6). If the damage is distal to the nerve root and affects a peripheral nerve (Figure 4.5), the symptoms will be felt in the area of cutaneous innervation of that particular nerve (Figure 4.7). In most cases sensory symptoms are felt distal to the site of nerve compression. Affected dermatomes and cutaneous innervation diagrams are provided in Chapters 5–11.

Motor symptoms from compression or tension damage include weakness or atrophy in muscles innervated by the affected nerve. Tables at the end of Chapters 5–11 list the nerves innervating the major muscles of that body region. Not all muscles innervated by a nerve are affected when the nerve is injured because of the location of the compression site. The more distal the compression site, the fewer muscles are affected (Figure 4.8).

Most large peripheral nerves of the extremities carry both motor and sensory signals, although the proportion of motor and sensory fibers varies by nerve. Some nerves, such as the median nerve at the carpal tunnel, are composed of a much higher percentage of sensory fibers.[24] Consequently, symptoms of carpal tunnel syndrome

usually begin with sensory impairment. Other nerves, such as the posterior interosseous nerve in the forearm, are composed primarily of motor fibers.[24] Compression or tension injury to this nerve produces mostly motor weakness. The section on nerve compression syndromes in each chapter describe the percentage of motor and sensory fibers in the affected peripheral nerves when there is a significant difference.

History

Identify the mechanics of the injury to determine the type of forces, compressive or tensile, sustained by nerves in the region. In an acute nerve injury the client reports a sudden forceful incident that produces either compressive or tensile forces on the nerve. Nerve pain is described as sharp, burning, or shooting, and frequently involves numbness or paresthesia. Keep in mind that pain from other pathologies, such as muscle strains or ligament sprains, can also be described as sharp or shooting. Make an effort to elicit further descriptions that more clearly explain the nature of the client's symptoms.

In a chronic compression or tension injury the client may not be able to pinpoint a particular activity as the cause of the pain, but describes motions that increase or decrease the symptoms. When possible, ask the client to be specific about the location of symptoms. When symptoms can be matched to a particular dermatome or region of cutaneous innervation, the affected nerve(s) can more easily be identified. It is then easier to match the anatomical pathway and mechanics of the nerve to determine if it is exposed to compression or tension in the movements or activities that increase or decrease symptoms.

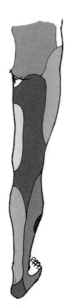

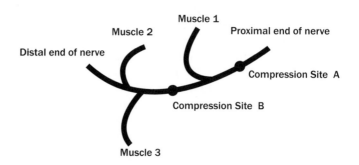

Figure 4.8 **The more distal the compression site, the fewer the muscles affected. Compression at Site A affects muscles 1-3. Compression at Site B only affects muscles 2 & 3.**

Figure 4.7 **Each shade of grey indicates the areas of cutaneous innervation of the peripheral nerves. Diagrams are provided in Chapters 5-11.**

Ask the client if there is any sensation of weakness or giving way in any motion or activity. Also identify if weakness is associated with pain or other sensory neurological symptoms. Weakness is indicative of motor impairment.

Observation

If the damage primarily affects sensory fibers in the nerve, there will be no significant observable responses to nerve compression or tension pathologies. If motor fibers are affected, there may be visible atrophy in the muscles supplied by the affected nerve. For example, visible atrophy of the adductor pollicis may be evident from compression of the ulnar nerve in the elbow or wrist. See the tables at the end of Chapters 5–11 for a list of muscles and the nerves that supply them. Some biomechanical compensation may result from pain avoidance, and patterns of dysfunction from these compensations are visible during ROM evaluation.

Palpation

Once nerves are injured from excess compression or tension they may become hypersensitive. Palpation of a compromised nerve reproduces the client's symptoms. If compression pathology exists, the nerve is tender where it is compressed. If there is adverse neural tension, a longer section of the nerve may produce symptoms when palpated.[22]

Range-of-Motion and Resistance Testing

AROM: Active motions are not likely to cause discomfort unless they further compress or stretch an affected nerve. Consider the path and mechanics of the nerve as well as

adjacent anatomical structures to determine if the suspected nerve is stretched or compressed with the motion being evaluated.

PROM: The same principles apply as for AROM.

MRT: Pain is not common with MRTs. However, if motor fibers are involved, muscle weakness might be evident. See the list of muscles, resisted actions, nerves, and nerve roots in the tables at the end of Chapter 5–11 for reference. Depending on the location of the pathology, weakness may be apparent in all or some of the muscles innervated by a particular nerve or nerve root during an MRT.

Suggestions for Treatment

The primary goal in treating nerve compression or tension pathology is to relieve adverse forces on the nerve. If soft tissue is binding or entrapping the nerve, reduce tension in that tissue so the nerve is no longer restricted. Use caution during treatment to ensure that additional pressure is not applied to the affected nerve, thereby aggravating symptoms. Soft-tissue treatment helps reduce the adverse compression or tension, but does not speed the healing of nerve pathologies, which are very slow to heal.[24] However, creating an optimum environment for the body's healing process is essential for the most efficient recovery process. Massage is an effective adjunct treatment to neural mobilization techniques, which are used to free bound or restricted nerves in neural tension disorders.[27]

TENDINOSIS, TENDINITIS, & TENOSYNOVITIS

Tendons are designed to withstand tensile stress as they transmit a muscle's contraction force to the bone when producing movement. *Overuse tendon pathologies* (tendinopathies) are **common soft-tissue disorders caused by repetitive or excessive stress**. While there are some physiological differences between tendinosis, tendinitis, and tenosynovitis, the causes, symptoms, clinical findings, and treatment approaches are similar. Because most overuse tendon pathologies are not tendinitis, this discussion focuses on tendinosis and tenosynovitis.

Characteristics

Chapter 2 discusses the physiological processes of tendinosis, tendinitis, and tenosynovitis. **Tendinitis** is actually **a rare condition involving tearing of tendon fibers**, although the term continues to be used to refer to general tendon pathology.[28-30] Tendon shapes are variable, but all are designed to withstand strong tensile loads (Figure 4.9). Some tendons withstand repetitive loads better than others due to the ratio of tendon size to load being withstood. Tendinosis and tendinitis can develop in any tendon, but are usually limited to tendons that have extensive overuse, biomechanical vulnerability, or are exposed to exceptionally high force loads.

Repetitive overuse can lead to **tendinosis**, which is **collagen degeneration in the tendon**. Tendinosis is most prevalent in tendons under high tensile load or those exposed to repetitive stress. The tendons most frequently affected include the Achilles, patellar, rotator cuff, bicipital, and forearm flexor and extensor tendons. Constant tensile loads, even if moderate, can also cause tendon damage. An example is the development of wrist extensor tendinosis (tennis elbow) from long periods of isometric contraction from using a computer mouse. It is tendinosis that affects the Achilles tendon, not tenosynovitis because the tendon lacks a synovial sheath.[31, 32]

Medications may adversely affect tendon function and lead to tendinosis. The fluoroquinolone family of antibiotics in particular is implicated as a cause for numerous tendon pathologies.[34] Corticosteroid treatment of tendons can weaken them and make them susceptible to further damage.[35] Long term use of these medications is associated with tendinosis and tendon ruptures. The Achilles tendon is usually the tendon affected.

Tenosynovitis only occurs in tendons surrounded by a synovial sheath. Tendons that must make large angular turns around joints, usually in the distal extremities, are surrounded by a synovial sheath (Figure 4.10). The function of the sheath is to reduce friction between the tendon and the adjacent joint structures, such as retinacula. Tenosynovitis develops when **chronic overuse of the tendon causes inflammation or adhesion to develop between the tendon and its synovial sheath**. Most of these tendons appear in the distal extremities. Common tendons affected include the toe extensors and tendons on the radial side of the wrist. The bicipital tendon is affected because while not in a distal extremity, it is surrounded by a synovial sheath to reduce friction while sliding through the bicipital groove.

History

All three conditions produce similar symptoms. The client reports pain in the tendon that usually increases with activity. In many cases pain reduces somewhat during activity and reappears at a later point. The pain reduction during activity is associated with increased endorphin levels and a blocking of pain by sensory signals associated with proprioception and movement.[33] There is little or no discomfort at rest.

Ask about activities that produce chronic stress on the tendon, such as repetitive activities, a sudden overload of the tendon, or a long period of isometric contraction. Occupational and sports activities are commonly involved with the development of these conditions. Identify the mechanics of offending activities to determine which tendons are exposed to the heightened stress levels. Also ask about any history of medication use, including fluoroquinolone antibiotics or corticosteroids.

Observation

There are no clear visible signs in most tendinosis, tendinitis, and tenosynovitis complaints. If a true tendinitis exists, there is some inflammatory activity, but it is rarely visible. Unlike other tendons in the body, thickening may be visible and palpable in the Achilles tendon.

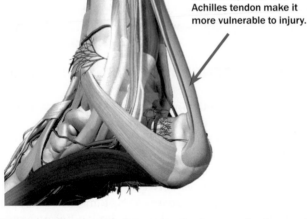

Constant, high load demands placed on the Achilles tendon make it more vulnerable to injury.

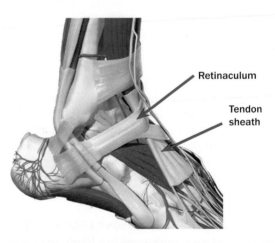

Retinaculum

Tendon sheath

Figure 4.9 Medial view of the ankle. Tendons vary in shape and the ability to withstand overload. (3-D image courtesy of Primal Pictures Ltd. www.primalpictures.com.)

Figure 4.10 Lateral view of the ankle. Angular pathways require the tendon to have a synovial sheath to reduce friction. (3-D image courtesy of Primal Pictures Ltd. www.primalpictures.com).

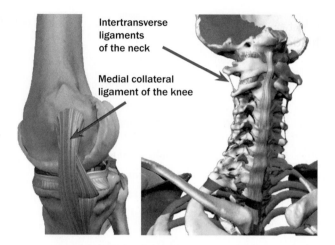

Intertransverse
ligaments
of the neck

Medial collateral
ligament of the knee

Figure 4.11 Ligament sizes vary, but all provide stability. (3-D image courtesy of Primal Pictures Ltd. www.primalpictures.com.)

Palpation

Pain is felt when the injured tendon is palpated. The pain reproduces the client's primary complaint. Pain also increases if the affected tendon is palpated during a simultaneous isometric muscle contraction as the increased tensile load on the tendon exacerbates the symptoms.

Range-of-Motion and Resistance Testing

AROM: Active motions usually do not cause discomfort unless there is significant tendon damage or an additional load during the active movement. For example, tendinosis in the Achilles tendon is rarely painful with plantar flexion in a non-weight-bearing position, but is likely painful if the client stands on tip-toes.

PROM: Passive movement that shortens the muscle-tendon unit (movement in the direction of the muscle's concentric action), decreases pain due to a reduction in tensile load on the tendon. Increased pain is felt when the affected tendon is stretched.

MRT: Pain is felt with any manual resistive test that engages the action of the affected muscle-tendon unit. See the list of muscles and their corresponding primary actions in Chapters 5–11 to determine which motions put a tensile load on the affected tendon.

Suggestions for Treatment

Most overuse tendon disorders are improved with conservative treatments that include rest from the offending activity, stretching, strength training, braces, and soft-tissue manipulation. Tendinosis is effectively treated with methods that help stimulate fibroblast activity and speed healing, such as deep friction. Massage has demonstrated positive results in accomplishing these goals.[36-38] Deep friction massage is also effective for decreasing adhesions that develop between a tendon and the surrounding synovial sheath in tenosynovitis.[39] Recent studies have suggested that eccentric strength training is also effective in treating overuse tendon disorders.[40]

LIGAMENT SPRAINS

An excessive tensile stress injury to a ligament is called a *sprain*. Ligaments are designed to connect bones to each other and resist a certain amount of tensile load. Sudden loads that overwhelm the ligament's tensile strength cause fiber failure and the ligament is stretched or torn.

Characteristics

Ligaments are dense connective tissue structures composed of elastin and collagen. Elastin provides a degree of pliability, while collagen gives them tensile strength. Ligaments are designed to withstand tensile loads along the direction that their fibers run.[41] Some ligaments, such as the medial collateral ligament of the knee, are large and designed to withstand high tensile loads. Others are much smaller because they are not exposed to high tensile forces (Figure 4.11). Regardless of their size, ligaments give stability to the skeleton's bony architecture.

Identifying ligament damage relies on an understanding of the ligament's location and the motions it is designed to resist. In many cases it is moderately easy to infer the resisted motions simply from the location. For example, it is easy to see that the medial collateral ligament of the knee resists valgus forces to the knee due to its position. With other ligaments it is not as easy to identify the primary motions they resist and greater understanding of anatomy and biomechanics is necessary.

An overwhelming sudden tensile load is the cause of a ligament sprain. For example, twisting the ankle or getting hit on the knee produces the type of forces that would sprain a ligament. Ligament sprains occur frequently in sporting activities, due to high and rapid force loads. However, prolonged stress on the ligaments can weaken them and make them more susceptible to injury from smaller loads. Ligament sprains are more prevalent in people with systemic disorders such as Ehlers-Danlos or Marfan syndromes, because these conditions involve connective tissue weakness.[42] Women in the later stages of pregnancy experience a greater number of ligament sprains due to increased ligamentous laxity resulting from elevated levels of the relaxin hormone.

A discussion of the physiology of ligament sprains is included in Chapter 2. To classify the level of tissue damage, sprains are divided into three categories: **first**, **second**, and **third degree**. Box 4.2 lists the characteristics of the grades of ligament sprain.

History

The client reports a sudden movement or force to the joint accompanied by mild to severe pain. If the injury is to a lower extremity ligament the client is likely to report difficulty in weight-bearing or locomotion. Pain subsides with rest and is aggravated by motions that stretch the ligament at the affected joint. If the ligament is relatively superficial, the client may be able to directly press on the area and indicate the primary location of pain.

Box 4.2 GRADES OF LIGAMENT SPRAIN

First Degree	Second Degree	Third Degree
Few ligament fibers torn	More fibers torn, up to half	Ligament severely torn or ruptured
Mild stretching possible, but not permanent	Ligament overstretched	Fibers need surgical repair
Minor joint instability	Moderate to major joint instability	Permanent changes in joint stability likely
Pain mild to moderate when stretched	Pain moderate to severe with ligament stretched	Pain severe at injury
Minor swelling	Moderate swelling around joint	Moderate to major swelling
Local muscle spasm possible	Local muscle spasm	Local muscle spasm
Decreased ROM	Decreased ROM	ROM increased or decreased
Joint intact	Joint intact	Joint dislocation or subluxation possible

---

Observation

Most ligament sprains produce varying degrees of swelling. Depending on the location of the ligament sprain, swelling may or may not be visible. Superficial ligaments in the distal extremities, such as ankle ligaments, routinely produce profuse visible swelling because of the difficulty in removing excess fluid from such a distal region through the lymphatic system. Swelling from deep ligament damage, such as the cruciate ligaments of the knee, is not always visible. In some joints severe ligament damage produces visible alteration in position of the bones. An example is the positional deformity that develops from second or third degree acromioclavicular and coracoclavicular ligament sprains.

Palpation

If the damaged ligament is superficial, swelling is palpable near the injury site. The damaged ligament is also tender to palpation. Many ligament sprains produce palpable spasm in nearby muscles.

Range-of-Motion and Resistance Testing:

AROM: Active motions cause pain if the affected ligaments are stretched. In severe sprains, pain may be produced if the ligament is moved at all, even short of stretching the ligament fibers.

PROM: The same principles apply as for AROM.

MRT: No pain is felt with resisted isometric contractions in most cases. There are a few unique situations where strong muscle contractions may pull on damaged ligament fibers. For example, in resisted knee extension the quadriceps group pulls on the anterior cruciate ligament and pain presents if it is damaged.

Suggestions for Treatment:

Deep friction massage is often advocated for treatment of ligament sprains because it is beneficial in stimulating collagen production in the damaged tissue.[37] Many ligaments, such as the anterior sacroiliac ligaments, are not accessible. In most cases these ligaments heal on their own. It is important that the client rest from offending activities or motions that further stress the ligaments.

Massage and stretching are effective in addressing muscle spasm that results from the injury. However, caution is advised in stretching procedures as overly aggressive stretching can irritate torn ligament fibers. Muscle tightness may be protecting the region against excess movement and therefore some hypertonicity is helpful, especially in the early stages of injury.

OSTEOARTHRITIS

Osteoarthritis is the most common type of joint disease and **involves degenerative changes at synovial joints** in the body.[43] By definition arthritis means inflammation of the joint, but other destructive processes precede the inflammatory activity. It is a challenging condition to treat and is becoming an economic burden to the health care systems in many countries. In the U.S. for example the number of adults with arthritis is projected to increase from 42.7 million in 2002 to around 65 million in 2030, due to the aging population.[44]

Characteristics

Synovial joints are the joints affected in osteoarthritis. Each has similar anatomical structures, even if the size of the joint's bones or the contact surface differs significantly. Within the synovial joint are the articulating bones, articular cartilage, a fibrous joint capsule and synovial membrane, synovial fluid, and joint cavity (Figure 4.12). These structures work together to create smooth gliding movement where adjacent bones contact each other. Maintaining this surface is especially important in the weight-bearing joints, such as the hip or knee, as excessive compressive stress can lead to bone degeneration in the joints.

Highly specialized cells called **chondrocytes** provide **articular (hyaline) cartilage** with the unique properties of friction reduction, cushioning, and protection of the articulating surface of bones.[45] Excess friction, age-related degeneration, or impact trauma can produce disintegration in the hyaline cartilage of adjacent bones, which is followed by an inflammatory reaction in the joint. The degeneration and subsequent inflammatory reaction is the condition of osteoarthritis.

Osteoarthritis has traditionally been divided into two categories: **primary** and **secondary**. Primary osteoarthritis appears to develop gradually from excessive wear on the joints, but the specific factors that lead to the condition are not well understood. There is an indication that repetitive stress to the joints of the hips, knees, and hands in certain occupations could play a role in creating earlier onset of the problem.[46]

Secondary osteoarthritis develops as the result of some other disease or pathological condition. Traumatic injury to the joint can initiate joint damage that leads to cartilage degeneration. In other cases surgery, obesity, or various activities are directly related to the condition's onset.[47] The condition is prevalent in soccer players due to impact trauma and in weight lifters because of their increased body weight.[48, 49] Increased weight and joint degeneration can also increase the likelihood of lower extremity postural distortions, such as genu varum and genu valgum. Both these distortions lead to greater joint wear and increased chance of developing osteoarthritis.

In both primary and secondary variations, the problem originates with the articular cartilage of the joint surfaces. Loss of cartilage causes repetitive wear, degeneration, and flaking of the cartilage. An inflammatory reaction results, with limitations in joint mobility and range of motion. In some cases inflammation stimulates **bone spurs** to form around the joints causing further pain and dysfunction. The spurs are common in the interphalangeal joints of the fingers. They are called **Heberden's nodes** when they develop at the distal interphalangeal joints and **Bouchard's nodes** at the proximal interphalangeal joint.[43] Spurs that develop from spinal osteoarthritis (also called spondylitis) can press on adjacent nerve roots and mimic intervertebral disc herniation.[43]

Congenital abnormalities in bone formation can predispose one to osteoarthritis. For example, altered patterns of weight-bearing occur in persons with abnormal bone growth or dysplasia of the hip. The alteration in joint mechanics associated with congenital disorders is likely to be a primary cause of osteoarthritis.[50]

Osteoarthritis produces pain in the joints that is aggravated with movement. Due to continual use, pain is usually worse later in the day. Joint swelling may increase with activity. Pain sometimes arises from long periods of immobility or even from changes in weather, although the association between weather and arthritis symptoms is still not clear.[51] Unlike systemic forms of arthritis, such as rheumatoid arthritis, there are no effects to organs or

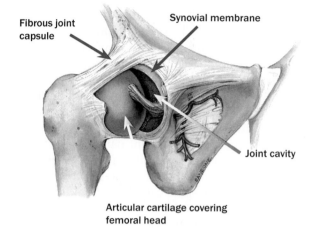

Figure 4.12 Anterior view of the hip showing components of a synovial joint. (Mediclip image copyright, 1998 Williams & Wilkins. All rights reserved.)

other remote tissues. The tissue damage is confined to the surfaces of the affected joints, although pain can be referred to other locations.

Osteoarthritis typically affects the fingers, spine, hips, and knees. While it periodically occurs in other joints, it is not common in the shoulder, elbow, wrist, or ankle. It does appear to have a hereditary pattern, but a direct congenital cause of osteoarthritis has not been established. There is a greater incidence in younger males and females over 45 years of age.[52]

History

The client reports pain in the affected joint(s), especially with continued use. Pain is usually worse in the later part of the day, and the client may also complain of swelling, heat, and crepitus in the joint. Reports of aggravated pain with changes in the weather are common. The client might also report an increase in symptoms as a result of long periods of immobility, especially if the condition is more advanced.

Observation

Joint swelling is evident in many cases, but absence of visible swelling does not indicate absence of the condition. Evaluate any postural disorders involving the affected joint(s) as postural disorders or bony alignment problems routinely accompany osteoarthritis. Bone spurs, such as Bouchard or Heberden's nodes, in the fingers may be visible.

Palpation

The affected joints may be tender to palpation due to increased swelling in the area. Tenderness is more common if the condition is advanced or if palpation presses the affected joint surfaces together. Bone spurs, if present, can sometimes be felt around the affected joint, especially in the fingers.

Range-of-Motion and Resistance Testing

AROM: Active motions can cause pain in any direction the joint is moved. However, pain can fluctuate with the time of day or the degree of aggravation of the joint. If the affected joint is a weight-bearing joint, pain is worse when active movement is performed while bearing weight. Edema, muscle spasm, or bone spurs could all prematurely limit the available range of movement.

PROM: As with active movement pain can occur in any direction and could fluctuate with the degree of the condition's irritation. Range of motion may end prematurely due to edema, muscle spasm, or bone spurs. The end feel for joint motions tends to be a bit leathery and a capsular pattern of restriction is typically evident (see Chapters 5–11 for that joint's capsular pattern.

MRT: Pain and weakness may be evident with MRT.

Suggestions for Treatment

While cartilage degeneration can not be reversed, massage and stretching can be used to reduce muscle spasm and decrease compressive forces associated with the joint disorder. These approaches are also helpful in reducing edema resulting from inflammation. Avoiding activities that increase joint irritation, compression, or inflammation is important. Weight reduction, dietary alteration, rest, supportive braces, and some exercise can be helpful, especially for osteoarthritis in the weight-bearing joints. Anti-inflammatory medication is commonly used to address the problem, although there are concerns about the long term health effects of anti-inflammatory medications.

References

1. Freedman KB, Bernstein J. Educational deficiencies in musculoskeletal medicine. J Bone Joint Surg Am. Apr 2002;84-A(4):604-608.
2. Craton N, Matheson GO. Training and clinical competency in musculoskeletal medicine. Identifying the problem. Sports Med. 1993;15(5):328-337.
3. Simons D, Travell J, Simons L. Myofascial Pain and Dysfunction: The Trigger Point Manual. Vol 1. 2nd ed. Baltimore: Williams & Wilkins; 1999.
4. Mani L, Gerr F. Work-related upper extremity musculoskeletal disorders. Prim Care. 2000;27(4):845-864.
5. Pascarelli EF, Hsu YP. Understanding work-related upper extremity disorders: clinical findings in 485 computer users, musicians, and others. J Occup Rehabil. Mar 2001;11(1):1-21.
6. Punnett L, Gold J, Katz JN, Gore R, Wegman DH. Ergonomic stressors and upper extremity musculoskeletal disorders in automobile manufacturing: a one year follow up study. Occup Environ Med. Aug 2004;61(8):668-674.
7. Winzeler S, Rosenstein BD. Orthopedic problems of the upper extremities. Assessment and diagnosis. Aaohn J. Apr 1997;45(4):188-200; quiz 201-183.
8. Huguenin L. Myofascial trigger points: the current evidence. Physical Therapy in Sport. 2004;5:2-12.
9. Simons DG. Review of enigmatic MTrPs as a common cause of enigmatic musculoskeletal pain and dysfunction. J Electromyogr Kinesiol. 2004;14(1):95-107.
10. Treaster D, Marras WS, Burr D, Sheedy JE, Hart D. Myofascial trigger point development from visual and postural stressors during computer work. J Electromyogr Kinesiol. Apr 2006;16(2):115-124.
11. Juhan D. Job's Body. Barrytown, NY: Station Hill Press; 1987.
12. McPartland JM. Travell trigger points--molecular and osteopathic perspectives. J Am Osteopath Assoc. Jun 2004;104(6):244-249.
13. Freedman KB, Bernstein J. The adequacy of medical school education in musculoskeletal medicine. J Bone Joint Surg Am. 1998;80(10):1421-1427.
14. Travell JS, D. Myofascial Pain and Dysfunction: The Trigger Point Manual. Vol 1. 1st ed. Baltimore: Williams & Wilkins; 1983.
15. Chaitow L, DeLany J. Clinical Application of Neuromuscular Techniques. Vol 1. Edinburgh: Churchill Livingstone; 2000.
16. Garrett WE, Jr., Safran MR, Seaber AV, Glisson RR, Ribbeck BM. Biomechanical comparison of stimulated and nonstimulated skeletal muscle pulled to failure. Am J Sports Med. 1987;15(5):448-454.
17. Garrett WE. Muscle strain injuries. Am J Sports Med. 1996;24(6 Suppl):S2-8.
18. Brockett CL, Morgan DL, Proske U. Predicting hamstring strain injury in elite athletes. Med Sci Sports Exerc. Mar 2004;36(3):379-387.
19. Cooper J. Throwing Injuries. In: Donatelli R, ed. Physical Therapy of the Shoulder. 3rd ed. New York: Churchill Livingstone; 1997.
20. Liebenson Ce. Rehabilitation of the Spine. Baltimore: Williams & Wilkins; 1996.
21. Ellenbecker TS. Clinical Examination of the Shoulder. St. Louis: Elsevier Saunders; 2004.
22. Butler D. Mobilisation of the Nervous System. London: Churchill Livingstone; 1991.

23. Turl SE, and George, K. P. Adverse Neural Tension - A Factor in Repetitive Hamstring Strain. J Orthop Sport Phys Therapy. 1998;27(1):16-21.

24. Dawson D, Hallett M, Wilbourn A. Entrapment Neuropathies. 3rd ed. Philadelphia: Lippincott-Raven; 1999.

25. Butler DaG, L. The Concept of Adverse Mechanical Tension in the Nervous System- Part 1: Testing for 'Dural tension'. Physiotherapy. 1989;75(11):622-628.

26. Breig A. Adverse Mechanical Tension in the Central Nervous System. Stockholm: Almqvist & Wiksell; 1978.

27. Shacklock M. Clinical Neurodynamics. Edinburgh: Elsevier; 2005.

28. Khan KM, Cook JL, Taunton JE, Bonar F. Overuse tendinosis, not tendinitis - Part 1: A new paradigm for a difficult clinical problem. Physician Sportsmed. 2000;28(5):38+.

29. Depalma MJ, Perkins RH. Patellar tendinosis. Physician Sportsmed. 2004;32(5).

30. Nirschl RP. Elbow tendinosis/tennis elbow. Clin Sports Med. 1992;11(4):851-870.

31. Jarvinen TA, Kannus P, Maffulli N, Khan KM. Achilles tendon disorders: etiology and epidemiology. Foot Ankle Clin. Jun 2005;10(2):255-266.

32. Soila K, Karjalainen PT, Aronen HJ, Pihlajamaki HK, Tirman PJ. High-resolution MR imaging of the asymptomatic Achilles tendon: new observations. AJR Am J Roentgenol. Aug 1999;173(2):323-328.

33. Melzack R. From the gate to the neuromatrix. Pain. Aug 1999;Suppl 6:S121-126.

34. Khaliq Y, Zhanel GG. Musculoskeletal injury associated with fluoroquinolone antibiotics. Clin Plast Surg. Oct 2005;32(4):495-502, vi.

35. Blanco I, Krahenbuhl S, Schlienger RG. Corticosteroid-associated tendinopathies: an analysis of the published literature and spontaneous pharmacovigilance data. Drug Saf. 2005;28(7):633-643.

36. Davidson CJ, Ganion LR, Gehlsen GM, Verhoestra B, Roepke JE, Sevier TL. Rat Tendon Morphologic and Functional-Changes Resulting from Soft-Tissue Mobilization. Med Sci Sport Exercise. 1997;29(3):313-319.

37. Gehlsen GM, Ganion LR, Helfst R. Fibroblast responses to variation in soft tissue mobilization pressure. Med Sci Sport Exercise. 1999;31(4):531-535.

38. Pellecchia GL, Hamel H, Behnke P. Treatment of Infrapatellar Tendinitis - A Combination of Modalities and Transverse Friction Massage Versus Iontophoresis. J Sport Rehabil. 1994;3(2):135-145.

39. Chamberlain GL. Cyriax's friction massage: a review. J Orthop Sport Phys Therapy. 1982;4(1):16-22.

40. Ohberg L, Lorentzon R, Alfredson H. Eccentric training in patients with chronic Achilles tendinosis: normalised tendon structure and decreased thickness at follow up. Br J Sports Med. Feb 2004;38(1):8-11; discussion 11.

41. White A, Panjabi M. Clinical Biomechanics of the Spine. 2nd ed. Philadelphia: Lippincott Williams & Wilkins; 1990.

42. Magee D. Orthopedic Physical Assessment. 3rd ed. Philadelphia: W.B. Saunders; 1997.

43. Stacy G, Basu AP. Osteoarthritis, Primary. eMedicine. 11-4-2005. Available at: www.emedicine.com. Accessed March 31, 2006.

44. Bolen J, Sniezek J, Theis K, et al. Racial/Ethnic Differences in the Prevalence and Impact of Doctor-Diagnosed Arthritis --- United States, 2002. MMWR. 2005;54(05):119-123.

45. Buckwalter JA, Mankin HJ, Grodzinsky AJ. Articular cartilage and osteoarthritis. Instr Course Lect. 2005;54:465-480.

46. Rossignol M, Leclerc A, Allaert FA, et al. Primary osteoarthritis of hip, knee, and hand in relation to occupational exposure. Occup Environ Med. Nov 2005;62(11):772-777.

47. Feller J. Anterior cruciate ligament rupture: is osteoarthritis inevitable? Br J Sports Med. Aug 2004;38(4):383-384.

48. Kujala UM, Kettunen J, Paananen H, et al. Knee osteoarthritis in former runners, soccer players, weight lifters, and shooters. Arthritis Rheum. Apr 1995;38(4):539-546.

49. Drawer S, Fuller CW. Propensity for osteoarthritis and lower limb joint pain in retired professional soccer players. Br J Sports Med. Dec 2001;35(6):402-408.

50. Lievense AM, Bierma-Zeinstra SM, Verhagen AP, Verhaar JA, Koes BW. Influence of hip dysplasia on the development of osteoarthritis of the hip. Ann Rheum Dis. Jun 2004;63(6):621-626.

51. Aikman H. The association between arthritis and the weather. Int J Biometeorol. Jun 1997;40(4):192-199.

52. Stitik TP, Foye P. Osteoarthritis. eMedicine. 4-8-2005. Available at: www.emedicine.com. Accessed March 30, 2006.

5 Foot, Ankle, & Leg

The foot and ankle are designed to withstand numerous stresses due to their unique biomechanical features and architecture, which produce locomotion while simultaneously managing shock absorption. Given the forces and stress placed on this region, structural or functional impairments are common.

The *ground reaction force* on the lower extremity is several times the weight of the body when running and produces considerable stress on the lower extremity.[1] Problems develop from activities that require long hours of standing or walking, particularly if done on hard surfaces such as concrete. Shoes can play a role in these conditions and may even produce injuries. High-heeled shoes have long been a source of foot pain, but even unsupportive or unyielding footwear can create complications.[2,3] In many cases, it is not immediately apparent that certain activities or foot-wear are stressful.

The foot, ankle, and leg region has some of the largest and strongest tendons in the body in order to handle the extreme tensile loads of locomotion and shock absorption. Consequently, injury conditions involving tendon overuse are frequent in this region. There are numerous high-profile conditions that occur in the foot, ankle, and leg. Many problems encountered in this region result from muscular overuse, such as muscle tightness and myofascial trigger points.

Movements and Motion Testing

SINGLE PLANE MOVEMENTS

The foot, ankle, and leg function as one complex unit with movement occurring at the ankle. There are four single-plane movements: dorsiflexion, plantar flexion, inversion, and eversion. Foot mechanics are intricate and movement does not always occur exclusively in a single plane. There are two additional multi-planar movements at the ankle, pronation and supination. Although there are four single-plane movements in the toes, only two are measured for clinical significance. In this text, movement occurring past full extension or anatomical position is considered hyperextension. The associated motions, planes, axes of rotation, and range-of-motion values for each joint are listed in Table 2 at the end of the chapter.

Ankle and Foot

Dorsiflexion and **plantar flexion** occur in the **sagittal plane** at the **talocrural joint** (Figures 5.1, 5.2). Dorsiflexion occurs when the dorsal surface of the foot moves toward the anterior surface of the leg; in plantar flexion the movement is away from the anterior surface of the leg. Average range of motion for dorsiflexion is 20^0–30^0; plantar flexion is 30^0–50^0.

Inversion and **eversion** occur at the ankle's **subtalar joint** in the **frontal plane** (Figure 5.3). Inversion occurs as the plantar surface of the foot moves toward the midline of the body; in eversion the movement is away from the midline of the body. Average range of motion at the subtalar joint is 20^0 for inversion; 15^0 for eversion.

Pronation is a **diagonal-plane** movement occurring around an **oblique axis** and includes **dorsiflexion, eversion,** and **abduction** of the foot (Figure 5.4). Pronation occurs normally during walking or running. **Supination** also occurs in a **diagonal plane** and combines **plantar flexion, inversion,** and **adduction** (Figure 5.4). Eversion and inversion are sometimes used as synonyms for pronation and supination. Because supination and pronation are combined movements in different planes, they are generally not included in single-plane movement evaluation of the foot and ankle.

Abduction and **adduction** occur in the **horizontal plane** (Figure 5.5). The distal end of the foot is turned laterally in abduction and medially in adduction. When the knee is flexed, abduction and adduction occur as a result of external or internal rotation of the tibia respectively. When the knee is extended, abduction and adduction

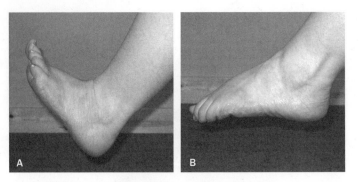

Figure 5.2 Ankle dorsiflexion (A) and plantar flexion (B).

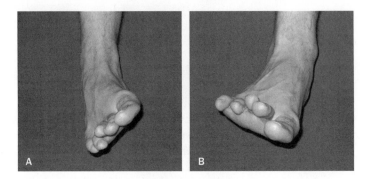

Figure 5.3 Sub-talar inversion (A) and eversion (B).

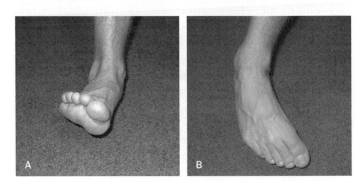

Figure 5.4 Foot pronation (A) and supination (B).

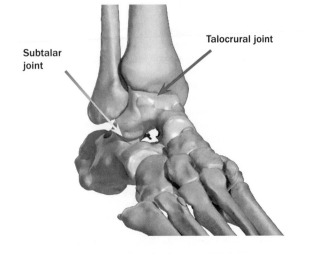

Figure 5.1 Right ankle showing the talocrural joint. (3-D anatomy image courtesy of Primal Pictures Ltd. www.primalpictures.com.)

result from external or internal rotation of the femur at the hip joint respectively. Range-of-motion evaluations for these motions are rarely used clinically as they depend on movement of other joints, making evaluation difficult.

Toes

Toe and hallux **flexion** and **extension** occur in the **sagittal plane** at the **metatarsophalangeal (MTP)** as well as the **proximal** and **distal interphalangeal (PIP & DIP) joints** (Figure 5.6). Returning the toes to anatomical position is extension and movement past anatomical position is considered hyperextension. Average range of motion in the toes is 30^0–40^0 in flexion; 50^0–60^0 in extension. **Abduction** and **adduction** of the toes is not evaluated because the motions are difficult to control.

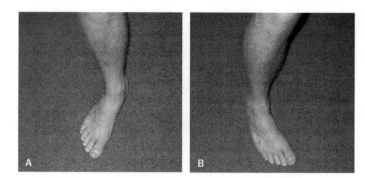

Figure 5.5 Foot abduction (A) and adduction (B).

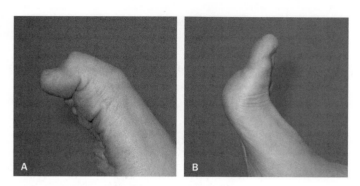

Figure 5.6 Hallux and toe flexion (A) and extension (B).

Capsular patterns

When evaluating joint function it is important to consider the role of the joint capsule. Pathological problems in the capsule, such as *fibrosis*, may be visible with the joint's *capsular pattern*. The capsular pattern is a pattern of movement restriction characteristic to each individual joint. It is present in both active and passive motion. It is represented by a sequential listing of the movements from most likely to least likely limited. See the description of capsular patterns for this region in Box 5.1.

RANGE-OF-MOTION & RESISTIVE TESTS

Results from single-plane movement analysis form the basis for further evaluation procedures. Movement testing should be performed in a certain order, allowing for an efficient evaluation and the least amount of accumulated discomfort or pain to develop. It is also general practice to leave movements known or expected to be painful to the end of the evaluation. When possible, the pain-free side is evaluated first.

   Active range-of-motion (AROM) movements are performed first to establish the client's movement abilities and pain symptoms. Passive range of motion (PROM) is performed next and manual resistive tests (MRT) follow. AROM results may make PROM assessment procedures unnecessary. If no pain occurs with active movement, pain is unlikely with passive movement. The practitioner should be familiar with the full step-by-step instructions and guidelines for how to interpret (ROM) and resistive test results explained in Chapter 3.

Active Range of Motion

Pain with active movement indicates problems in either the contractile or inert tissues associated with that movement. Factors that prematurely limit active movement in the foot and ankle include *hypertonicity, myofascial trigger points, strains, ligamentous or capsular damage, muscle contractures, pain from nerve compression or tension, tendinosis, tenosynovitis, fibrous cysts, or joint disorders* such as *arthritis*.

Box 5.1 Capsular Patterns for the Foot & Ankle

Talocrural Joint
   Plantar flexion is more limited than dorsiflexion.

Subtalar joint
   Pronation and supination usually equally limited.

MTP joints
   For the 1st MTP, extension is more limited than flexion. Limitations in the remaining four joints vary.

General Instructions for ROM & Resistive Tests

Overall
   • Determine motions possible at the joint to be tested.
   • Select the motion to be evaluated.
   • Determine the tissues involved in the motion.
   • Leave motions expected to be painful to the last.
   • Test the uninvolved side first.
   • Ask about, note any reported pain or discomfort.

AROM
   • Demonstrate the movement to be performed.
   • Have the client perform the movement.

PROM
   • Establish the joint's normal end feel.
   • Have the client relax as much as possible.
   • Use gentle and slow movements.

MRT
   • Test one action at a time.
   • Position should isolate the action/ muscles involved.
   • If pain is suspected, start in a mid-range position.
   • Client uses a strong, but appropriate amount of effort.

Box 5.2 Muscle Actions of the Ankle & Foot

Ankle (Talocrural joint)	**Dorsiflexion**		**Plantar flexion**
	Tibialis anterior		Gastrocnemius
	Extensor hallucis longus		Soleus
	Extensor digitorum longus		Tibialis posterior
	Peroneus tertius		Peroneus longus
			Peroneus brevis
			Plantaris
			Flexor hallucis longus
			Flexor digitorum longus
Ankle (Subtalar joint)	**Inversion**		**Eversion**
	Tibialis posterior		Peroneus longus
	Tibialis anterior		Peroneus brevis
	Extensor hallucis longus		Peroneus tertius
	Flexor hallucis longus		
	Flexor digitorum longus		
Hallux	**Flexion**		**Extension**
	Flexor hallucis longus		Extensor hallucis longus
	Flexor hallucis brevis		Extensor hallucis brevis
			Extensor digitorum brevis
Toes	**Flexion**		**Extension**
	Flexor digitorum longus		Extensor digitorum longus
	Flexor digitorum brevis		Extensor digitorum brevis
	Lumbricales		
	Quadratus plantae		

Compare AROM test results with those from passive and manual resistive tests to identify possible reasons for movement restriction. The muscles used to perform actions of the foot and ankle are listed in Box 5.2. Note that other muscles can contribute to the motion and subsequent dysfunction.

Passive Range of Motion

Passive motion is performed after active. Pain during passive movement predominantly implicates inert tissues. However, muscles and tendons that contract in the opposite direction are stretched at the end range of passive movement.

PROM testing also evaluates end feel. Box 5.3 lists the primary joint locations and their normal end feel. Review Chapter 3 for a discussion of normal and pathological end feel descriptions. Factors that could prematurely limit passive movement are the same as for active movement.

Manual Resistive Tests

A manual resistive test (MRT) produces pain when there is a mechanical disruption of tissue. Pain with an MRT indicates that one or more of the muscles and/or tendons performing that action are involved. Testing all of a muscle's actions is not necessary, as a muscle's secondary actions recruit other muscles and make the test results less accurate. Palpation elicits more information if the test alone does not produce pain or discomfort. Refer to Box 5.2 for the list of primary muscles involved with each action. Table 1 at the end of the chapter lists actions commonly used for testing muscles in the foot and ankle.

In some cases weakness is evident with MRTs. Factors that produce weakness include *lack of use, fatigue, reflex muscular inhibition,* and possibly a neurological pathology (*radiculopathy, peripheral neuropathy,* or a *systemic neurological disorder*). The nerves or nerve roots that may be involved are listed in Table 1 at the end of the chapter.

Box 5.3 Joints, Associated Motion, & Normal End Feel		
Ankle (Talocrural)	Dorsiflexion	Tissue stretch (soft)
	Plantar flexion	Tissue stretch (firm)
Ankle (Subtalar)	Inversion	Tissue stretch (soft)
	Eversion	Tissue stretch (firm)
Toes (all)	Flexion	Tissue stretch (soft)
	Extension	Tissue stretch (soft)

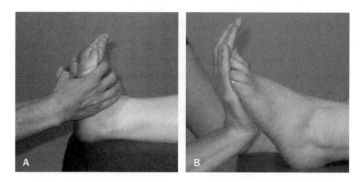

Figure 5.7 Resisted dorsiflexion (A) and plantar flexion (B).

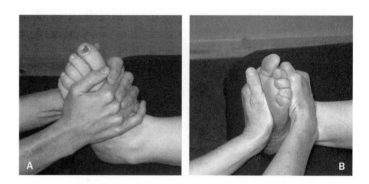

Figure 5.8 Resisted inversion (A) and eversion (B).

Ankle and Foot

RESISTED DORSIFLEXION AND PLANTAR FLEXION

To test dorsiflexion, the client is supine with the foot in neutral. The practitioner places both hands on the dorsal surface of the client's foot, as the client holds the position. The practitioner attempts to pull the client's foot into plantar flexion. Placing the hand over the toes engages the toe extensors more. If the resistance is placed on the dorsal surface of the foot and not the toes, greater action of the **tibialis anterior** is required and the test more effectively isolates that muscle (Figure 5.7).

To test plantar flexion, the client assumes the same starting position as for dorsiflexion. The practitioner places a palm on the plantar surface of the client's foot near the metatarsal heads. The client holds the position as the practitioner attempts to push the foot into dorsiflexion (Figure 5.7). Due to the mechanics of the triceps surae muscle group, pain may not be felt with an MRT even with muscle/tendon unit damage because not enough force is recruited. Evaluation of plantar flexor tissue damage may require a stronger MRT. Have the client stand on the toes of the affected side to generate greater force.

RESISTED INVERSION AND EVERSION

The client is supine with the foot in neutral. The practitioner grasps the dorsal and plantar surface of the foot and interlocks the fingers to control motion at the subtalar joint. The client holds the position as the practitioner attempts to move the foot into eversion or inversion (Figure 5.8).

Hallux and Toes

RESISTED FLEXION AND EXTENSION

The client is supine with the hallux or toes in a neutral position. To test flexion, the client holds the position as the practitioner attempts to push the distal end of the hallux or toes into extension (Figure 5.9). To test extension, the client holds the position as the practitioner attempts to move the distal end of the hallux or toes into flexion (Figure 5.9).

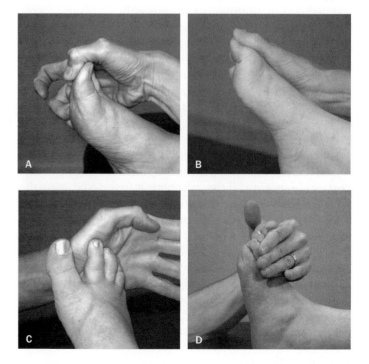

Figure 5.9 Resisted hallux flexion (A), hallux extension (B), toe flexion (C), and toe extension (D).

Structural and Postural Deviations

The following section covers common structural or postural deviations unique to the foot and ankle. Under each condition there is a brief description of its characteristics followed by HOPRS findings. If applicable, orthopedic tests are included in the special tests section. If there is no special orthopedic test listed for that condition, evaluation should focus on other portions of the assessment process, such as range-of-motion testing.

CALCANEAL VARUS

Calcaneal varus is a structural deviation that involves a *varus angulation* in which the distal end of a bony segment deviates in a medial direction.

Characteristics
In calcaneal varus, the distal end of the calcaneus deviates medially at the subtalar joint and is associated with inversion. (Figure 5.10). Calcaneal varus may result from an injury, such as *ankle fracture,* or from a chronic period of *faulty ankle biomechanics*. Resulting bony displacements or ligament damage alter the proper alignment in the subtalar joint leading to the postural distortion. The faulty biomechanical patterns of calcaneal varus may lead to *excessive supination* of the foot during gait.

Calcaneal varus affects the entire kinematic chain. The foot needs to stay in neutral for proper shock absorption. Valgus and varus angulations in the calcaneus alter this biomechanical alignment and unevenly distribute forces throughout the lower extremity and sometimes into the axial skeleton.

Calcaneal varus is sometimes caused by tightness in the **invertors** of the foot. The condition can also result from childhood foot and *lower extremity postural problems*. In some cases, previous *systemic neurological disorders* produce dysfunctional activity in the foot muscles leading to calcaneal varus.

Because the ankle is inverted during calcaneal varus, an individual with this postural distortion is prone to *lateral ankle sprains*.[4] If the calcaneus is inverted during the weight-bearing stance, there is a greater chance of rolling off the lateral side of the foot and spraining the lateral ankle ligaments.

History
The client may report foot pain or discomfort, but may not be aware of the postural distortion. Identify any history of ankle sprains or injuries. Ask about other conditions that might arise from or contribute to this distortion.

Observation
In many cases, calcaneal varus is not evident while the individual is standing and is better evaluated in a non-weight-bearing position. In severe cases, it is also evident in a weight-bearing position. When viewed from behind,

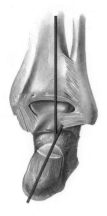

Figure 5.10 Posterior view of the right ankle showing medial deviation of the distal calcaneus in calcaneal varus. (Mediclip image copyright, 1998 Williams & Wilkins. All rights reserved.)

the distal calcaneus is seen to deviate in a medial direction. The deviation is evident by comparing a ruler or straight edge perpendicular to the ground with the midline of the posterior calcaneus. A slight degree of calcaneal varus in a non-weight-bearing position is normal.

One way to evaluate the functional effects of calcaneal varus is to evaluate the wear pattern on the bottom surface of the shoes. An individual that has calcaneal varus normally has greater supination during normal gait, which causes an exaggerated wear pattern on the lateral side of the shoe sole. Evaluating the wear pattern is only effective with shoes that have been worn for a sufficient period of time.

Palpation
There are no specific findings with palpation. However, there may be corresponding hypertonicity or myofascial trigger points in the invertor muscles of the foot.

Range-of-Motion and Resistance Testing
AROM: Active range of motion may not be impaired, but there could be restriction in foot eversion due to hypertonicity of the invertor muscles. If the calcaneal varus has resulted from an injury to the ankle, restrictions in active motion may be evident.
PROM: The same principles apply as for active motion.
MRT: No unusual findings are present with manual resistive tests.

Suggestions for Treatment
Massage techniques aimed at reducing tightness in the invertor muscle group may be helpful. Also, reducing tightness or myofascial trigger points in the peroneal muscles is beneficial. The best results for changing this structural condition are through the use of orthotics and movement re-education. Muscles and other soft tissues must be taught different patterns of coordination. The client may need to be referred to an orthopedist or podiatrist for a proper course of treatment.

CALCANEAL VALGUS

Calcaneal valgus is a structural deviation that involves a *valgus angulation* in which the distal end of a bony segment deviates in a lateral direction.

Characteristics

In calcaneal valgus, the distal end of the calcaneus deviates laterally at the subtalar joint and is associated with eversion (Figure 5.11). Calcaneal valgus may result from traumatic injury, but typically occurs as an acquired structural distortion. The condition typically results from poor biomechanical patterns in gait. Calcaneal valgus is a primary component of *overpronation*. Valgus angulations of the calcaneus occur with greater frequency than varus because it is more customary to overpronate than to oversupinate the foot.[5]

The condition could have its origins in a childhood podiatric problem. Causes also include improper footwear, excess weight, or conditions that produce ligamentous laxity, such as *Marfan* or *Ehlers-Danlos syndromes*.[6] In a traumatic injury, *ankle fractures* or *ligament sprains* may result in a permanent deformation or alter the mechanics of the ankle.

Calcaneal valgus is related to other postural distortions in the lower extremity as well, such as *genu valgum* (knock knees), *femoral anteversion,* or a *large Q angle* (see Chapter 6). The subtalar eversion of calcaneal valgus produces **internal tibial rotation**, which may contribute to other disorders, such as *shin splints, meniscal injury,* or *ligamentous stress*.[5] Hypertonicity in the **evertor** muscles of the foot (the peroneal group) may contribute to calcaneal valgus, but will not cause the condition. The **tibialis posterior** is frequently overstressed during calcaneal valgus and excessive pronation.

History

The client may report foot pain or discomfort, but may not be aware of the postural distortion. Ask if they have

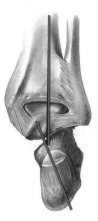

Figure 5.11 Posterior view of the right ankle showing lateral deviation of the distal calcaneus in calcaneal valgus. (Mediclip image copyright, 1998 Williams & Wilkins. All rights reserved.)

experienced any of the postural problems, injuries, and the other factors listed above, such as posterior shin splints or knee problems.

Observation

Calcaneal valgus is best observed from behind with the client barefoot and standing, which allows the practitioner to observe the angle of the calcaneus in relation to the Achilles tendon. Calcaneal valgus causes what is called a *peek-a-boo heel*. When the foot is viewed from the anterior direction, the heel is generally not visible. In calcaneal valgus, the heel can be slightly observed from the lateral side of the foot when viewed from the anterior direction (Figure 5.12).

Palpation

There are usually no specific findings with palpation. The peroneal muscles of the foot may be hypertonic and the plantar surface tender where the tibialis posterior attaches. Mild alteration in bony contours of the foot, especially on the medial side, may be palpable.

Range-of-Motion and Resistance Testing

AROM: Active range of motion is generally not impaired. Excessive fibrosity may develop and maintain the postural distortion. Inversion may or may not be limited. There may be a slight restriction in inversion of the foot due to hypertonicity of the evertor muscles.
PROM: The same principles apply as for active motion.
MRT: No unusual findings with manual resistive tests.

Suggestions for Treatment

The entire kinematic chain of the lower extremity should be assessed for involvement in this condition. Massage for the evertor muscle group is helpful if their tightness contributes to the condition. Changing calcaneal valgus requires orthotics and movement re-education directed at the entire lower extremity.

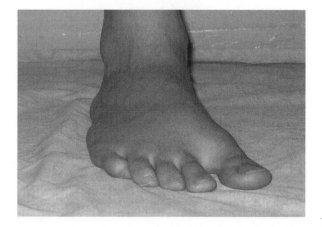

Figure 5.12 Peek-a-boo heel. When the foot is viewed straight from the anterior direction, the heel is visible to the lateral side of the foot.

EXCESSIVE SUPINATION

Excessive supination is a postural disorder that interferes with proper function of the foot and can lead to a number of other problems in the lower extremity.

Characteristics

Excessive supination is considered a *dynamic* postural disorder, because it involves the foot's movement through the weight-bearing phases of locomotion rather than in a static position. Supination is motion around an oblique or diagonal axis and is a combination of inversion, adduction and plantar flexion. The ability of the foot to supinate and pronate is particularly important for adapting to variations in ground surface. The effects of supination, especially the subtalar inversion, can be evident in a standing position (Figure 5.13). The foot is in a slight degree of supination during the swing-through phase of the normal gait and begins to pronate immediately after contacting the ground.

During excessive supination, the body's weight is placed on the outside lateral edge of the foot rather than spread equally across the plantar surface. Excessive supination causes an unequal distribution of weight and shock absorption. Consequently, numerous lower extremity problems can result due to altered biomechanics. Individuals who oversupinate are more susceptible to *lateral ankle sprains* because the foot is in a greater degree of inversion during the weight-bearing phase.

Gradual postural change, such as tightness in the **invertors,** is the usual cause. A severe ankle sprain that prevents the ankle from moving through full pronation can also leave the individual with greater supination. Excessive supination can result from childhood orthopedic disorders, such as clubfoot (also called *talipes equinovarus*). The exact cause of clubfoot has not been determined, but proposed explanations include a neuromuscular disorder acquired during development, a ligamentous deficiency, or a result of an awkward position of the fetus in the womb.[7]

History

Ask the client about acute injuries prior to their developing the condition and any increased incidence of ankle sprains. In many cases the client does not describe any pain or discomfort from the problem.

Observation

Supination of the foot must be observed throughout the gait cycle and the condition is best viewed from behind and while the individual is walking, such as on a treadmill. Due to the subtalar inversion there may be a discrepancy in the degree of visible supination between weight-bearing and non-weight-bearing positions. A non-weight-bearing position will make the subtalar inversion visible. An exaggerated wear pattern on the lateral edge of the shoe may be evident.

Palpation

There are no specific findings during palpation for excessive supination, although there may be tenderness in the peroneal muscles due to overstretching. There may also be tenderness in the tibialis posterior due to hypertonicity. In severe cases, callus formation is palpable on the lateral edge of the bottom of the foot due to uneven weight distribution on the foot.

Range-of-Motion and Resistance Testing

AROM: There may be limitation in active eversion of the foot due to hypertonicity in the invertors.
PROM: The same principles apply as for active motion.
MRT: No unusual findings with manual resistive tests.

Suggestions for Treatment

Excessive supination is treated with neuromuscular re-education and postural correction during gait. An orthotic worn in the shoe is successful in achieving the correction in many cases. Massage treatment should focus on the invertor muscles.

OVERPRONATION

Although the term *pronation* is routinely used to describe dysfunctional foot mechanics, a more accurate reference is *overpronation.* The condition is also called *hyperpronation* or *excessive pronation.*

Characteristics

Similar to excessive supination, overpronation is a dynamic postural deviation which means it does not occur in a static position, but rather as a movement dysfunction during the weight-bearing phase of gait. Pronation is an

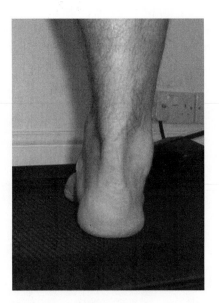

Figure 5.13 Excessive supination, especially the subtalar inversion, is sometimes evident in a standing position. (Image courtesy of Primal Pictures Ltd. www.primalpictures.com).

important part of the normal gait pattern and includes abduction, eversion, and dorsiflexion. **Overpronation results when the foot moves either too far or too fast through the phases of pronation, placing more weight on the medial side of the foot during gait.**

Unless there is a severe, acute injury, overpronation develops as a gradual biomechanical distortion. Several factors contribute to developing overpronation, including *tibialis posterior weakness, ligament weakness, excess weight, pes planus, genu valgum, subtalar eversion, or other biomechanical distortions in the foot or ankle.* Overpronation often includes a combination of factors.

Tibialis posterior weakness is one of the primary factors leading to overpronation. Pronation is primarily controlled by the architecture of the foot and eccentric activation of the tibialis posterior.[6] If the tibialis posterior is weak, the muscle cannot adequately slow the natural pronation cycle.

Another primary cause of overpronation is calcaneal valgus (subtalar eversion). When the calcaneus is everted, weight is forced onto the medial edge of the foot. The subtalar eversion of pronation is visible in a standing position and it is evident that increased weight is placed on the medial side of the foot (Figure 5.14). Obesity can cause overpronation, producing subtalar eversion and forcing the longitudinal arch to collapse.

Overpronation can be a contributing factor in other lower extremity disorders, such as *foot pain, plantar fasciitis, ankle injuries, medial tibial stress syndrome, periostitis, stress fractures,* and *myofascial trigger points.* Overpronation increases the degree of internal tibial rotation, thereby contributing to various knee disorders such as *meniscal injury* or *ligament sprains.*

The effects of the postural deviation are exaggerated in athletes due to the increase in foot strikes while running and the greater impact load experienced. When running, three to four times the body weight is experienced with each foot strike.[8] If overpronation exists, the shock force is transmitted further up the kinetic chain.

History

The client describes pain in the foot, ankle, leg, or knee that is aggravated by repeated stress such as walking or running for long distances, or standing for long periods. Identify previous or concurrent lower extremity problems, which are associated with or caused by overpronation.

Observation

Overpronation is best viewed from the posterior while the individual is walking, such as on a treadmill. When viewed with the client in a standing position, the overpronated foot looks similar to calcaneal valgus because subtalar eversion is a fundamental component of overpronation. Examine the shoes for evidence of excessive pronation. If the shoes have had sufficient use, there will be an exaggerated wear pattern toward the medial side of the shoe bottom.

Palpation

Some bony landmarks may be exaggerated if subtalar eversion is severe. Increased tenderness of the tibialis posterior or its attachment sites is a regular finding during palpation.

Range-of-Motion and Resistance Testing

AROM: Active inversion could be limited due to hypertonicity of the muscles that maintain pronation. Range of motion in inversion is generally not affected.

PROM: The same principles apply as for active motion.

MRT: There are no unusual findings with manual resistive tests.

Suggestions for Treatment

Muscular weakness in the tibialis posterior is often addressed with strength training. Massage treatment can relieve myofascial trigger points in the tibialis posterior and other muscles and address resulting neuromuscular dysfunction in the leg or foot. Lengthening the evertors is beneficial as well. Biomechanical correction of overpronation is important and may require orthotics, neuromuscular re-education, or gait retraining methods. Stretching the gastrocnemius and soleus muscles will reduce hypertonicity in these muscles.[6]

PES PLANUS

Pes planus is a structural foot disorder that interferes with proper function of the foot and can lead to a number of other problems in the lower extremity. The condition is referred to as *flat foot.*

Characteristics

Pes planus is characterized by a dropped or **fallen medial longitudinal arch.** Pes planus can impair the shock-absorbing capabilities of the foot. Many soft tissues play important roles in maintaining the longitudinal arch of the foot and helping in shock absorption, includ-

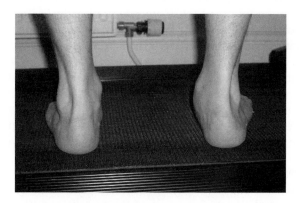

Figure 5.14 The effects of overpronation can be visible in a standing position. Greater weight is borne by the medial side of the foot. (Image courtesy of Primal Pictures Ltd. www.primalpictures.com).

ing the **intrinsic foot muscles, the plantar fascia, tarsal ligaments,** and leg muscles such as the **tibialis posterior**. Additional soft-tissue supports include the **deltoid ligament** and **calcaneonavicular ligament,** also called the *spring ligament*.[9] Weakness or laxity in these tissues causes the longitudinal arch to lose its structural integrity.

Of these muscles, the tibialis posterior is considered the primary dynamic structural support for the arch. When other support tissues are weakened, even greater load is placed on the tibialis posterior in order to maintain the arch. Fatigue and dysfunction of this muscle is a common cause of pes planus and can lead to other problems such as *shin splints, stress fractures*, and *plantar fasciitis*.

The condition may appear earlier in life as a congenital deformity, but is often the result of age, increasing weight, and gradual loss of residual strength in the soft tissues that support the arch. Pes planus does not always lead to other disorders of the lower extremity. Many people have pes planus and experience no symptoms.

History

The client may complain of pain in the foot or lower extremity. They might report that the pain is relieved when wearing orthotics or shoes with significant arch support. Because this condition can be congenital, ask about whether other family members have the condition. Additional soft-tissue disorders may co-exist, such as those mentioned above, but it may be difficult to trace their origin specifically to pes planus.

Observation

Pes planus is best viewed from the medial side of the foot with the client barefoot and standing on a rigid surface. If the medial side of the foot comes close to the ground it is apparent that the arch is low (Figure 5.15). Exact measurements for how high the arch should be are rarely provided. Whether the arch is low enough to cause problems is usually subjective.

If the condition is an inherited disorder, the dropped arch is visible in both a weight-bearing and non-weight-bearing position. If pes planus results from other factors, the arch will appear normal when non-weight-bearing, but flatten with weight. Compare the height of the arch in both a weight-bearing and non-weight-bearing position to determine if there is a significant difference in arch height.[10] If the arch collapses at the onset of loading the foot with body weight, a problem may exist. In severe cases of pes planus, the navicular bone may have dropped low enough to cause friction irritation and callus development in the skin producing a visible callus on the underside of the foot.

Palpation

Calluses or skin irritations mentioned above may be palpable on the bottom surface of the foot. It is difficult to slip a finger under the medial edge of the foot when the individual is weight-bearing.

Range-of-Motion and Resistance Testing

AROM: No specific findings with active motion.
PROM: The same principles apply as for active motion.
MRT: In some cases the tibialis posterior muscle may appear weak due to muscular fatigue, dysfunction, or rupture. In other cases the condition exists with no apparent weakness or pain during manual resistance.

Suggestions for Treatment

Orthotics or arch supports are used to support the arches. Exercise therapy is sometimes used to strengthen the intrinsic muscles of the foot and the tibialis posterior, thereby aiding the integrity of the arch. Massage applications may be helpful in normalizing muscular balance of the muscles that act on the foot and ankle, but the primary problem in pes planus is muscular weakness and connective tissue laxity (such as in the plantar fascia). The most effective treatment emphasizes strengthening those tissues.

PES CAVUS

Pes cavus is a structural foot disorder that interferes with proper function of the foot and can lead to a number of other problems in the lower extremity. The condition is referred to as a *high arch* and does not occur with the same frequency as the pes planus deviation.

Characteristics

Pes cavus indicates an exaggerated and high longitudinal arch of the foot (Figure 5.16). There is no standard as to how high an arch has to be in order to be called *pes cavus*. In this condition the soft tissues of the foot are shortened, making the entire foot appear somewhat shorter. **Intrinsic foot muscles**, as well as the **tibialis anterior and posterior,** may be hypertonic and maintain the distorted position of the arch. The **plantar fascia** is in a shortened position causing increased tensile loads at its attachment points, especially at the **anterior calcaneus**.

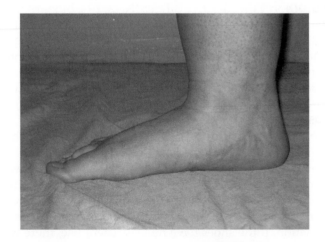

Figure 5.15 Pes planus is a loss of the longitudinal arch, which may eventually lead to other foot and lower extremity disorders.

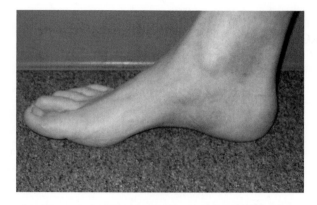

Figure 5.16 Pes cavus is an exaggerated or high longitudinal arch. It is relatively easy to slide a finger underneath the arch in pes cavus.

With the increased arch height, the metatarsal heads are less horizontal in relation to the ground and force loads from body weight are exaggerated at the metatarsal heads, which can lead to a host of other disorders.

Pes cavus usually occurs as an acquired postural distortion, but can also result from certain neuromuscular disorders such as ***Charcot-Marie-Tooth disease***.[11] The condition can also be congenital. It is normal to see an increased incidence of other foot, ankle, or leg disorders that the pes cavus has contributed to, such as ***metatarsal stress fractures or Morton's neuroma***. Pes cavus is often a precursor to ***plantar fasciitis***.

History
The client may complain of pain in the foot or lower extremity, especially with repetitive motion while bearing weight. Pain or discomfort is sometimes felt at the metatarsal heads on the underside of the foot, due to their increased angle. If there is increased tension on the plantar fascia, pain may be reported at the anterior base of the calcaneus. There may also be pain on the lateral edge of the foot due to increased weight-bearing in this region.[12] The client may report pain relief from orthotics that support the arch. Ask if other family members have the condition. In many cases pes cavus has no symptoms, as client has adapted to the foot structure.

Observation
The foot is best viewed from the medial side, with the client barefoot and standing on a rigid surface. An increased degree of space under the metatarsal arch is indicative of pes cavus. There is no standard for what constitutes too much space under the arch. If a finger can be slid easily under the metatarsal arch, the client is considered to have a foot with a high arch. In a severe form of pes cavus, the pads of the toes may not touch the ground when the client is in a standing position.

Palpation
The metatarsal heads may be more prominent on the underside of the foot because of the increased height of the arch. There could be callus formation under the metatarsal heads because of friction from increased weight-bearing on the forefoot. In some cases, the navicular bone is prominent on the dorsal surface of the foot. Roughened skin or callus formation may also be apparent on the dorsal side of the toes as they rub on the shoe.

Range-of-Motion and Resistance Testing
AROM: Unless the condition is severe, there are no specific findings in pes cavus. When severe, limitations are possible in active toe flexion and extension due to connective tissue shortening.
PROM: The same principles apply as for active motion.
MRT: There are no specific findings if the condition is not severe. In severe cases, weakness may be apparent during resisted toe flexion or extension due to chronic neuromuscular distress. Weakness in other muscles of the lower extremity could result if Charcot-Marie-Tooth disease is responsible for the pes cavus.

Suggestions for Treatment
One of the primary perpetuating factors with pes cavus is tightness in the flexor muscles and soft tissues on the plantar surface of the foot. These tissues respond well to massage treatments such as deep stripping techniques. Stretching and massage are helpful for muscles such as the tibialis anterior and posterior, peroneal muscles, and flexors of the foot and toes. If conservative treatments are ineffective, surgery is sometimes used to decrease the height of the arch.

MORTON'S FOOT

Morton's foot is a structural anomaly in which the 2nd toe appears longer than the **hallux** (great toe) (Figure 5.17).

Characteristics
Morton's foot (also called *Grecian foot*) can result from either a short first metatarsal or a long 2nd metatarsal. It is a common anatomical variation appearing in about 40% of the population.[13] Morton's foot is not necessarily pathological and many individuals with this postural deviation never experience symptoms. A Morton's foot will be most problematic when the first metatarsal is shorter than the 2nd and the hallux is shorter than the 2nd toe.

When the first metatarsal is shorter than the 2nd, there is a change in the distribution of weight in the foot and lower extremity. Greater weight is placed under the 2nd metatarsal head from the point at which the heel rises off the ground all the way through the toe-off phase of gait, which may cause calluses. The impact of greater weight loads may not be significant for someone who is engaged in normal daily activities, but when activity levels increase, problems can occur. For example, symptoms resulting from Morton's foot are seen in military recruits who suddenly increase their levels of activity. Problems

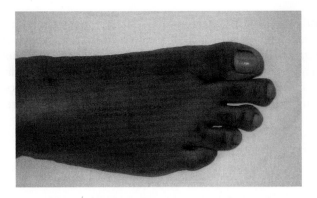

Figure 5.17 Morton's foot is evident with the 2nd toe appearing longer than the hallux.

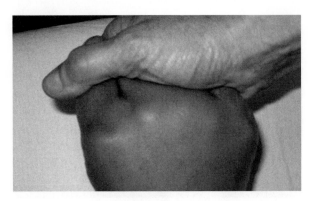

Figure 5.18 Metatarsal head evaluation to indicate Morton's foot. Note the prominence of the metatarsal heads, visibly indicating the second metatarsal longer than the first.

are also seen in athletes engaged in running activities.

The Morton's foot structure is likely to have numerous biomechanical ramifications not only in the foot but throughout the body. *Biomechanical compensations* or *myofascial trigger points* develop in response to the postural strain caused by Morton's foot. Trigger points are often observed in the **peroneal muscles, knee extensors,** as well as **gluteus medius** and **minimus.** Pain avoidance and altered muscular function from trigger point activity may produce pain or alterations in gait. In addition, trigger points can develop in the shoulders, head, and neck due to the myofascial trigger points in the foot and leg.[13]

History

The client may not have symptoms related specifically to Morton's foot. The altered biomechanics of the foot, ankle, and leg can lead to other postural compensations that produce pain. Identify any recent changes in activity level that are associated with increased lower extremity pain. Ask about other lower extremity pain complaints as they may be caused by the biomechanical compensations of Morton's foot.

Observation

In most cases of Morton's foot, the 2nd toe extends further distally than the hallux making the condition easy to identify. In other cases, the 2nd toe is short in relation to the hallux, even though the 2nd metatarsal is longer than the first and the condition is not immediately apparent.

One method of identifying Morton's foot is to look at the space between the toes when any two toes are pulled away from each other. If the client has a Morton's foot, the web of skin between the 2nd and 3rd toes may be larger than that between the 1st and 2nd toes. In some cases calluses are visible on the bottom surface of the foot under the 2nd metatarsal head.

Palpation

Calluses may be palpable. Palpating the metatarsal heads can help determine their relative length. They are best evaluated with the metatarsal head evaluation test.

Range-of-Motion and Resistance Testing

AROM: Active motion has no specific limitations.
PROM: Passive motion has no specific limitations.
MRT: Neither pain or weakness are present with MRTs.

Special Tests
Metatarsal Head Evaluation
The practitioner grasps the client's toes and bends them into full flexion. When the toes are fully flexed, the metatarsal heads are prominent on the dorsal surface of the foot (Figure 5.18). The relative lengths of the metatarsal heads are evaluated at this point. The 1st metatarsal is visibly shorter than the 2nd.

Explanation: When the toes are pulled forward into flexion the metatarsal heads become prominent and their relative length is easier to evaluate.

Suggestions for Treatment
Manual therapy does not correct the bone length problem in Morton's foot. Soft-tissue stresses created by this condition may be addressed through the use of orthotics or pads on the plantar surface of the foot. Massage, stretching, and other forms of soft-tissue manipulation may be helpful for correcting myofascial trigger points or muscular imbalances that have occurred in reaction to the Morton's foot.

HALLUX VALGUS

Hallux Valgus is a structural deviation that involves a *valgus angulation* and is sometimes called a *bunion*.

Characteristics
In a hallux valgus deformity, the distal end of the hallux deviates in a lateral direction (Figure 5.19). The deformity is caused by a variety of biomechanical, structural, or genetic factors including poor footwear, *lax ligaments, weak muscles, or abnormal bone structure*.[10]

The most frequent explanation for hallux valgus deformity is that it is caused by wearing shoes with a narrow toe box.[14] As the foot is forced into the narrow shoe, the

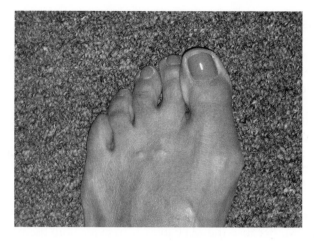

Figure 5.19 Hallux valgus deformity; sometimes called a *bunion*.

distal phalanges are pushed toward the midline of the foot and a valgus angulation results. As the distal end of the hallux is pushed laterally (toward the foot's midline), the proximal end pushes the first metatarsal head medially against the edge of the shoe, resulting in *callus* formation and *subcutaneous inflammation*. The term *bunion* is used to refer to either the callus formation or the hallux valgus deformity.[15] The biomechanical distortion resulting from hallux valgus can produce a host of lower extremity disorders, such as *shin splints, stress fractures, myofascial trigger points, overpronation,* and others.

Biomechanical problems, such as *pes planus, ligament laxity,* and *overpronation* can also lead to the development of hallux valgus. For example, overpronation causes a drift in the position of the metatarsal heads and forces the first metatarsal head in a medial direction.[16] As the first metatarsal head is forced in a medial direction, it pushes the proximal hallux with it, causing the distal hallux to deviate in the opposite direction (laterally). Hallux valgus deformities occur more often in women than men, but it is undetermined if this is due to a structural cause or associated with a particular type of shoe.[14]

There is appears to be a genetic pattern for developing the condition. It is undetermined whether the disorder is actually inherited or if what is passed down is a foot structure that makes one vulnerable to developing the condition. If the foot structure is inherited, various factors (footwear, pressure on the metatarsal heads, etc.) would also need to be present to develop the condition. Familial patterns of development in the absence of narrow footwear suggest there may be other causes, such as *biomechanical factors, metabolic disorders, or neuro-muscular disease.*

History
The client may report wearing shoes with a narrow toe box. The period of time the person will have worn the shoes prior to experiencing symptoms will vary with the their propensity for developing the disorder. Ask the client if they have worn high-heel shoes as they make the

condition worse.

Determine if there is a familial history of hallux valgus deformity. Ask about metabolic or arthritic disorders, such as *gouty arthritis, rheumatoid arthritis,* or connective tissue problems such as ligamentous laxity, *Marfan* or *Ehlers-Danlos syndromes.* It is also important ask about neuromuscular disorders that may be related such as *multiple sclerosis, cerebral palsy,* or *Charcot-Marie-Tooth disease.*

Observation
Observe the client's bare foot in a neutral standing position. The distal end of the hallux deviates in a lateral direction (angling toward the other toes). The deviation can be so severe the hallux *rides up* over the other toes.

Palpation
There may be pain and tenderness over the outside edge of the first metatarsal head, especially if a callus has developed. The tissue covering the first metatarsal head feels thick and fibrous from the constant pressure against the inside of the shoe.

Range-of-Motion and Resistance Testing
AROM: Hallux flexion or extension may be limited due to connective tissue buildup. Flexion may also be limited if the hallux has ridden up over the 2nd toe.
PROM: Hallux flexion and extension are sometimes limited. Passive abduction of the hallux (pulling it away from the other toes) will usually be restricted due to connective tissue remodeling around the dysfunctional articulation.
MRT: Resisted hallux flexion or extension may appear weak from neuromuscular components of the disorder or because of mechanical binding around the joint.

Suggestions for Treatment
If there is a mechanical cause of the deformity, such as narrow shoes, it is difficult to reverse the process because the hallux must be pulled in the opposite direction. In some cases, gradual movement of the hallux and metatarsal heads is encouraged with pads between the hallux and 2nd toe or orthotics. Massage techniques can relax tissues that are shortened. Soft-tissue manipulation is unlikely to reverse the valgus angulation. A surgical procedure called an *osteotomy* may be performed to realign the bones.

HAMMER TOES

Hammer toes are a structural distortion caused by contractures or chronic shortening in the toe flexor muscles. This condition can cause other biomechanical problems throughout the kinetic chain.

Characteristics
A *contracture* is a permanent or semi-permanent contraction due to spasm or paralysis.[17] They typically

affect muscles that produce flexion and are also called *flexion contractures*. In hammer toes, **the dysfunctional contractures hold the metatarsophalangeal (MTP) and distal interphalangeal (DIP) joints in extension and the proximal interphalangeal (PIP) joint in flexion** (Figure 5.20). This position causes excess friction between the top of the toes and the inner surface of the shoe, causing calluses or friction blisters.

Hammer toes are associated with a *pes cavus* foot. The high arch in a pes cavus foot can produce contraction of the **toe flexors**, creating other postural compensations such as the hammer toe. A hammer toe is most common in the **2nd toe**, but can develop in any of the toes except the hallux. The condition does not occur in the hallux because it has only one interphalangeal joint and two are needed to produce the hammer toe deformity.

Hammer toes can be hereditary, caused by muscular imbalance, or develop from other mechanical factors such as improper shoes. There is an association between hammer toes and a **2nd ray** in the foot that is longer than the **first ray**. A *ray* is defined as one metatarsal and its associated set of phalanges.[5] A relatively long 2nd ray also occurs in the *Morton's foot* deformity. Other causes of hammer toes include *muscular hypertonicity, neuromuscular or joint disorders* such as *gout* or *rheumatoid arthritis*, or metabolic factors.

In some cases a variation of the hammer toe deformity develops called *claw toe*. It also involves flexion contractures of the MTP and PIP joints. In the claw toe deformity the DIP is in flexion rather than extension (Figure 5.21). Its causes are the same as hammer toe.

History

The client with a hammer toe may complain of pain over the dorsal aspect of the PIP joint and could also have pain on the plantar aspect of the metatarsal heads. The client might have a pes cavus foot.

Observation

The hammer toe alignment is clearly visible. Sometimes there are visible calluses on the dorsal surface of the toes or the plantar surface of the foot under the metatarsal heads.

Palpation

Hypertonicity is often palpable in the flexor and extensor muscles of the toes due to excess levels of contraction. Palpable calluses may have developed from rubbing the dorsal surface of the phalanges against the shoe.

Range-of-Motion and Resistance Testing

AROM: Because the MTP joint is in extension, there will be little ability to further extend it actively. Flexing this joint may be difficult as well. Active movement difficulties are not easily evident at the IP joints because control is difficult even in a normal foot.

PROM: Limited passive flexion of the MTP joints and extension of the proximal IP joints is characteristic.

MRT: Pain is unlikely with manual resistive tests, but muscle weakness is possible when attempting resisted extension of the MTP and IP joints. Muscle weakness results from active insufficiency (inability to further contract an already shortened muscle).

Suggestions for Treatment

Hammer toes are usually treated conservatively. Pain is reduced by placing pads on the top surface of the toes to reduce friction against the shoe or strapping the toe with tape or slings.[18] Orthotics are used to change foot biomechanics. Massage of the toe flexors and extensors is encouraged to achieve muscular balance in the foot. Changing footwear can be helpful. If pes cavus is contributing, it will need treatment as well. If conservative treatment is not helpful surgery can be performed to change the faulty alignment.

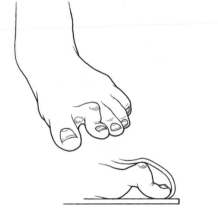

Figure 5.20 Hammer toe deformity with the DIP in extension. (Used with permission from Richardson J, Iglarsh ZA. Clinical Orthopaedic Physical Therapy. Philadelphia: W.B. Saunders; 1994).

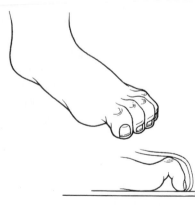

Figure 5.21 Claw toe deformity with the DIP in flexion. (Used with permission from Richardson J, Iglarsh ZA. Clinical Orthopaedic Physical Therapy. Philadelphia: W.B. Saunders; 1994).

Common Injury Conditions

LATERAL ANKLE SPRAIN

Lateral ankle sprains are the most widespread lower extremity, soft-tissue injury.[19] It is estimated that 85% of all ankle injuries involve a form of ligament sprain.[20] These sprains occur frequently in sports such as basketball, volleyball, football, and soccer.[21]

Characteristics

Due to the greater range of motion with inversion, and the subsequent instability that follows, there are more **lateral ankle ligament** sprains than **medial ankle ligament sprains. It is** *excess inversion* **that causes lateral ankle sprains**. The **fibula**, located on the lateral side of the ankle, extends further distally than the **tibia** on the medial side of the ankle. Eversion is restricted because of the tarsal bone's contact with the fibula. Because the tibia does not extend as far distally, it does not provide the same degree of resistance to inversion.

Lateral ankle sprains are also more common due to the strength of the ligaments that resist forces that would cause injury. Three primary ligaments on the lateral side of the ankle provide stability against inversion. From weakest to strongest they are the **anterior talofibular, calcaneofibular,** and **posterior talofibular** (Figure 5.22).[22] The anterior talofibular is the weakest and the ligament typically injured in a sprain. The anterior talofibular ligament is even more susceptible to damage when plantar flexion is involved. When the foot is inverted and plantar flexed, the **anterior talofibular** is in its most vulnerable position. For example stepping off a curb and twisting the ankle puts the ankle in plantar flexion and inversion, causing a lateral sprain. If the injury is severe, the **calcaneofibular ligament** is typically involved.

Lateral ankle sprains are listed as **grade 1 (mild), grade 2 (moderate),** or **grade 3 (severe).** Refer to Chapter 2 for the characteristics of the different grades of sprain. In a grade 1 sprain, generally only the **anterior talofibular ligament** is involved. In serious grade 2 and grade 3 sprains, the **anterior talofibular** and **calcaneofibular ligaments** may both be injured and a greater degree of instability is present.[23]

Lateral ankle sprains produce profuse swelling that can linger in the area for weeks after the initial injury. Swelling remains because the lymphatic system has to fight gravity to move the fluid from the distal lower extremity. The supporting ligaments of the ankle are essential for proper biomechanical function in the foot. Consequently, instability resulting from injury to these ligaments may seriously limit mobility and predispose the person to similar injuries in the future.

History

The client reports a sudden motion that caused sharp pain on the lateral side of the ankle. Obtain an accurate

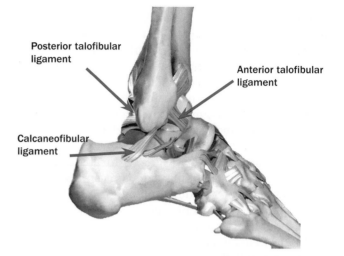

Figure 5.22 Lateral view of the right ankle showing stabilizing lateral ligaments that provide resistance to inversion. (3-D anatomy image courtesy of Primal Pictures Ltd. www.primalpictures.com.)

description of the mechanics of the injury to determine if the lateral ligaments are involved. Ask the client if they have had previous sprains to the injured ankle. Prior injuries make the ligaments vulnerable to re-injury. Previous participation in sports may indicate former injury or predisposition to ankle sprains. In addition to immediate pain, the client reports swelling that increased immediately after the injury.

Observation

Swelling is a prominent visual sign and sometimes remains in the area for weeks after the injury, especially if the injury is a 2nd or 3rd degree sprain. The client characteristically walks with a limp, if bearing weight on the injured ankle is even possible. If capillary disruption occurred, bruising may be visible as well.

Palpation

The area around the lateral ankle is tender to touch. Inflammation is characteristically present and applying pressure on the swollen tissues produces additional pain. The tissue has a puffy feeling and movement of the subcutaneous fluid is often visible when palpating the area. Other muscles, such as the peroneal group, could be hypertonic from reflex muscle spasm following the injury. These muscles tighten to compensate for lost joint stability due to the ligament damage.

Range-of-Motion and Resistance Testing

AROM: Active movements are likely to be painful, especially if the injury is severe. While there may be pain in single-plane movements, the greatest pain is felt with inversion because it stretches the damaged ligament fibers. Pain may also be increased in eversion or dorsiflexion due to increased pressure from edema surrounding the lateral ankle.

PROM: Passive movements can be painful because

of swelling in the joint or tensile stress on damaged ligaments. Inversion is most painful as it stretches the damaged ligament fibers. With complete rupture of the ligament, it is possible for passive inversion to be performed that does not cause additional pain because the ligament fibers have been totally disrupted, although instability and hypermobility are evident. If the injury is severe, nerve fibers may also be torn or disrupted leading to a decrease in pain signals.

MRT: Pain is characteristic with an MRT for ankle eversion if the peroneal tendons are injured. Pain can result from muscle or fascia near the joints pulling on the damaged ligament fibers or attachment sites. In many cases the primary injury is ligamentous and MRT does not increase pain. Muscle weakness due to reflex muscular inhibition generally exists whether pain is present or not.

Special Tests
Ankle Drawer Test
The ankle drawer test is designed to determine the integrity of the anterior talofibular ligament. It is easiest to perform with the client seated on the edge of the treatment table. The practitioner stabilizes the anterior distal tibia with one hand while pulling the posterior calcaneus in an anterior direction with the other hand (Figure 5.23). Forward shifting or a soft, mushy end feel suggests ligamentous laxity. The procedure may cause pain with a 1st or 2nd degree sprain. In a 3rd degree sprain there is significant movement, but limited pain due to complete rupture of the affected ligament. Do not mistake the slight amount of dorsiflexion that occurs during the test for forward translation of the foot.

With some clients there is ligamentous laxity in numerous ligaments and it will be unclear if the perceived movement results from normal laxity or a damaged ligament. Compare the amount of movement on the injured side with that on the unaffected side.

Explanation: When the ankle is in a neutral position, the anterior talofibular ligament has a primary role in resisting forward translation of the foot. If the foot is allowed to move forward, it is because there is laxity or a tear in the anterior talofibular ligament. If the ligament is damaged but not fully torn, the tensile stress on the injured ligament fibers produces pain.

Talar Tilt Test
The talar tilt test emphasizes the calcaneofibular ligament. This test can be performed in several positions, but is easiest with the client in a side-lying position. The affected ankle is off the edge of the table and the foot is in a neutral position (in relation to plantar flexion and dorsiflexion). The practitioner grasps the ankle with the thumbs on each side (anterior and posterior) of the lateral malleolus and attempts to move the client's foot into inversion to evaluate pain and mobility (Figure 5.24).

Explanation: When the foot is in a neutral position the calcaneofibular ligament resists pure inversion. The inversion force to the ankle in this test position puts greater stress on the calcaneofibular ligament. This test should be performed in addition to the ankle drawer test so the integrity of both ligaments can be evaluated.

Differential Evaluation
Tendon avulsion, peroneal tendon injury, ankle fracture, syndesmosis sprain, capsular tearing, ankle impingement syndrome.

Suggestions for Treatment
Ankle sprains are best treated in the initial stage with **PRICE (protection, rest, ice, compression, and elevation)**. Once the severity of the sprain is determined, treatment can be further defined. Most ligament sprains are managed by conservative treatment, but a severe ligament sprain may warrant surgical intervention.[24] Physical therapy treatment for ankle sprains includes range-of-motion exercises, stretching muscles around the ankle joint, strengthening, and proprioceptive exercises using a wobble board, also called a *BAPS (biomechanical ankle plat-*

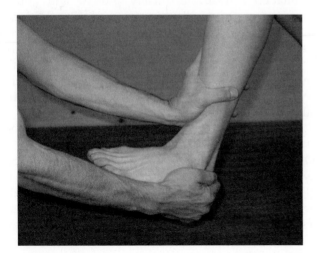

Figure 5.23 Ankle drawer test.

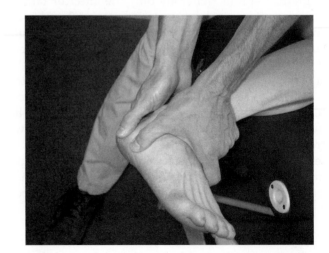

Figure 5.24 Talar tilt test.

form system) board.[25] Drawing letters of the alphabet in the air with the toes is an exercise to help return movement in all planes. Movement exercises should be performed within the client's comfort range.

Massage applications are useful at certain stages of healing. General applications to the calf will help reduce protective spasms in the muscles. Special attention to the peroneal muscles is indicated for lateral ankle sprains. These muscles enhance the stability of the ankle to compensate for the injured ligament(s).

Once the acute phase of the injury has subsided, deep transverse friction to the injured ligaments enables proper alignment of scar tissue so that a functional scar can develop. Deep friction massage is also important to prevent the healing ligament from adhering to underlying or adjacent tissues during the healing process.[26] Massage can eventually be combined with active and passive range-of-motion to improve mobility.

MEDIAL ANKLE SPRAIN

Medial ankle sprains are less common than lateral ankle sprains and generally indicate a greater degree of trauma to the ankle. Car accidents can produce this type of sprain. Sporting activities may also involve forces strong enough to produce this injury.

Characteristics
The primary function of the **medial ankle ligaments** is to prevent *excessive eversion*. The ligaments are aided in that role by the fibula. Bony stability against excess eversion and the strength of the ligaments are the primary factors that make this injury so rare. Medial ankle sprains involve the group of ligaments collectively referred to as the **deltoid ligament**, and include, from posterior to anterior, the **posterior tibiotalar, tibiocalcaneal, tibionavicular,** and **anterior tibiotalar** (Figure 5.25).

Due to the strength of the deltoid ligament, a greater force is required to produce stretching or tearing of the ligaments. Deltoid ligament sprains are seen in injuries that also involve *ankle fractures* or *tendon avulsions*, indicating very high force loads placed on the ankle. The extent of trauma needed to produce a sprain of the deltoid ligament frequently produces a large amount of scar tissue in the region following the injury. Permanent movement limitations due to severe bone damage may also result.

Prior injuries to the medial ankle complex may produce instability and cause future injury. If a medial ankle sprain is suspected, the client should be referred to a physician to evaluate for fractures or dislocations.

History
The client reports an excessive force to the ankle, such as having the foot crushed against the floorboard in an automobile accident. If a sports injury, the client describes a sudden motion that causes sharp pain on the medial side

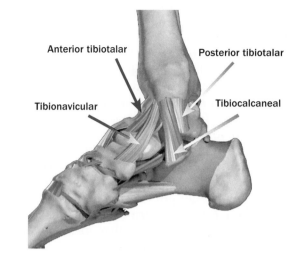

Figure 5.25 Medial view of the right ankle showing the deltoid ligament complex that provides resistance to eversion. (3-D anatomy image courtesy of Primal Pictures Ltd. www.primalpictures.com.)

of the ankle. If possible, explore whether the described impact is one that would put tensile force on the deltoid ligament complex. Ask about prior injuries to the medial ankle complex as instability in the region may be a factor in the current injury.

Observation
Swelling is a prominent visual sign and immediately follows the injury. Swelling can remain in the area for weeks after the injury, especially if the injury is a 2nd or 3rd degree sprain. The client walks with a limp, if bearing weight on the injured ankle is even possible. If capillary damage has occurred, bruising is expected. In severe injuries where there is a fracture or dislocation, misplacement of bony contours may be noticeable.

Palpation
The area around the medial ankle is tender. Inflammation is sometimes felt and applying pressure on the swollen tissue causes additional pain. The area has a puffy feeling and movement of subcutaneous fluid may be visible when palpating the area. Other tissues may hurt when palpated, due to tendon or ligament avulsions or fractures. Dislocations or fractures produce altered contours of bone around the medial malleolus that are palpable.

Range-of-Motion and Resistance Testing
AROM: Active movements are painful and restricted, especially if the injury is severe. There may be pain in single-plane movements, but the greatest amount of pain is felt with eversion due to stretch of the damaged ligament fibers. If fractures or dislocations accompany the sprain, movement will be limited.

PROM: Passive movements are painful due to swelling that causes pressure on free nerve endings. Eversion will be painful. With complete rupture of the ligament, passive eversion may not cause additional pain but there will be a moderately firm end feel as the fibula prevents further eversion.

MRT: Because tendon and ligament avulsions frequently occur with medial ankle sprains, MRTs in multiple directions are routinely weak and painful. Pain is caused by muscles and tendons pulling on damaged connective tissues. Weakness from reflex muscular inhibition may be present with numerous MRTs.

It is unlikely that an MRT will place additional tensile stress on the deltoid ligament itself. However, the presence of pain with this test should alert the practitioner to investigate all possible structures in the area for damage and refer out for further evaluation. Deltoid ligament sprains typically occur with more severe injuries, so damage to muscular tissues is likely.

Differential Evaluation

Tendon avulsion, tendon damage to tibialis posterior, flexor hallucis longus, or flexor digitorum longus, fracture, syndesmosis sprain, capsular tearing.

Suggestions for Treatment

The methods of treatment are the same as for *lateral ankle sprain* with the major difference being the site of injury. Site specific treatments such as deep friction massage are aimed at the medial ankle region instead of the lateral ankle region.

SYNDESMOSIS ANKLE SPRAIN

While the lateral ankle sprain is the most common ankle ligament injury, other ligaments should be considered in ankle injuries. Failure to recognize other types of ligamentous injury, such as a *syndesmosis ankle sprain*, may lead to inappropriate treatment and prolonged disability.

Characteristics

A *syndesmosis* is a fibrous joint with little mobility located where two bones are directly connected by ligaments or another connective tissue membrane. The ankle's *distal tibiofibular syndesmosis* is the tough fibrous connection that holds the distal ends of the tibia and fibula together and is another site for ligament sprains. Because the location of the distal tibiofibular syndesmosis is superior to the **ankle (talocrural) joint**, it is often called a *high ankle sprain*.

The distal tibiofibular syndesmosis is connected by several ligaments and connective tissues, including the lower margin of the **interosseous membrane and ligament** and the **anterior, posterior, and transverse tibiofibular ligaments** (Figure 5.26). Sprains to the distal tibiofibular syndesmosis characteristically involve the anterior or posterior tibiofibular ligaments or the interosseous ligament. Sprains occur when the distal tibia and fibula are forced apart.[27]

There are two primary biomechanical situations in which these bones might be forced apart to create a syn-

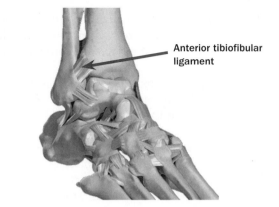

Anterior tibiofibular ligament

Figure 5.26 The right ankle showing the distal tibiofibular syndesmosis. The anterior tibiofibular ligament is most superficial. (3-D anatomy image courtesy of Primal Pictures Ltd. www.primalpictures.com.)

desmosis sprain. In normal mechanics, the ankle has only a slight degree of rotational movement. In the ankle these rotary motions are described as adduction and abduction, although some authors describe them as medial or lateral rotation respectively. **If the ankle is rotated into the extremes of adduction or abduction, the distal tibia and fibula will be forced apart and a syndesmosis tear will result.**

A similar situation occurs with extremes of **dorsiflexion**. During dorsiflexion, the talus rolls under the distal tibia and fibula. The inferior portion of the talus is wider than the superior portion. When the inferior portion of the talus rolls up between the tibia and fibula at the end of dorsiflexion, the wide body of the talus may force the bones to separate. The amount of separation is usually within the normal degree of ligamentous pliability. However, syndesmosis sprain is likely if the ankle is forced into extreme dorsiflexion, or is rotated while dorsiflexed. Such a mechanical stress might occur in activities where the person turns the body on a planted foot while squatting.

In some cases a syndesmosis sprain will exist for some time before it is accurately identified, the initial assumption being that a lateral ankle sprain has occurred. Treatment aimed at a lateral ankle sprain may not resolve the problem because the true site of injury is the syndesmosis.

History

The client describes an inciting event where the ankle is forced into extreme dorsiflexion, a rotary movement, or a combination of the two. The injury generally results when rotary stress and extreme dorsiflexion are simultaneous. The client describes pain in the ankle region, but may have difficulty pointing to the primary site of pain because some syndesmosis ligaments are deep. Conversely, if a lateral ankle sprain exists, it will be easy for the client to point to and press on the painful structures because they are superficial.

Observation

Syndesmosis sprains do not show the same degree of swelling that is present with lateral or medial ankle sprains. Therefore, they are harder to visually identify. Some swelling may be visible above the malleoli on either side. With serious capillary damage, bruising is evident.

Palpation

The area around the distal tibiofibular joints may be tender, especially near the anterior or posterior tibiofibular ligaments.[28] The site of actual ligamentous damage could be hard to reach, so pain from ligament damage may not be easily reproduced with palpation. With swelling, palpation of the area causes pain.

Range-of-Motion and Resistance Testing

AROM: Pain is felt with external rotation (abduction) of the foot. Active external rotation should be performed with the knee flexed so the internal knee ligaments are slackened. If they aren't, more rotation will occur at the hip and confuse results of the evaluation. Having the client sit on the edge of the treatment table is the best position to evaluate this movement. Pain may also be felt near the end of dorsiflexion as the tibia and fibula are forced apart.

PROM: Passive movement causes pain in the same directions as active movement: primarily dorsiflexion and external rotation (abduction) of the ankle.

MRT: Resisted muscle contractions do not increase pain when performed in a neutral position and without maximal muscular effort. Some weakness can be experienced from reflex muscular inhibition.

Special Tests

Squeeze Test

The practitioner grasps the tibia and fibula at about the proximal or mid-calf region and squeezes them together (Figure 5.27). If pain is felt in the region of the distal tibiofibular joint, then syndesmotic injury may be responsible. It is important to note that some fractures or compartment syndromes are painful with this procedure, so ruling these other problems out is important.

   Explanation: Squeezing the tibia and fibula together in the mid-calf or a more proximal region causes them to be separated at the distal syndesmosis.[29] The tensile stress on the ligaments is greater in the external rotation stress test below, making it a more accurate test.

External Rotation Stress Test

The client is seated on the edge of the treatment table with the knee flexed to 90° and the ankle in a neutral position. The practitioner places a hand under the plantar surface of the client's foot. The foot is then passively, externally rotated (abducted) to the end range of motion (Figure 5.28). If this motion reproduces the client's pain, there is a good likelihood of syndesmosis injury.

   Explanation: Rotation (abduction) is not a normal

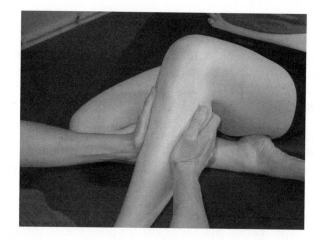

Figure 5.27 **Squeeze test to evaluate syndesmosis sprain.**

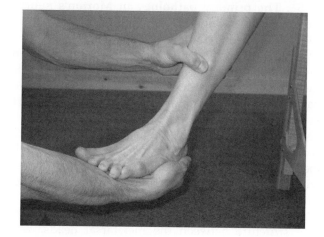

Figure 5.28 **External rotation stress test.**

motion of the ankle, so little motion occurs in this direction. By attempting to rotate the ankle, the tibia and fibula are spread apart and stress on the damaged ligaments produces pain.[30] Additional tensile stress is applied by moving the foot into more dorsiflexion, further spreading the tibia and fibula apart, before applying rotational stress.

Differential Evaluation

Tendon avulsion, tenosynovitis, tendon damage to muscles of dorsiflexion, distal tibial or fibular fracture, capsular tearing, medial or lateral ankle ligament sprain.

Suggestions for Treatment

Syndesmosis sprains are treated much like medial or lateral ankle sprains, with the initial stage treated with **PRICE.** Once the severity of the ligament sprain is determined, treatment can be defined. Bracing is used to improve stability and enhance earlier weight-bearing. Healing times of a syndesmosis sprain tend to be longer than for lateral ankle sprains.

   Massage reduces corresponding muscle spasms or hypertonicity. It is difficult to reach the damaged ligament fibers, so treatment may be indirect.

MORTON'S NEUROMA

Morton's neuroma is a mechanical compression condition that causes pain in the forefoot and toes. A *neuroma* is an inflamed or irritated nerve. The condition is also called *Morton's metatarsalgia* or *interdigital neuroma*.

Characteristics

The **plantar nerves** are an extension of the **tibial nerve**, which itself is a division of the **sciatic nerve**. As the tibial nerve passes through the **tarsal tunnel**, it divides into the **medial** and **lateral plantar nerves**. Both nerves course along the plantar surface of the foot and terminate in the toes. The medial plantar nerve supplies the 1st through 3rd digits, while the lateral plantar nerve supplies the 4th and 5th. **The primary pathology in Morton's neuroma involves compression of the plantar nerves, which pass between the metatarsal heads.**

Morton's neuroma presents with greatest frequency between the 3rd and 4th metatarsal heads because the space between the heads is smallest here.[31] The condition can also occur between the 2nd and 3rd metatarsals because the intermetatarsal space is also narrow.

Morton's neuroma develops for several reasons. The nerve can be aggravated by wearing narrow toe-box shoes, which compresses the metatarsal heads. In addition, in some people fibers from the medial and lateral plantar nerves converge close to the heads of the 3rd and 4th metatarsals (Figure 5.29). This junction creates a larger nerve structure between the metatarsal heads, which makes them more vulnerable to compression.

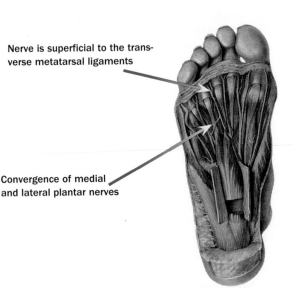

Nerve is superficial to the transverse metatarsal ligaments

Convergence of medial and lateral plantar nerves

Figure 5.29 Convergence of the medial and lateral plantar nerves near the space between the 3rd and 4th metatarsal heads. In certain cases, the convergence is closer to the metatarsal heads than illustrated here. The nerves are also superficial to the transverse metatarsal ligaments making them further susceptible to neural tension. (Mediclip image copyright, 1998 Williams & Wilkins. All rights reserved).

Another factor that can cause irritation is tensile stress on the nerve as it is pulled against the **transverse metatarsal ligament**, which is deep in the foot and connects adjacent metatarsal heads (Figure 5.29).[31] The branches of the digital nerves extending into the toes are superficial (closer to the skin on the plantar surface) to the ligaments. The nerves are pulled taut against these ligaments at the extremes of toe extension, such as in the final stages of push-off or squatting with the weight on the balls of the feet, and pain can be produced.[32, 33] This same neural tension may occur from wearing high-heeled shoes, as they also maintain the toes in hyperextension.

Less commonly, a previous injury, such as a fracture or ligament damage, could produce scar tissue that reduces the space between the metatarsal heads. Scar tissue could also bind the nerve to adjacent structures, including the ligament, impairing proper movement of the nerve.

History

The client reports sharp, shooting pain, numbness, or paresthesia in the forefoot and extending distally into the toes, typically in the region of the 3rd and 4th toes. Pain is aggravated with certain shoes (those with a narrow toe box or high heels) and reduced while barefoot or when wearing low-heeled shoes with a wider toe box. Pain may also be felt with certain shoes that are tied too tight. There may be pain at the end of the push-off phase when walking or running, but generally only when the client is wearing shoes as opposed to being barefoot. Clients may also report a relief of symptoms by massaging the foot, as it may spread the metatarsal heads and mobilize the entrapped nerve.

Observation

There are no visible signs of Morton's neuroma. The presence of a hallux valgus deformity may indicate a history of wearing narrow toe-box shoes.

Palpation

There are no significant signs of pain with palpation unless the practitioner applies pressure to the intermetatarsal space between the metatarsal heads, furthering compression of the nerve.

Range-of-Motion and Resistance Testing

AROM: Active motion generally does not cause pain. Pain might be felt at the end of dorsiflexion with the toes in extension due to neural tension. Pain in this position is aggravated if the entire sciatic nerve is stretched, as in a straight leg raise test.

PROM: Passive motion may cause pain when the toes are pulled into hyperextension. Pain is more likely if there is also tension on the sciatic nerve. See the section on neurological problems in the low back region and discussion of the straight leg raise and slump tests for information on how to stretch the sciatic nerve.

MRT: There are no specific findings with MRTs.

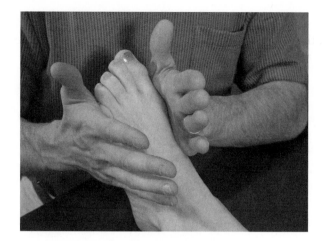

Figure 5.30 Morton's test.

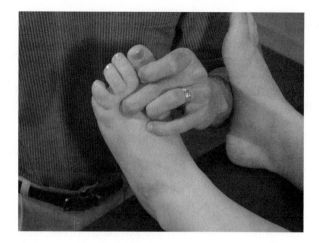

Figure 5.31 Interdigital squeeze test.

Special Tests
Morton's Test
The client is supine on the treatment table. The practitioner grasps the client's forefoot from both sides and applies moderate pressure, squeezing the metatarsal heads together (Figure 5.30). If this action reproduces the client's symptoms (primarily sharp, shooting pain into the toes, especially the 3rd and 4th), Morton's neuroma may exist. Make sure pressure is delivered straight toward the center of the foot so the transverse arch is not exaggerated, which would decrease pressure on the nerve and make the test less accurate.

Explanation: Pressure applied to the medial and lateral sides of the foot increases compression on the irritated nerve structure between the metatarsal heads. If the condition is present, the client's pain is reproduced.

Interdigital Squeeze Test
The client is supine on the treatment table. The practitioner uses the thumb and index finger to compress the space between the involved metatarsal heads—normally the space between the 3rd and 4th (Figure 5.31). Moderate pressure is used. If the characteristic neurological pain is created, there is a good indication of Morton's neuroma.

Explanation: Pressure is applied to the affected nerve between the metatarsal heads. If the condition is present, the client's pain is reproduced. This test is more likely to produce a positive result than the Morton's test if the primary problem is the nerve being pulled taut against the transverse metatarsal ligament.

Differential Evaluation
Stress fracture, arthritis, gout, tarsal tunnel syndrome, other proximal neuropathies, lumbo-sacral radiculopathies, arthritis.

Suggestions for Treatment
Changing footwear is a crucial part of treatment for this problem. Sometimes a cushioned dome pad can be worn inside the shoe and helps spread the metatarsal heads and decrease pressure on the nerve. Massage is helpful, but should not be deep and invasive between the metatarsal heads. The best results are achieved with massage techniques that encourage spreading and mobilizing the metatarsal heads, which stretch the intrinsic foot muscles and reduce compression of the nerve. If conservative treatment is not successful, surgical excision of the nerve can be performed.

PLANTAR FASCIITIS

Plantar fasciitis is a recurrent overuse condition affecting the foot, especially in the athletic population.[34] It occurs from repetitive microtrauma that is exaggerated by various biomechanical factors such as a *pes planus or pes cavus* foot.

Characteristics
The **plantar fascia** is composed of both superficial and deep layers. It is the deep layer that is of greatest interest in this condition. The plantar fascia attaches proximally to the **anterior calcaneus** and distally blends into the ligaments surrounding the **MTP joints** and **flexor tendon sheaths** of all five metatarsals (Figure 5.32). It provides the primary soft-tissue support for the longitudinal arch and its impairment can reduce arch stiffness by 25%.[35] The plantar fascia is an important shock absorber, decreasing the impact forces of foot strike. Reducing these impact forces is particularly important in sporting activities because **ground reaction force** can be 2–3 times the body's weight when running.[36] Without tissues such as the plantar fascia mitigating these forces, the body is susceptible to a host of problems such as *stress fractures, joint disorders*, or *shin splints*.

The plantar fascia performs its function by acting as a spring that maintains the arch. A mechanical analogy called a *windlass* is often used to describe this function (Figure 5.33). The windlass works to maintain tension on the arch even as the arch shortens, which it does during push-off or landing from a jump.[37] An individual with *pes planus* (flat foot) has a poor longitudinal arch, which decreases the shock absorbing capability of the windlass structure of the plantar fascia.[38] This is one reason why plantar fasciitis characteristically appears in people who have pes planus. It also occurs in people with *pes cavus* (high arch) because tension on the plantar fascia is increased and stress is placed on its attachment site on the anterior calcaneus.[39]

Plantar fasciitis is routinely **considered an inflammatory condition involving the attachment site of the plantar fascia on the calcaneus.** Recent studies suggest that inflammation may not always be involved, and the primary tissue irritation could be *collagen degeneration* in the fascia akin to that experienced in overuse *tendinosis.*[40] Both processes are likely to be involved in the condition.

Plantar fasciitis frequently involves fiber degeneration of the plantar fascia. Fiber degeneration can occur anywhere along its course, but the primary site of involvement is the **proximal attachment** at the **anterior calcaneus.** The attachment site is particularly tender because plantar fasciitis places tensile stress on the periosteum surrounding the bone. The periosteum is one of the most pain-sensitive tissues in the body, so tensile stress on it can produce significant pain.[8] Due to repetitive tensile stress on the calcaneal attachment site, an *exostosis (bone spur)* may develop on the anterior calcaneus. Plantar fasciitis may exist without calcaneal spurs and vice versa.

Several factors can play a role in the onset of the condition. *Overpronation* is a biomechanical dysfunction that is a recognized cause of plantar fasciitis.[41] Ordinarily the **tibialis posterior** muscle aids the plantar fascia in shock absorption. The muscle's function is compromised in overpronation and the plantar fascia has to take on a greater role of shock absorption in the lower extremity. *Hypertonicity* or *myofascial trigger points* in the **triceps surae** (gastrocnemius and soleus) muscles may set up dysfunctional tension patterns in the foot muscles and contribute to plantar fasciitis as they limit movement of the windlass mechanism in the foot.

A sudden change in activity levels, such as that seen in new military recruits, is linked to plantar fasciitis.[42] Significant weight gain, especially if recent, may put additional stress on the plantar fascia and longitudinal arch. For example, plantar fasciitis is increasingly common in the later stages of pregnancy when rapid weight gain occurs over a short period of time and relaxin levels are elevated in the blood stream, decreasing connective tissue strength.

Footwear and ground surface play an important role in cumulative trauma of the plantar fascia. Certain types of shoes, such as high-heeled shoes, decrease the shock-absorbing quality of the plantar fascia because they alter foot mechanics. Likewise, steel-shanked construction boots decrease flexibility of the foot and may lead to cumulative trauma, especially if the person walks or

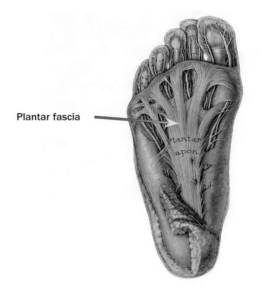

Plantar fascia

Figure 5.32 The plantar fascia, also called the plantar aponeurosis, on the bottom of the foot. (Mediclip image copyright, 1998 Williams & Wilkins. All rights reserved).

stands on a hard surface all day. Activities that require repetitive impact loading on the foot are usually responsible for the condition.

History

The client reports sharp, intense pain at the heel or plantar surface of the foot. Pain is normally exaggerated when first getting out of bed and starting to walk in the morning.[43] The pain usually subsides, but may not be alleviated altogether, after some period of walking. Symptoms are aggravated by repetitive motion on hard, unyielding surfaces, such as running on pavement.

Find out if the client is involved in repetitive activities such as running, jumping, or dancing. Ask about the ground surface involved in these activities, as a harder surface can aggravate the problem.

Observation

There are no visible signs to indicate this condition. Inflammation, when present, is rarely visible due to the subcutaneous fat pads and thickness of the skin on the plantar surface of the foot. The practitioner should consider the presence of certain structural problems as possible precipitating factors, such as pes cavus and pes planus foot. Excessive pronation can cause plantar fasciitis, so look for factors such as calcaneal valgus that may indicate its presence.

Palpation

The client feels tenderness when the sole of the foot is palpated. Pain is exaggerated near the anterior region of the calcaneus at the proximal plantar fascia insertion, but can be present anywhere on the plantar fascia. Inflammation is rarely palpable. Hypertonicity or myofascial trigger point activity is sometimes palpable in the triceps surae

---

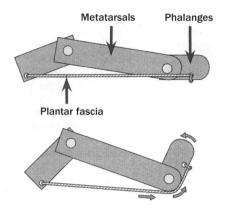

Figure 5.33 The plantar fascia functioning as a windlass mechanism in the foot. (Used with permission from Lowe W. Orthopedic Massage: Theory and Technique. Edinburgh: Mosby; 2003).

muscles. A bone spur on the anterior calcaneus could be palpable, but not always.

Range-of-Motion and Resistance Testing

AROM: Active dorsiflexion may be painful with the toes hyperextended, as the plantar fascia stretches and pulls on the irritated calcaneal insertion site. Dorsiflexion may be limited by tightness in the triceps surae. There may be pain when standing on the ball of the affected foot with the toes in hyperextension.

PROM: The same principles apply as for active motion.

MRT: No specific MRTs elicit pain. Pain is possible with strongly resisted plantar flexion, as mentioned in the AROM section. Weakness in plantar flexion may be evident from reflex muscle inhibition when weight is placed on the affected forefoot.

Differential Evaluation

Morton's neuroma, tarsal tunnel syndrome, proximal neuropathies or radiculopathies, tendon avulsions or dysfunctions (especially tibialis posterior), myofascial trigger points within intrinsic foot muscles, stress fracture, sprains to ligaments of metatarsal or tarsal bones, entrapment of medial or lateral plantar nerves.

Suggestions for Treatment

Conservative treatment is usually successful in addressing this problem. The individual should modify or cease offending activities that caused or contributed to the condition. Orthotics are prescribed in some cases. A tension night splint, which holds the foot in dorsiflexion during the night, is beneficial and decreases pain when first loading the foot with weight in the morning.[44, 45]

Massage, such as deep longitudinal stripping, reduces tension in the deep flexor muscles of the foot and may aid in pain relief. To prevent further stretching or pulling of the plantar fascia attachment site, stripping techniques should be done toward the calcaneus. Caution is advised

with deep pressure techniques near the anterior calcaneus to prevent further compression on a bone spur that might be present, which could irritate or damage the tissues.

Massage and stretching methods should focus on the kinetic chain of soft tissues that maintain and control the longitudinal arch, including the tissues on the plantar surface of the foot, the tibialis posterior, and triceps surae muscles due to their action on the calcaneus. Myofascial trigger points in the triceps surae can be addressed with massage as well.

STRESS FRACTURE OF THE FOOT

A *stress fracture* **is an overuse condition that develops as a result of repetitive stress loading on the bone**. They are common in the foot, especially the metatarsals, because of the weight and force loads placed on the small bones in this region (Figure 5.34).[46]

Characteristics

A stress fracture is not an acute injury. Rather, the condition results from levels of compressive stress that accumulate gradually. Bone gradually cracks when placed under repeated loads. Stress fractures can occur from relatively few repetitions of a high load, or many repetitions of a low or normal load.[8] Bone can remodel and recover from a particular load, given enough time. A stress fracture only occurs when the amount and frequency of loading exceeds the bone's remodeling capability.

Stress fractures also occur due to *muscular fatigue*. The **tibialis posterior** and **plantar fascia** play an important role in maintaining the longitudinal arch and preventing stress fractures of the foot. If these tissues become fatigued and weakened there is greater stress on the bones as they become the structure that absorbs the shock.

There are several biomechanical factors to consider

Box 5.4 CLINICAL NOTES

Tarsal tunnel syndrome and plantar fasciitis

Sharp pain in the plantar surface of the foot could result from a number of causes. Two conditions that produce similar symptoms in the foot are *tarsal tunnel syndrome* and *plantar fasciitis*. In some cases it may be easy to mistake these conditions, but they have some distinguishing aspects.

Plantar fasciitis is most painful first thing in the morning when weight is put on the foot after being in a non-weight-bearing position all night. The pain is due to sudden tensile loads on the plantar fascia attachment at the calcaneus. It is particularly tender to the touch at the calcaneal attachment of the fascia.

Pain from tarsal tunnel syndrome is also felt along the plantar surface of the foot. It is exacerbated when pressure is applied to the medial ankle directly over the tarsal tunnel. Pay close attention to all different aspects of the assessment process as a number of evaluation procedures may produce pain with both conditions.

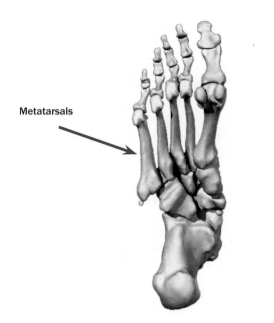

Metatarsals

Figure 5.34 The long, thin metatarsal bones are susceptible to stress fractures (3-D anatomy image courtesy of Primal Pictures Ltd. www.primalpictures.com.)

if stress fractures in foot and ankle bones are suspected. The geometry and architecture of the bones is particularly important. For example long thin bones, such as the **metatarsals,** are susceptible to loads that produce a fracture. Larger, shorter, and thicker bones, such as the **talus**, are resistant to fractures. The talus is also protected in that there are other bones and ligaments that help absorb shock and decrease the likelihood of fracture. However, some larger foot bones that are exposed to direct compressive loads, such as the calcaneus, may sustain stress fractures.

Recent changes in training surface, such as changing from running on grass to running on concrete may be sufficient to cause stress fractures. Footwear can lead to additional stress on the bones. While a stress fracture can occur in children, the condition is more common in adults due to the loss of density in bones and the slowing of the remodeling process.

Sudden increases in activity levels are typically at fault. For example, stress fractures are a frequent injury in military recruits and some estimates suggest that 5% of new recruits will develop stress fractures, especially in the lower extremity.[47] Stress fractures also occur in activities requiring repetitive loading of normal force amounts, such as track and field athletics.[48]

Physical examination can identify some symptoms of stress fracture, but if the condition is suspected the client should be referred to a physician for proper evaluation. Unlike other fractures, a stress fracture may be difficult to identify even with x-ray because the bone disruption can be minor. In many cases a bone scan is necessary. It is important to identify potential risk factors or symptoms indicating stress fracture early on because if left untreated, stress fractures can become debilitating and greatly lengthen the rehabilitation process.

History

The client complains of pain near the fracture site that is associated with activity. Inquire into activities that either place repetitive high or normal stresses on the foot or ankles. Pain will be aggravated by repetitive loading such as running, especially on hard surfaces. The pain subsides with rest. Ask the client about recent changes in activity levels prior to the onset of symptoms. Ask about changes in footwear.

Observation

There are no specific visual findings to indicate a stress fracture. Postural distortions such as pes planus or over-pronation could indicate unequal stress placed on the lower extremity that may affect the bone. Examine the entire lower extremity kinematic chain for postural factors that lead to biomechanical dysfunction. It may be helpful to examine the client's shoes for wear patterns that indicate tissue overload.

Palpation

Point tenderness is present at the site of the fracture. The pain is localized in a small area directly on the bone, as opposed to diffuse soft-tissue pain in the general area. In some cases the bone with the stress fracture is not directly palpable, but pressing on adjacent tissues may elicit the pain. If the stress fracture has existed for some time and the bone is easy to palpate, periosteal thickening may be evident with palpation.[49]

Range-of-Motion and Resistance Testing

AROM: There are no specific findings if motion evaluation is performed in a non-weight-bearing position. There may be tenderness when active motion is performed in a weight-bearing position due to compressive loads on the bone or tensile forces from muscle attachments near the site of the fracture.

PROM: The same principles apply as for active motion.

MRT: In some cases there is tenderness with MRTs if the muscle being tested has an attachment site near the fracture. The tendon can pull on the periosteum near the fracture site and if the periosteum is disrupted from a stress fracture, tensile stress from a contracting muscle may reproduce pain.

Special Test
Bone percussion

Strongly tapping the bone with the fingertips reproduces pain from some stress fractures. The vibration along the bone irritates the damaged tissue and periosteum thereby reproducing the client's pain. Placing a vibrating tuning fork on the bone or, in some instances, ultrasound administered over the area may create the same results. Note that these evaluation methods are not considered highly reliable.

Differential Evaluation

Morton's neuroma, tarsal tunnel syndrome, proximal neuropathies, plantar fasciitis, tendon avulsions, myofascial trigger points within intrinsic foot muscles, sprains to ligaments of metatarsal or tarsal bones, apophysitis, Freiberg disease.

Suggestions for Treatment

Stress fractures are best addressed through rest and activity modification. Rest from the offending activity may be lengthy, sometimes as long as 4 – 8 weeks.[49] Modalities, such as electrical stimulation, are used with some success in speeding the healing of fracture sites.[50] Massage may be helpful in normalizing biomechanical stresses in the region of the stress fracture, but does not directly improve healing.

TARSAL TUNNEL SYNDROME

Nerve entrapment syndromes do not occur with as much frequency in the lower extremity as they do in the upper extremity. Some authors consider *Tarsal tunnel syndrome (TTS)* to be a rare condition, leading to it being overlooked as a source of foot pain.[51] The location of pain on the plantar surface of the foot produced by TTS may also cause it to be mistaken for *plantar fasciitis*. Like carpal tunnel syndrome in the wrist, it involves a nerve passing through a **fibroosseous tunnel** created by a binding **retinaculum**.

Characteristics

The **tibial nerve** (sometimes called the *posterior tibial nerve*) runs through the lower leg in the **deep posterior compartment**. As the nerve exits the deep posterior compartment it passes around the medial side of the ankle on its way to termination in the toes. Near the **medial malleolus** the tibial nerve divides into three branches. The **medial calcaneal nerve** is primarily a sensory branch that serves the posterior and bottom surface of the heel. The other branches, the **medial** and **lateral plantar nerves,** carry motor and sensory signals to the plantar surface of the foot and into the toes.

Just after the tibial nerve divides into these three branches, they all pass under a fascial band on the medial side of the ankle called the **flexor retinaculum** or **laciniate ligament** (Figure 5.35). The retinaculum is connected superiorly to the medial malleolus and inferiorly to the medial side of the calcaneus. This space under the retinaculum is the **tarsal tunnel**. In some people, the nerve branches after passing through the tunnel. There are several other structures that pass through the tunnel, including the tendons of **tibialis posterior, flexor digitorum longus,** and **flexor hallucis longus**, and the **posterior tibial artery** and **vein.**

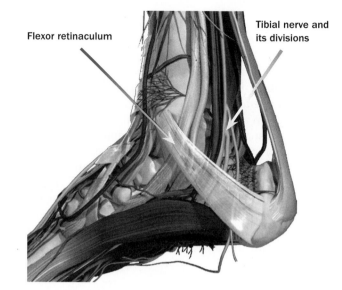

Figure 5.35 Divisions of the tibial nerve as they pass underneath the flexor retinaculum. (3-D anatomy image courtesy of Primal Pictures Ltd. www.primalpictures.com.)

Tarsal tunnel syndrome results when the tibial nerve is exposed to compressive or tensile stress within the tarsal tunnel. Any of the branches of the nerve may be affected. Branching of the tibial nerve inside the tunnel or prior to entering it increases the likelihood of symptoms from nerve pathologies.[52] A number of factors could create these stresses. Compression can occur from extrinsic factors coming from outside the tunnel. For example, a direct blow to the medial side of the ankle or fractures or dislocations that compress the nerve.

Nerve compression also occurs from intrinsic factors, such as *space-occupying lesions* or *ganglions,* which press on the nerve within the tunnel.[53, 54] Anatomical anomalies, such as bony prominences that protrude into the tunnel, can also compress the nerve. Each of the tendons that pass through the tunnel is encased within its own **synovial sheath.** A swelling of the tendon and synovial sheath (tenosynovitis) may compress either the **tibial nerve** or the nearby **vascular structures**. *Tenosynovitis* results from repetitive overuse of the involved tendons. The tunnel's contents may be compressed in a *calcaneal varus* foot alignment as the overall space in the tarsal tunnel is decreased leading to nerve compression. Compression of the tendons within the tunnel in a varus foot alignment may lead to tenosynovitis and additional nerve pressure.

Tensile forces on the nerves in the tarsal tunnel may also be a cause of symptoms. Neural tension results from either a sudden stretch of the nerves or from biomechanical distortion, such as a *calcaneal valgus* foot alignment.[55] TTS is prevalent in runners with altered foot mechanics during gait.[56]

Significant compression or tension within the tunnel may not be required to create symptoms in TTS. Because the tarsal tunnel is at the distal end of the lower extremity, the nerves have a long path prior to entering the tunnel.

The tibial nerve is susceptible to compression pathologies in a number of locations along its length before entering the tunnel. Distal compression or tension pathologies are more likely if there is a proximal pathology of the same nerve. This principle is referred to as the *double or multiple crush phenomenon* (see Chapter 2).[57] For example TTS may occur in a situation where proximal nerve compression exists, such as *piriformis syndrome* or *disc herniation* pressing on nerve roots in the lumbar region.

Peripheral neuropathies like TTS are linked to conditions such as *diabetes, muscular sclerosis, rheumatoid arthritis,* and *hyperthyroidism.*[58] Note that some medications may cause sensitivity in the distal lower extremity nerves that could be mistaken for compression pathologies in the tarsal tunnel.

History

The client reports sharp, shooting pain sensations around the medial ankle and along the plantar surface of the foot. In addition to pain there may be paresthesia, numbness, or motor weakness in the muscles of the foot. Symptoms are ordinarily worse after long periods of standing or walking, but may also be aggravated during the night if the nerve is in a compromised position for prolonged periods. Ask about recent trauma involving sudden compressive or tensile loads on the nerve, as recent injuries may be responsible for the symptoms. It is important to screen for proximal nerve conditions and ask about systemic disorders that may cause TTS or be related to it.

Observation

There are no visible signs specifically for tarsal tunnel syndrome, but certain postural disorders such as calcaneal varus or valgus can play a role in nerve dysfunction. Although uncommon, if TTS is severe or has been present for a long time, some atrophy of the muscles innervated by the divisions of the tibial nerve may be apparent.

Palpation

Placing pressure directly on the tarsal tunnel is one of the most valuable ways of identifying this condition and is sometimes called the tarsal compression test. If the pressure reproduces the client's primary pain, it is a good indication of tarsal tunnel syndrome. Determine whether the sensations are primarily neurological, as irritated tendon sheaths in the area may also cause pain with palpation. If nerve compression is the problem, symptoms are felt in the medial ankle and along the plantar surface of the foot. If the problem results from tendon irritation, such as tenosynovitis, pain occurs in the medial ankle region where pressure is applied.

Range-of-Motion and Resistance Testing

AROM: Pain or discomfort may be present at the far extremes of active dorsiflexion, inversion, or eversion, but this finding is not consistent. Pain might be evident when dorsiflexion and eversion are performed simulta-

neously (see Dorsiflexion-eversion test below). Due to the continuity of the tibial nerve, pain from active movement may be aggravated if more proximal parts of the sciatic nerve are also stretched simultaneously.

PROM: The same principles apply as for active motion.

MRT: MRTs rarely produce pain or discomfort. Weakness with MRTs may be apparent in some of the intrinsic foot muscles supplied by the distal branches of the tibial nerve.

Special Tests

Dorsiflexion-Eversion Test

The client is in a supine position. The ankle is passively moved into maximum dorsiflexion and eversion while the toes are held in hyperextension (Figure 5.36). The position is held for 5–10 seconds. If symptoms develop, it is a positive sign for TTS.

Explanation: When the foot is in this position the tibial nerve is stretched beneath the flexor retinaculum, pulling the nerve taut and causing compression. This is a relatively new special test for tarsal tunnel syndrome, but it

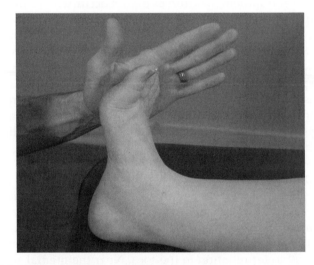

Figure 5.36 **Dorsiflexion-eversion test.**

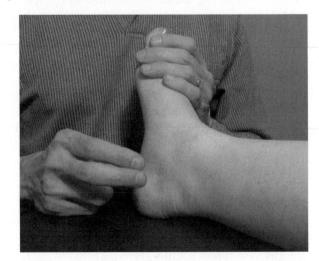

Figure 5.37 **Tinel's sign at the ankle.**

has shown clinical success and improved accuracy over other procedures such as the Tinel's sign.[59]

Tinel's Sign

Tapping directly over the region of a neuropathy to reproduce symptoms is known as Tinel's sign (Figure 5.37). If there is a short, sharp neurological sensation on each tap it indicates hypersensitivity of the nerve and may indicate TTS. Tinel's sign is not highly accurate and should be used in conjunction with other tests when possible.

Explanation: Compression makes the irritated nerve hypersensitive to pressure, even when applied briefly, and can produce the symptoms.

Differential Evaluation

Morton's neuroma, plantar fasciitis, proximal neuropathies, lumbar radiculopathy, tendon avulsions, myofascial trigger points within intrinsic foot muscles, sprains to ligaments of metatarsal or tarsal bones, rheumatoid arthritis, diabetic or systemic neuropathy, complex regional pain syndrome.

Suggestions for Treatment

TTS is first treated with conservative measures. Orthotics may be beneficial. If the primary problem involves overpronation, which stretches the tibial nerve in the tunnel, an orthotic can be built for the medial side to prevent the foot rolling into excessive eversion.

Massage can be helpful for nerve pathologies such as TTS, but should be performed carefully because massage that further compresses the nerve will aggravate the condition. Techniques are aimed at reducing the factors that lead to TTS, but do not specifically treat the damaged nerve. For example, reducing tension in the muscles of the deep posterior compartment will improve mobility of the tibial nerve and its branches so they are not unnecessarily bound in the region.

Anti-inflammatory medications such as NSAIDS are sometimes used to reduce swelling in the flexor tendons' synovial sheaths, if tenosynovitis is a factor. Corticosteroid injections into the region of the tarsal tunnel are also used to address inflammation, although controversy exists about the safety and effectiveness of this procedure.

If conservative treatment is unsuccessful, surgery is used to divide the flexor retinaculum and increase the space for the structures under the tunnel. There are detrimental biomechanical effects to cutting the flexor retinaculum, including the development of scar tissue, so conservative approaches are generally preferred.

RETROCALCANEAL BURSITIS

The primary function of a **bursa** is to reduce friction between adjacent tissues. Inflammation and irritation of one of the bursa on the posterior heel is called *retrocalcaneal bursitis* or *Haglund's disease*.[60] Note that Haglund's disease is different than *Haglund's deformity*.[61]

Characteristics

Due to high friction loads in the posterior heel, there are two bursae here that decrease compression on the distal **Achilles tendon** and the **posterior calcaneus**. The bursa on the posterior aspect of the calcaneus that is deep to the Achilles tendon is called the **retrocalcaneal** or **subtendinous bursa** (Figure 5.38). The other bursa is just under the skin and superficial to the Achilles tendon and is called the **subcutaneous calcaneal** or **Achilles bursa**.[62] Technically, retrocalcaneal bursitis refers only to bursitis of the subtendinous bursa and not the subcutaneous calcaneal bursa. Inflammation of the subcutaneous calcaneal bursa is sometimes called *Achilles bursitis*, although both conditions can be lumped together under the term *retrocalcaneal bursitis*. Of the two, subtendinous bursitis is more common and this discussion focuses on that pathology.

The retrocalcaneal bursa is likely to be irritated from compression by the heel counter of the shoe. The pressure occurs from shoes that are either too small, tied too tight, or made of stiff and unyielding material. As the heel counter of the shoe presses the bursa against the posterior calcaneus, irritation develops and can lead to inflammation. In some cases, certain systemic conditions may increase the likelihood of retrocalcaneal bursitis, such as *gout, Reiter syndrome, or rheumatoid arthritis*.[62]

Other structural problems of the heel increase the chance of developing bursitis. In some cases there are numerous factors, such as those that make up *Haglund's syndrome*, that lead to the problem.

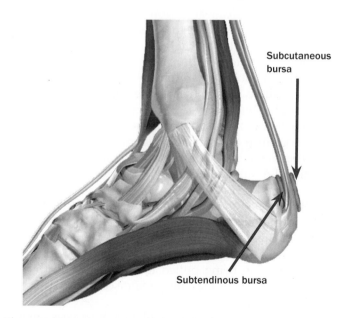

Subcutaneous bursa

Subtendinous bursa

Figure 5.38 Medial view of the right ankle showing the subtendinous and subcutaneous bursae. (3-D anatomy image courtesy of Primal Pictures Ltd. www.primalpictures.com.)

Haglund's syndrome is identified as a swelling in the posterior heel that includes retrocalcaneal bursitis, thickening of the Achilles tendon, convexity of the soft tissues around the Achilles tendon insertion, and an enlargement of the bone where the Achilles tendon inserts.[63] The enlargement of the bone and tissue in the region near the retrocalcaneal bursa is often referred to as a *pump bump* or *Haglund's deformity*.[61] When this bump is present, retrocalcaneal bursitis may develop as the bursa is pressed against the protruding surface.

History

The client describes a painful sensation on the posterior aspect of the heel that is aggravated with walking or running. The pain is relieved when shoes are removed. Ask about recent changes in footwear or increased activity levels. For example, individuals accustomed to wearing high-heeled shoes may experience retrocalcaneal bursitis after switching to flat shoes. The Achilles tendon becomes accustomed to a shortened position in the high-heel and then is stretched in the flat shoe, putting additional pressure on the retrocalcaneal bursa.[62]

The client may report pain relief with anti-inflammatory medication such as NSAIDS. Ask about recent problems with the systemic conditions listed above as they may aggravate the symptoms.[62]

Observation

There is an enlarged area just over the posterior calcaneus, which could either represent tissue swelling or only be indicative of a pump bump. With inflammation, redness may also be apparent. In some instances the skin overlying the bursa looks rough and irritated as well.

Palpation

The posterior calcaneal region is tender to palpation. Pressure here reproduces the client's pain. In some cases it is possible to determine if the primary problem is in the subcutaneous calcaneal bursa or the subtendinous bursa through palpation. If the problem is in the subcutaneous calcaneal bursa, puffiness and swelling may be palpable. If the subtendinous bursa is affected, pinching the area anterior to the Achilles tendon near its insertion point may reproduce the primary discomfort. Note that pain near the Achilles tendon insertion is also present with insertional Achilles tendinitis.

Range-of-Motion and Resistance Testing

AROM: The client should be evaluated with the shoes off so additional pressure by the shoes can be ruled out. Pain at the end range of dorsiflexion may occur due to the Achilles tendon being pulled taut against a protruding pump bump. There may be some discomfort felt in full plantar flexion, but not often.
PROM: The same principles apply as for active motion.
MRT: There are no significant findings with manual resistive tests.

Differential Evaluation

Achilles tendinosis/tendinitis, tendon avulsions, referral from myofascial trigger points, blister, callus, Reiter's syndrome, rheumatoid arthritis, plantar fasciitis, gout, calcaneal bone injuries.

Suggestions for Treatment

Retrocalcaneal bursitis, like most other bursitis conditions, is treated with rest and activity modification. Anti-inflammatory medication or cold applications are also used. Stretching exercises for the gastrocnemius and soleus are recommended. A heel-lift in the shoe can shorten the gastrocnemius and soleus, taking tension off the Achilles tendon and reducing pressure on the bursa. Massage to the posterior calf muscles can be helpful in reducing overall tension in these muscles, thereby decreasing the amount of irritation on the bursa. Massage does not directly relieve compression on the bursa and should not be performed on the posterior heel.

ACHILLES TENDON DISORDER

The **Achilles tendon (AT)** is the strongest tendon in the body and requires this strength because of the high force loads required during motions such as walking, running, or landing from a jump. *Achilles tendon disorders* are prevalent lower extremity injuries, especially among runners.[64,65] The condition can develop at any age, but there is an increased frequency in older populations.

Characteristics

The AT has a poor mechanical advantage in controlling plantar flexion movements in the foot. Strong contractions of the **gastrocnemius** and **soleus muscles** are required to perform the normal motions of the foot and ankle and place high tensile loads on the AT. As a result, the tendon is susceptible to a variety of pathologies such as *tendinosis, paratendinitis* (also spelled *paratendonitis*), and *tendinitis*.

The gastrocnemius and soleus muscles insert into the calcaneus by way of the AT. Because the gastrocnemius has two heads and the soleus has one and they share an attachment tendon, the muscles are sometimes called the **triceps surae**.

The AT is surrounded by a membrane called the **paratenon**. This membrane, which is sometimes erroneously labeled a synovial sheath, surrounds other tendons of the distal extremities. The difference between the AT and these other tendons is that the AT does not pass under a retinaculum. Other tendons such as the toe extensors or tibialis anterior are bound close to the joint by the extensor retinaculum and require a synovial sheath to reduce friction between the tendon and the retinaculum. The paratenon is not a synovial sheath, but in the AT this membrane is thicker and therefore looks like a true synovial sheath.[26] The AT derives a great deal of its blood supply from small capillary vessels within the paratenon.

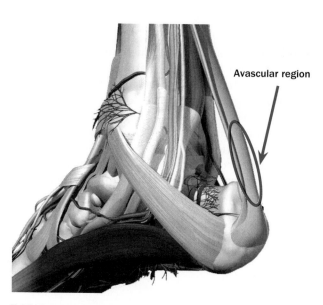

Figure 5.39 Posterior-medial view of the right ankle showing the avascular region in the distal Achilles tendon. (3-D anatomy image courtesy of Primal Pictures Ltd. www.primalpictures.com.)

There is an **avascular zone** of the tendon near the distal insertion into the calcaneus that can become the site of degenerative changes and damage to the AT (Figure 5.39).[66, 67]

The term *tendinitis* is used extensively to describe overuse tendon problems throughout the body. Numerous authors find the term inappropriate because most overuse tendon pathologies do not involve inflammation.[68-71] Yet the AT is one tendon that does appear to have inflammatory activity resulting from overuse in the tendon as well as the paratenon. Consequently, the terms ending in *–itis* appear clinically accurate when referring to the AT.

Several pathologies could be called Achilles tendinitis. The first two conditions are *insertional* and *non-insertional tendinitis*. Both forms arise from similar factors including overuse, previous corticosteroid treatment, systemic disorders, use of other medications, or lack of proper conditioning. Structural or biomechanical factors such as *overpronation, calcaneal varus or valgus,* and *genu valgum* are structural characteristics that may lead to Achilles tendon degeneration.[72]

Insertional tendinitis involves disorders that occur at the insertion of the AT into the calcaneus. It is prevalent in older individuals and those who engage in activities without proper conditioning. Because the avascular zone of the AT is near the insertion, lack of tendon healing due to ischemia can contribute to this disorder.[67]

High tensile loads placed on the AT insertion are likely to cause microtrauma in the structural framework of the bone at the attachment site. In addition, the periosteum that surrounds the calcaneus is pain sensitive and irritations of the attachment site can be very painful. The main complaint from individuals with insertional tendinitis is heel pain. Sufficient evaluation will be necessary as several conditions produce similar pain sensations near the tendon insertion, such as *retrocalcaneal bursitis* and

Haglund's deformity.

Non-insertional tendinitis typically affects athletes and those engaged in vigorous physical activity. **The pathologies included under the umbrella of non-insertional tendinitis include** *paratendinitis, tendinosis,* and *tendinitis*. Tendinosis is grouped with these inflammatory conditions mainly for convenience and because tendinosis frequently precedes inflammation in the AT. The distinction of whether or not inflammatory activity is present in the tendon is important because it guides clinical treatment decisions.

By name **paratendinitis suggestions inflammation of the paratenon**. As the condition advances, it can involve inflammation of the tendon. Paratendinitis is divided into three stages: acute (less than 2 weeks), subacute (2-6 weeks), and chronic (more than 6 weeks).[73] There may be diffuse edema around the tendon along with thickening of the tendon. Crepitation, tenderness, and morning pain are common. Pain increases during plantar flexion and dorsiflexion as the tendon slides within the paratenon. If tendinitis occurs along with the paratendinitis, there may be palpable nodules in the tendon.

Tendinosis is degeneration of the collagen matrix within the tendon, which leads to pain and loss of function. The collagen degeneration of tendinosis is the most widespread form of overuse pathology seen in other tendons of the body.[69, 74] The degenerative changes of tendinosis are caused by age, repetitive microtrauma, or other factors that lead to collagen breakdown.

Inflammation of the tendon is tendinitis. It can be acute or chronic and primarily affects the avascular zone near the base of the tendon. There is tenderness throughout the tendon and fibrous thickening near the distal end, which is apparent when the tendon is compared to the unaffected side (assuming the other side is not affected). If not treated properly, tendinitis causes further tendon weakening and can lead to either partial or complete tendon ruptures.[75]

Recent studies show a link between certain medications and the onset of Achilles tendon degeneration and ruptures. Especially implicated are medications in the fluoroquinolone family of antibiotics, such as ciprofloxacin (brand named Cipro).[76-78] These medications appear to produce tendon pathology in large tendons of the body, even in the absence of vigorous repeated activity. In addition, systemic disorders such as *hyperthyroidism, renal insufficiency, gout,* or *rheumatoid arthritis* can also contribute to tendinitis in the AT.[79, 80]

History

The client describes pain near the posterior heel near the tendon insertion. There may be pain during activity or after it has ceased. Pain is usually felt directly on the calcaneus in insertional tendinitis and along the distal third of the tendon in non-insertional tendinitis. Ask about recent increases in activity levels, especially running or jumping.

Inquire about previous injuries or problems with calf muscle strength, foot pain, or posterior heel pain. These factors may indicate biomechanical deficiencies in the foot or ankle that aggravate Achilles tendon pathology.[81] When evaluating recent activities consider if there is a history of poor conditioning, improper shoes or training surfaces, inadequate flexibility, or increased duration of aggravating activities. Ask about recent medications, especially antibiotics in the fluoroquinolone family.

Observation

The Achilles tendon is often thickened and enlarged. Thickening is a fibrous reaction in the collagen matrix and does not necessarily indicate inflammation. In some cases, nodules are visible on the tendon. Perform an adequate visual analysis of biomechanical or structural problems in the lower extremity, such as overpronation, calcaneal valgus, or genu valgum, as many can lead to AT disorders.

Palpation

The tendon is tender to pressure, especially near the distal third of the tendon in the area with decreased vascularity. The tendon may feel dense and nodules are sometimes palpable along its length and tender. When palpating the tendon, move the skin back and forth over the tendon to identify sensations of crepitus or rubbing. Rubbing sensations may be described as similar to that felt when snow is rubbed together in the hands and squeaks.

Range-of-Motion and Resistance Testing

AROM: Active plantar flexion may be painful if performed in a weight-bearing position and is not likely in a non-weight-bearing position unless the condition is severe. There could be pain near the end range of dorsiflexion as the tendon is stretched. The client might report feeling crepitation or squeaking of the tendon during dorsiflexion or plantar flexion. The practitioner may also feel crepitation if the tendon is lightly palpated during

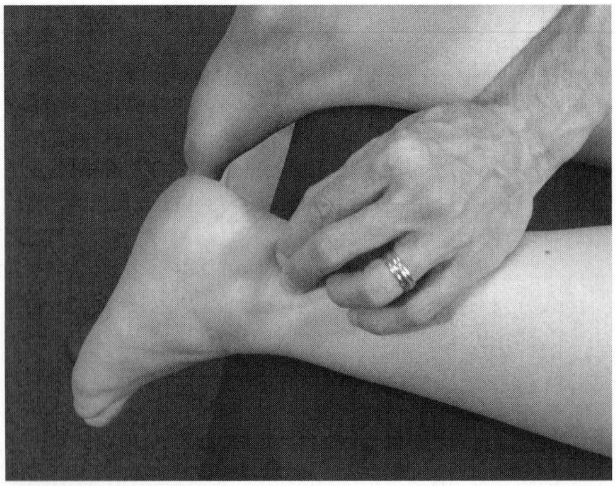

Figure 5.40 Achilles tendon pinch test.

movement.

PROM: Pain may be felt at the end range of dorsiflexion as the tendon is stretched. Pain is unusual during passive plantar flexion. In some cases there is discomfort at the end range of plantar flexion as inflamed tissues are crowded in the posterior heel region. The crepitation or tendon squeaking described in active motion may occur in passive motion.

MRT: Pain results from resisted plantar flexion. Because the Achilles tendon is so strong, an MRT performed with manual resistance alone may not generate sufficient force to produce pain unless the condition is severe. Greater force can be generated by having the client stand on the ball of one foot and hold the position. Weakness will be evident due to reflex muscular inhibition if the condition has progressed.

Special Test
Achilles Tendon Pinch Test

This test is helpful to discriminate between Achilles tendon disorders and retrocalcaneal bursitis. The client is prone. The practitioner squeezes the sides of the tendon superior to the calcaneus to attempt to reproduce the client's primary complaint (Figure 5.40). Pressure must be placed on each side of the Achilles tendon, squeezing towards the middle; pressure should not be placed straight down on top of the tendon (pressing from the posterior side in an anterior direction). Pressure should also be applied superior to the location of the retrocalcaneal bursae so the AT is the only structure being compressed.

Explanation: Squeezing the dysfunctional tendon reproduces the client's pain. All tendon fibers would be affected so squeezing from the sides puts pressure on the tendon, but decreases the chance that pain originates from structures directly posterior to the calcaneus, such as the retrocalcaneal bursa.

Differential Evaluation

Retrocalcaneal bursitis, tendon avulsions, referral from myofascial trigger points, blister, callus, strain to distal triceps surae musculotendinous junction, pain from Haglund's deformity, Achilles tendon rupture, ankle fracture, compartment syndromes, ankle ligamentous injury.

Suggestions for Treatment

Achilles tendon disorders are best controlled through rest and activity modification. Do not confuse rest with immobilization. Immobilization may lead to the development of fibrous adhesions. Rest means stopping offending activities. Cold applications and anti-inflammatory medication may be used to address inflammatory activity if present. As soon as stretching is tolerable, it is helpful to stretch the Achilles tendon several times per day.

Massage applications to the calf muscles reduce tension and decrease tensile forces on the tendon. Deep friction as tolerated in the problem area is beneficial in stimulating fibroblast proliferation in the tendon to repair the damaged collagen matrix. Cold applications prior to the deep friction reduce the intensity of the discomfort, and re-applying cold after treatment reduces the accelerated metabolic response to the friction. Heel lifts inside the shoe may be recommended to help reduce tension on the tendon. Corticosteroid injections were formerly used with greater frequency and are not recommended now because of long-term detrimental effects on the tendon, such as tendon rupture.[82]

ACHILLES TENDON RUPTURE

Not many tendons in the body are susceptible to complete rupture, but the **Achilles tendon** is and it is the strongest tendon in the body. Exceptionally high force loads, usually precipitated by chronic tendon degeneration, can cause rupture of the tendon. *Achilles tendon ruptures* are prevalent in the athletic population but occur in the absence of vigorous activity if certain risk factors are present. Surprisingly, despite the importance of the gastrocnemius and soleus in plantar flexion, complete rupture of the Achilles tendon does not prevent the individual from being able to walk.

Characteristics
The Achilles tendon is the distal attachment of the **gastrocnemius** and **soleus** muscles. Due to the biomechanical arrangement in the foot, these muscles generate exceptionally strong contraction forces. High forces result from sudden eccentric load on the tendon, such as landing from a jump. Ruptures result from poor conditioning, increased age, sudden activity level increases, or other risk factors such as changes in training surface, certain medications, or prior treatments for Achilles tendinitis.

It would seem that loss of gastrocnemius and soleus function with an Achilles tendon rupture would be obvious because these muscles are such an important part of generating plantar flexor strength. However, muscles such as the **tibialis posterior, flexor digitorum longus**, and **flexor hallucis longus** can still produce weak plantar flexion and allow the individual to walk, albeit with a limp. The ability of the client to plantar flex the foot, despite complete Achilles tendon rupture, may lead to misdiagnosis or delayed treatment.[83]

Previous chronic tendon degeneration increases the chance of ruptures. When *tendinosis, tendinitis,* or *paratendinitis* in the tendon are not properly addressed, a structural weakness develops. Once this weakness is present, the tendon is vulnerable to damage. Ruptures can occur in the **musculotendinous junction** or within the body of the tendon itself, but are seen regularly in the distal region of the tendon where the blood supply is poorest (Figure 5.41).[83]

In addition to various physical and activity factors, some medications are implicated as risk factors for producing tendon rupture, especially in the Achilles tendon. Achilles tendinitis has routinely been perceived as an inflammatory condition and has been treated with injection of **corticosteroids** as an anti-inflammatory agent. Corticosteroids are known to cause *collagen weakening* and have led to tendon ruptures.[82, 84, 85] Corticosteroids aren't the only group of medicines that may lead to Achilles tendon ruptures. The **fluoroquinolone** family of antibiotics appears to cause weakening in tendons whose function requires exposure to high force loads, such as the Achilles, patellar, and rotator cuff tendons. There is an established correlation between fluoroquinolones and Achilles tendon ruptures.[76, 77, 86]

Achilles tendon ruptures occur at any age, but present with greater frequency in 30–50 year-old men. As the client ages, tendon strength decreases while collagen degeneration matrix increases, resulting in less force being required to produce tendon rupture.

History
The client describes sudden onset of posterior calf or heel pain associated with difficulty in using the plantar flexor muscles. In some cases there is a loud popping sound at the time of injury. The client reports trouble walking and plantar flexing the foot. Plantar flexion may not be absent due to compensation by other muscles. If possible, identify the mechanics of movement that caused the injury. Usually there is forced eccentric dorsiflexion related to the onset of the injury. A rupture can also occur from a direct blunt trauma to the tendon. Ask about impact to the tendon at the time of injury. A thorough history should

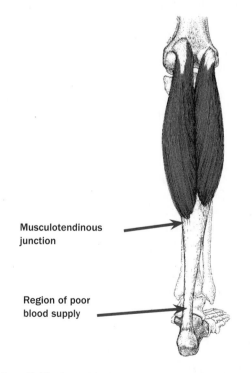

Musculotendinous junction

Region of poor blood supply

Figure 5.41 Posterior view of the right calf showing regions susceptible to Achilles tendon rupture. (3-D anatomy image courtesy of Primal Pictures Ltd. www.primalpictures.com.)

evaluate previous medications that may have precipitated the tendon rupture, in particular ask about anti-inflammatory medications or fluoroquinolone antibiotics.

Observation

As a result of complete rupture, the gastrocnemius and soleus may appear to bunch up toward their proximal ends. Depending on the location of the rupture, there may be bruising if enough capillary beds are disrupted. Because ruptures characteristically occur in the distal region of the tendon where blood supply is poor, bruising may not be evident. The client is likely to walk with a limp due to pain and loss of plantar flexor strength. Some calf swelling may be visible depending on the location of the rupture.

Palpation

An enlarged muscle mass may be palpable where the gastrocnemius has gathered toward its proximal end. There is also a palpable gap above the distal end of the tendon where it has detached. The calf muscles feel tight where they are bunched up toward their proximal ends.

Range-of-Motion and Resistance Testing

AROM: The client might be able to produce some active plantar flexion despite the total disruption of the gastrocnemius/soleus muscle-tendon unit, although the motion may not appear smooth and coordinated. If the tear still has fibers intact, performance of both plantar flexion and dorsiflexion produce pain. Weakness is evident, especially during plantar flexion.

PROM: With complete rupture, limitations in passive motion are rarely noticeable except passive dorsiflexion is normally increased in comparison to the unaffected side. If some fibers remain intact, passive dorsiflexion is painful as the tensile load pulls on the few remaining fibers at the tear site.

MRT: Weakness is evident with resisted plantar flexion and pain is produced if fibers are intact.

Special Test
Thompson Test

The client is prone on the treatment table. The practitioner grasps the calf muscles on each side near the musculotendinous junction and squeezes (Figure 5.42). If the gastrocnemius and soleus muscles have an intact connection with the Achilles tendon, the foot plantar flexes as the muscles are squeezed.

Explanation: Squeezing the calf muscles increases the tensile pulling force on the Achilles tendon. In an intact muscle-tendon unit, this force is sufficient to plantar flex the foot. If there is a rupture to the muscle-tendon unit, there is no plantar flexion of the foot.

Differential Evaluation

Achilles tendinosis, deep posterior compartment muscle strains, Achilles tendinitis, ankle fracture, ankle sprain,

gastrocnemius or soleus tear, plantaris tear.

Suggestions for Treatment

This condition usually requires surgery to reconnect the ruptured tendon and muscle fibers. Operative treatment is typically reserved for those individuals who have a greater chance for future rupture if the condition is not properly addressed. Those who are older, inactive, have systemic illnesses, or poor tissue integrity might not be good candidates for surgical treatment. Massage is helpful in the post-surgical phase to decrease tension of the muscle-tendon unit and improve the environment for optimum recovery. Massage treatment should be performed in consultation with the physician to determine when to initiate treatment and how much pressure the surgery site can withstand so that further damage is not caused.

ANTERIOR COMPARTMENT SYNDROME

Muscles in the extremities are contained within fascial compartments. *Anterior compartment syndrome* **results from intracompartmental pressure that increases due to muscular swelling**. When the muscles swell they compress other structures within the compartment causing neurovascular impairment. Compartment syndromes are not common, but one location where they do occur is the anterior compartment of the lower leg.[87] Although rare, compartment syndromes can also occur in the deep posterior compartment.[88]

Characteristics

The lower leg is divided into four compartments: the **deep posterior, superficial posterior, lateral**, and **anterior** (Figure 5.43). Each compartment is separated by strong fascial walls that run through its length, which are stiff and less pliable than the fascial tissues in other regions of the body.[89] The anterior compartment is bordered by the fascial walls, the tough interosseous membrane, and

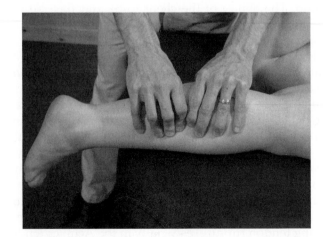

Figure 5.42 Thompson test.

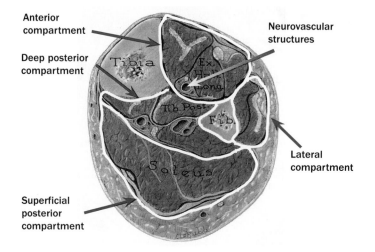

Anterior compartment

Deep posterior compartment

Superficial posterior compartment

Neurovascular structures

Lateral compartment

Figure 5.43 Cross-sectional view of the right leg showing the compartments. (Mediclip image copyright, 1998 Williams & Wilkins. All rights reserved.)

the tibia and fibula. The compartment contains the **tibialis anterior, extensor hallucis longus**, and **extensor digitorum longus** muscles, as well as the **deep peroneal nerve** and **anterior tibial artery and vein**.

Anterior compartment syndrome is more prevalent as a chronic condition and results from overuse, such as running on a hard surface or suddenly changing training intensity. This chronic form is often referred to as *exertional compartment syndrome (ECS)*. Repetitive stress of the lower leg causes the muscles to swell within the compartment. Because the walls of the compartment are stiff and unyielding, the expanding muscles are not allowed to enlarge appropriately. Pressure increases within the compartment as the muscles attempt to expand. This pressure compresses the **deep peroneal nerve** and/or the **arteries** and **veins** within the compartment. The client can experience pain, as well as symptoms of **nerve** or **vascular compression**.

In exertional compartment syndrome, symptoms will increase as the client engages in the aggravating activity. Once the activity is ceased, symptoms generally subside within about 30 minutes as pressure returns to normal. Exertional compartment syndrome is sometimes mistaken for *shin splints* and the reduction of symptoms when activity is ceased is one way to distinguish the two. Shin splint pain characteristically increases after the activity with **delayed onset soreness**.

Acute compartment syndromes can occur following a direct blow to the muscles of the lower leg, such as being kicked during a soccer game. Immediately after the blow, the muscles within the compartment swell in reaction to the impact trauma. One possible cause of acute compartment syndrome is **tibial fracture,** where bone fragments protrude into the compartment causing swelling.[87] High levels of lower leg activity can also produce an acute

compartment syndrome even in the absence of any direct trauma.[90]

An acute compartment syndrome is a serious disorder and needs immediate evaluation by a physician. Exertional compartment syndrome is not as dangerous as acute compartment syndromes because the increase in pressure is under the individual's control. Compartment syndromes are difficult to verify clinically and should be evaluated with an intracompartmental pressure reading.[91] Failure to recognize and treat this condition quickly may lead to permanent nerve or vascular damage and may even require limb amputation.

History

Clients with exertional compartment syndrome describe a repetitive activity performed on a regular basis. The client might also report sudden increase in activity levels that preceded the onset of symptoms. For example, chronic compartment syndromes often develop in military recruits when they begin basic training and drastically increase activity levels.[92] Neurological and vascular symptoms are similar to an acute compartment syndrome, but their severity depends on how much pressure develops within the compartment. Increases in pressure within the compartment, correspond with worse symptoms.

If the compartment syndrome is acute, the client reports a direct blow or other injury to the anterior leg. Pain and discomfort develop rapidly and may be accompanied by neurological or vascular symptoms. Neurological symptoms include paresthesia, numbness, or motor impairment. If there is motor impairment, it manifests as weakness in the dorsiflexor muscles causing a dysfunctional *drop-foot gait*. In drop-foot gait, the toes drag the ground during the swing-through phase, as if the individual was wearing shoes that were too long. The client may report symptoms such as coldness in the feet, pallor, or generalized aching pain from tissue ischemia.

Observation

Although compartment syndrome involves swollen muscles within the compartment, the swelling is unlikely to be visible because the compartmental walls prevent the muscles' expansion. Some color changes in the leg or foot may be evident due to vascular compression. In severe cases, weakness or atrophy in the dorsiflexors is apparent with gait changes such as the drop-foot gait.

Palpation

One of the most important indicators of either acute or chronic compartment syndrome is pain with palpation that is out of proportion to what would be expected with that level of pressure. Acute anterior compartment syndromes are tender to palpation in the entire region of the anterior compartment. Pain is strong and is felt throughout the muscles of the anterior compartment.

If the individual has ceased the activity several hours

prior to examination, chronic compartment syndromes may not be painful with palpation. For example, if the client last experienced symptoms during running the day before, there is unlikely to be any significant discomfort with palpation because the pressure has subsided during the intervening 24 hours. There could be general tenderness from muscular ischemia, nerve irritation, or irritation of the periosteum where the tibialis anterior attaches.

Range-of-Motion and Resistance Testing

AROM: In acute compartment syndrome, dorsiflexion or plantar flexion of the foot can cause pain if the condition is severe. If it is not severe, active movement does not cause discomfort. In a chronic compartment syndrome, the same is true if the motion is evaluated close to the time of irritation. If the range-of-motion evaluation is performed after compartmental pressure has subsided, pain and discomfort with active movement is not felt.

PROM: The same principles apply as for active motion.

MRT: If the compartment syndrome is severe, there might be pain with resisted dorsiflexion, but this is not characteristic. If compartmental pressures have impaired function of the nerve, weakness of the dorsiflexors may also be apparent.

Differential Evaluation

Anterior shin splints, stress fracture, proximal entrapment of peroneal nerve, proximal neuropathy, lumbar radiculopathy, circulatory disorder, strain to anterior compartment muscle(s), tenosynovitis, periostitis, proximal vascular entrapment, local tumors, medial tibial stress syndrome, and deep vein thrombosis.

Suggestions for Treatment

Conservative forms of treatment such as rest, activity modification, and stretching can be employed in an effort to treat compartment syndrome. Compartmental pressure has limited blood flow in the limb. Ice, compression, and elevation are contraindicated, especially in acute compartment syndromes, because they have detrimental effects on circulation and may increase the risk of tissue necrosis.

Activity modification, changing footwear, and using orthotics to address biomechanical problems may reduce aggravating factors of exertional compartment syndrome. Massage applications to the anterior leg are helpful for chronic compartment syndrome. Massage should not be performed immediately after activity when swelling is still present. Massage should also not be performed on an acute compartment syndrome.

In the event of an acute compartment syndrome, the client should be referred to a physician immediately. An emergency surgical procedure called a *fasciotomy* can be performed to relieve pressure on neurovascular structures. In this procedure, an incision is made in the fascial walls in order to allow the enlarged muscles to protrude.

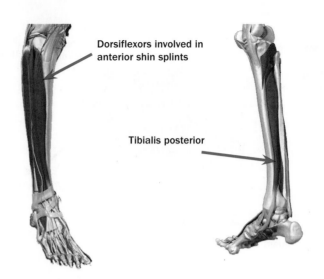

Dorsiflexors involved in anterior shin splints

Tibialis posterior

Figure 5.44 Primary muscles involved in anterior shin splints (A) and posterior shin splints (B). (3-D anatomy image courtesy of Primal Pictures Ltd. www.primalpictures.com.)

SHIN SPLINTS

Shin splints are an overuse condition producing chronic exertional shin pain in the leg.[93, 94] This condition is common among the athletic population, affecting dancers, runners, aerobics athletes, and others who engage in activities requiring repetitive loading of the lower extremity.

Characteristics

In the proximal anterior lateral region of the leg, the condition is called *anterior shin splints* and is attributed to overuse of the **dorsiflexor** muscles, such as the **tibialis anterior, extensor digitorum longus** and **extensor hallucis longus** (Figure 5.44). Overuse results from excessive eccentric loading on the dorsiflexors that might occur, for example, when walking or running downhill. Anterior shin splints are caused by **constant tensile stress on the tibial attachment of the involved muscles that produces irritation and inflammation in the periosteum**. For this reason, the problem is also called *periostitis*.[95] *Fascial tearing, ischemia, hypertonicity,* or *myofascial trigger points* can accompany anterior shin splints.

The condition is also seen regularly in the distal medial region of the leg, where it is called *posterior shin splints* or *medial tibial stress syndrome (MTSS)*. MTSS represents a stress reaction in the tibia due to chronic overloading and is typical in clients engaged in repetitive lower extremity activities, such as running, dancing, or jumping. In these activities, a strong tensile load is placed on the **tibialis posterior**, which is transferred to the muscle's attachment site along the tibial border (Figure 5.44). Constant tensile stress on the periosteum at the attachment site causes periostitis and can eventually lead to more serious conditions.

The **soleus** is another muscle that may have an important role in this condition.[96] This muscle's attachment sites are very close to those of the tibialis posterior. The majority of symptoms in MTSS are felt in the distal one-third of the tibia where both the tibialis posterior and soleus attach. There are conflicting viewpoints about how low the tibialis posterior attaches on the tibia and whether it contributes to MTSS pain.[97, 98]

Pes planus (flat feet), inadequate footwear, running on hard surfaces, or improper biomechanical function of the foot or leg, such as *overpronation,* may all be factors causing tibial stress. A forefoot running stride could be a primary factor in some cases of MTSS.[99] Landing on the forefoot places excessive tensile stress on the tibialis posterior muscle and other plantar flexors.

MTSS lies along a continuum of overuse conditions affecting the tibia and is frequently a precursor to *stress fractures* in the tibia.[94] The development of tibial stress is exacerbated by *hypertonicity* in the tibialis posterior or soleus muscles, which may cause a slight **bowing** of the tibia, eventually leading to stress fractures.[100] Consequently, stress fractures should always be considered a possible cause of pain for individuals suspected of having MTSS.

History

In either form of shin splints, the client reports a history of repetitive activity performed on a regular basis or a sudden increase in activity levels. With anterior shin splints, the activity preceding symptoms causes excessive loading (usually eccentric) on the dorsiflexor group, for example hiking down a long, steep slope. The client reports pain primarily in the proximal anterior lateral tibia near the upper margin of the tibialis anterior, during activity or after.

If MTSS is the primary concern, the client reports pain in the distal medial region of the tibia either during activity or after it has ceased. A runner with overpronation might acquire this form of the condition.

It is routine for the client with either anterior or medial shin splint pain in its early stages to report pain at the beginning of an activity that subsides as the activity progresses, with pain returning after the activity ceases. Pain may mimic delayed onset muscle soreness by coming on hours later. If the condition is a serious irritation of the periosteum or underlying bone, as in advanced cases of MTSS, pain is most prominent during activity when the tibia and the muscular attachment sites are stressed. Pain also occurs during normal activities or at rest.[94]

Observation

There are no specific visual findings for anterior or posterior shin splints, but other visual indicators should be considered. For example, flat feet or overpronation are often causes of MTSS. Evaluating the wear pattern on the bottom surface of the shoe may provide clues about foot mechanics. An increased wear pattern on the medial side of the shoe is indicative of overpronation.

Palpation

With anterior shin splints there is diffuse tenderness in the soft tissues of the proximal anterior compartment. Tenderness is exaggerated along the lateral tibia where the tibialis anterior tendon fibers pull on the periosteum. Pain from MTSS is felt with palpation in a diffuse area along the posterior medial border of the tibia regardless of whether this pain is originating from the soleus or tibialis posterior. Some thickening or fibrosis may also be palpable along the tibial border, which could result from the tibialis posterior or soleus attachment site.

Range-of-Motion and Resistance Testing

AROM: Active dorsiflexion or plantar flexion may cause pain with either type of shin splints, but for different reasons and in different locations. With anterior shin splints, pain may occur during contraction (dorsiflexion) or stretch (plantar flexion) of the affected muscles. If MTSS is present, pain might be felt in the posterior medial leg during contraction (plantar flexion) or stretch (dorsiflexion). In both conditions, the pain may not occur until either greater contraction forces (manual resistive test) or full stretching place enough tensile stress on the attachment sites of the affected muscles.

PROM: Passive plantar flexion may cause pain at the far end of motion with anterior shin splints, because the action stretches the dorsiflexors and pulls on the attachment sites. In MTSS, passive dorsiflexion may be painful as the tibialis posterior and soleus are stretched. In either case, passive shortening of the affected muscles is unlikely to produce pain.

MRT: Pain is felt in the proximal anterior leg with resisted dorsiflexion if anterior shin splints are present. With MTSS, pain may occur in the distal medial leg with resisted inversion or plantar flexion. Combining palpation with manual resistance may provide additional information about the affected tissues.

Box 5.5 Clinical Notes

Evaluating overuse shin pain

Two conditions that occur routinely in the athletic population are anterior shin splints and exertional anterior compartment syndrome. Both conditions produce pain on the anterior shin region and can be easily confused, but there are notable differences.

Compartment syndrome pain usually worsens as activity progresses and most of the pain is felt during activity. Anterior shin splint pain can occur as activity begins, but will frequently subside as activity progresses. Pain from shin splints is routinely most aggravated a day or so after activity has ceased.

Be careful to watch for signs of neurovascular compression that indicate the presence of a compartment syndrome, as the client should be referred to a physician for appropriate evaluation.

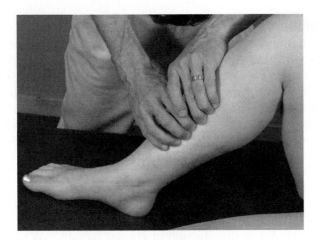

Figure 5.45 Tibialis posterior compression test.

Special Test
Tibialis Posterior Compression Test
This test identifies MTSS. The client is supine on the treatment table with the hip partially flexed and the knee flexed to about 90⁰, allowing the foot to rest flat on the table. Pressure is applied to the soft tissues along the posterior/medial border of the tibia (Figure 5.45). If pressure reproduces the pain experienced by the client, then MTSS is likely.

   Explanation: Pressure applied to the soft tissues in this region may reproduce pain as they pull on the irritated attachment sites. The soleus is easily accessible in this region, but the tibialis posterior is difficult to reach because it is in the deep posterior compartment and covered by other muscles. Pressure on the affected muscles increases pain from the irritated periosteum. Note that the actual attachment sites of the soleus and tibialis posterior can vary between individuals, so sometimes the pain is proximal and at other times more distal.

Differential Evaluation
Anterior compartment syndrome, stress fracture, proximal entrapment of peroneal nerve, proximal neuropathy, lumbar radiculopathy, circulatory disorder, strain to anterior compartment muscle(s), tenosynovitis, tendinitis, bone tumors.

Suggestions for Treatment
Both anterior and posterior shin splints are treated with conservative measures. Activity modification and rest normally allow this condition to subside without other intervention. Orthotics are frequently used to correct biomechanical deficiencies, especially in MTSS. Day-to-day activities of walking and movement may cause the condition to persist. In addition to modifying activities, massage applications can achieve very good results with both conditions. Massage techniques performed in conjunction with active and passive movements are especially helpful.

STRESS FRACTURE (LEG)

Repeated compressive loads on a bone may cause micro-failure of its intrinsic structure, producing a *stress fracture*. Stress fractures are normally due to a sudden increase in activity levels, such as starting a running program on hard pavement without proper conditioning. They are typically seen in the lower limbs, especially the tibia, as this structure must absorb the ground reaction force from activities like running or jumping (Figure 5.46).

Characteristics
In the leg, stress fractures affect the **tibia** because it is the **primary weight-bearing bone** in the lower leg, but they can occur in the **fibula** as well.[101] Soft tissues play an important role in absorbing impact forces from various activities, but ultimately these forces are transmitted to the skeletal structures. Without adequate mitigation, **repetitive loads lead to cumulative stress on the bone, causing small levels of damage or destruction and eventually failure**. The minor damage from repeated use may not be not detectable until it reaches a certain threshold; once the threshold is passed, structural failure ensues and a stress fracture results.[102]

   The impact of various activities on bones such as the tibia should not be underemphasized, especially if the activities are performed on an unyielding surface. For example, the ground reaction force may reach 12 times the body weight when landing from a jump.[102] Stress fractures occur in active individuals such as athletes, dancers, or military recruits due to the repetitive loading on lower extremities in their activities. Stress fractures routinely occur in clients with loss of bone mineral density. Even without vigorous activity, older persons are at greater risk for developing the condition. Women with the *female athlete triad* (amenorrhea, osteoporosis, and eating disorders) are also at higher risk due to loss of bone density.[94] If not properly treated, stress fractures can develop into more serious fractures and require longer rehabilitation.

   Overuse and fatigue of the lower extremity muscles reduce their shock-absorbing capacity, causing additional stress on the bones. Muscular overuse and structural disorders, such as *pes planus*, *leg length discrepancies*, or *overpronation* may be precipitating factors. Dietary, hormonal, or systemic factors may lead to loss of bone strength, and conditions such as *osteoporosis, calcium deficiency,* or *menstrual irregularities* may relate to condition onset.[102]

   Stress fractures are verified by high-tech diagnostic procedures and are not adequately evaluated with physical examination. If the practitioner suspects a stress fracture the client should be referred to a physician.

History
The client complains of pain localized to a small area on the bone that increases with activity and subsides with rest. The pain complaint begins shortly after a sudden

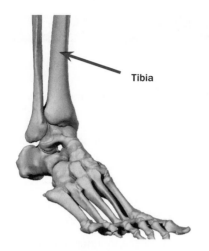

Tibia

Figure 5.46 Stress fractures in the leg are more common in the tibia as it is the primary weight-bearing bone in the lower leg. (3-D anatomy image courtesy of Primal Pictures Ltd. www.primalpictures.com.)

increase in activity level, such as initiating a new training regimen. If the condition progresses, the pain lingers for a longer period after each bout of activity has ceased. In advanced stress fractures the client may complain of night pain, due to painful bone remodeling. Ask about types of repetitive activities and evaluate for contributing disorders such as those listed above. Ask client if bone density has been tested or if they have bone loss issues.

Observation
There are no specific visual findings to indicate a stress fracture. Stress fractures are generally visible on a bone scan, but this is a high-tech diagnostic procedure that must be performed and evaluated by a physician. Visible postural distortions such as pes planus, leg length discrepancy, or overpronation may be indicators of unequal stress placed on the lower extremity.

Palpation
The client feels exaggerated point tenderness in a small localized area on the bone with palpation. The pain is directly on the bone as opposed to being in the surrounding soft tissues, as in shin splints.

Range-of-Motion and Resistance Testing
AROM: There are no specific findings in active motion unless the stress fracture is advanced and active muscle contraction or stretch pulls on an attachment site near the stress fracture.
PROM: There are no specific findings with passive motion unless muscle stretch pulls on a fracture site.
MRT: There are no specific findings unless the contraction of muscle pulls on a fracture site.

Special Test
Bone Percussion
Tapping strongly on the bone with the fingertips directly over the fracture site may reproduce pain from some

stress fractures. Placing a vibrating tuning fork on the bone may also reproduce the pain. However, these evaluations are not considered reliable.

Explanation: The vibration caused by the acoustic stimulus (tuning fork, tapping, etc.) travels along the bone and irritates the injury site thereby reproducing the client's pain.

Differential Evaluation
Anterior compartment syndrome, shin splints, proximal entrapment of peroneal nerve, proximal neuropathy, lumbar radiculopathy, strain to anterior compartment muscle(s), bone contusion, delayed onset muscle soreness, bone tumors.

Suggestions for Treatment
The most effective way to address stress fractures is through rest and activity modification. Some modalities, such as electrical stimulation, are used to speed the healing of fracture sites. Massage applications may be helpful in normalizing biomechanical stresses in the region of the stress fracture, but there is no evidence that massage directly affects the healing of a fracture. Clients with suspected stress fractures should be referred to a physician for proper evaluation.

GENERAL NEUROMUSCULAR DISORDERS

In many cases, soft-tissue dysfunctions are not given a specific name. Adequate assessment is required to determine the tissues most likely involved and to take into account pathologies that may or may not have specific titles. Chapter 4 provides a discussion of the pathological processes of hypertonicity, myofascial trigger points, muscle strains, nerve compression and tension, tendinosis, tenosynovitis, ligament sprains, and osteoarthritis in any region of the body. Chapter 4 also includes the history, observation, palpation, relevant tests, and treatment suggestions sections for these conditions. The principles are the same for these conditions wherever they occur in the body.

Included in this section are specific tables and graphics for the foot, ankle, and leg, including dermatomes, cutaneous innervation, trigger point referral patterns, and findings for MRTs. Sensory symptoms from a lumbar radiculopathy may be felt in the distal lower extremity and are experienced within the dermatome associated with that nerve root, see Figure 5.47. Sensory symptoms of peripheral neuropathy are felt in the region of cutaneous innervation for the nerve affected, see Figure 5.48. There are numerous locations in the distal lower extremity where peripheral neuropathies could occur; many are discussed as discrete conditions earlier in the chapter. Box 5.6 shows the other common locations where nerve compression might occur in the foot, ankle, and leg. Radiculopathies or peripheral neuropathies may cause motor dysfunction and produce weakness in the muscles innervated by the affected nerve (Box 5.7).

Neural tension tests affecting nerves in the lower extremity should only be considered adjunctive evaluation methods and not specific tests for lower extremity nerve pathology. A list of primary lower extremity motor nerves and the muscles they innervate is provided in Box 5.7. Table 1 provides a chart of muscles, their resisted actions, and potentially affected nerves or nerve roots.

Muscular hypertonicity occurs in the distal lower extremity as a result of overload such as repetitive motion stress or trauma. Common myofascial trigger point referral patterns for the major muscles in this region are shown in Figure 5.49.

Box 5.6 Regions of Possible Nerve Entrapment

Peroneal nerve
  Near the fibular head
  Within the anterior compartment in the leg

Sural nerve
  In the superficial posterior compartment

Tibial nerve
  Within the deep posterior compartment of the leg
  At the tarsal tunnel

Medial and/or lateral plantar nerves
  Passing between the metatarsal heads, underneath
  the transverse metatarsal ligaments

Table 1 Weakness with Manual Resistive Test and Possible Nerve Involvement

Muscle	Resisted Action	Possible Nerve Involvement if Action Weak
Extensor digitorum brevis	Extension of toes (resist proximal phalanx)	Deep peroneal nerve (L5, S1)
Extensor digitorum longus	Extension of toes (resist distal phalanx)	Deep peroneal nerve (L4, L5, S1)
Extensor hallucis longus	Extension of hallux (resist distal phalanx)	Deep peroneal nerve (L4, L5, S1)
Flexor digitorum brevis	Flexion of toes (resist proximal phalanx)	Medial plantar nerve (L4, L5)
Flexor digitorum longus	Flexion of toes (resist distal phalanx)	Tibial nerve (L5, S1)
Flexor hallucis brevis	Flexion of hallux (resist proximal phalanx)	Medial plantar nerve (L4, L5, S1)
Flexor hallucis longus	Flexion of hallux (resist distal phalanx)	Tibial nerve (L5, S1, S2)
Gastrocnemius	Plantar flexion with knee extended	Tibial nerve (S1, S2)
Peroneus brevis	Foot eversion	Superficial peroneal nerve (L4, L5, S1)
Peroneus longus	Foot eversion	Superficial peroneal nerve (L4, L5, S1)
Plantaris	Plantar flexion	Tibial nerve (L4, L5, S1)
Soleus	Plantar flexion with knee partially flexed	Tibial nerve (S1, S2)
Tibialis anterior	Dorsiflexion	Deep peroneal nerve (L4, L5, S1)
Tibialis posterior	Foot inversion	Tibial nerve (L5, S1)

Table 2 Joints, Associated Motions, Planes of Motion in Anatomical Position, Axis of Rotation, and Average ROM

Joint	Motion	Plane of Motion	Axis of Rotation	Avg. ROM (degrees)
Ankle (talocrural)	Dorsiflexion	Sagittal	Medial-lateral	20-30
	Plantar flexion	Sagittal	Medial-lateral	30-50
Ankle (subtalar)	Inversion	Frontal	Anterior-posterior	20
	Eversion	Frontal	Anterior-posterior	15
Toes	Flexion	Sagittal	Medial-lateral	30-40
	Extension	Sagittal	Medial-lateral	50-60

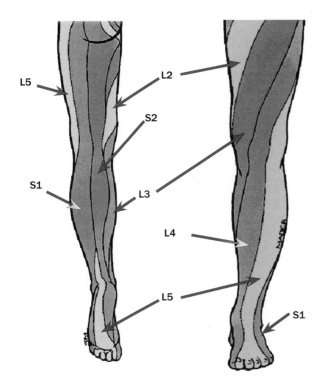

Figure 5.47 Dermatomes of the lower extremity (Mediclip image copyright, 1998 Williams & Wilkins. All rights reserved.)

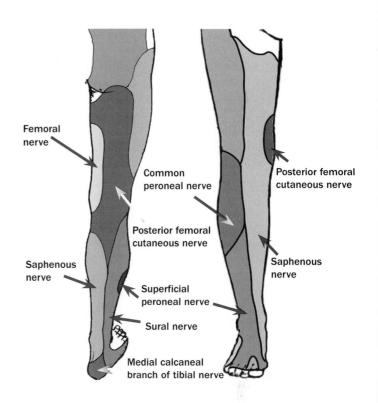

Figure 5.48 Cutaneous innervation of the distal lower extremity.

Box 5.7 Innervation of Distal Lower Extremity Muscles

Tibial Nerve	Lateral Plantar Nerve	Superficial Peroneal Nerve
Gastrocnemius	Quadratus plantae	Peroneus longus
Plantaris	Abductor digiti minimi	Peroneus brevis
Popliteus	Lumbricales	
Soleus	Adductor hallucis	Deep Peroneal Nerve
Tibialis posterior	Dorsal interossei	Tibialis anterior
Flexor digitorum longus	Plantar interossei	Extensor hallucis longus
Flexor hallucis longus	Flexor digiti minimi brevis	Extensor digitorum longus
		Extensor digitorum brevis
	Medial Plantar Nerve	Peroneus tertius
	Lumbrical, 1st	Dorsal interosseous, 2nd
	Abductor hallucis	
	Flexor hallucis brevis	
	Flexor digitorum brevis	

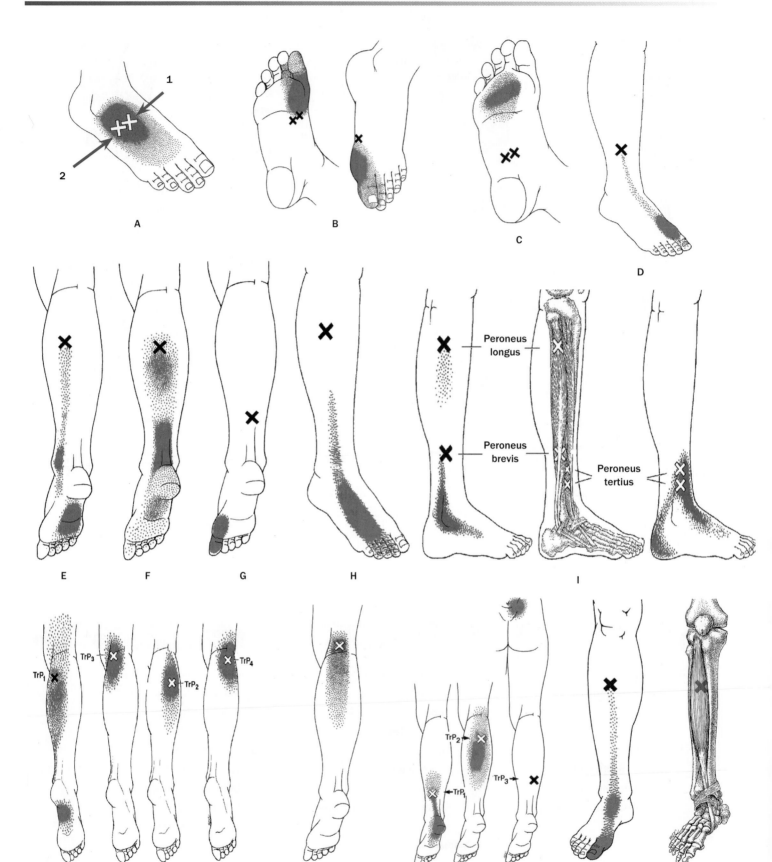

Figure 5.49 Myofascial trigger point referral patterns: Extensor hallucis brevis (A1), Extensor digitorum brevis (A2), Flexor hallucis brevis (B), Flexor digitorum brevis (C), Extensor hallucis longus (D), Flexor digitorum longus (E), Tibialis posterior (F), Flexor hallucis longus (G), Extensor digitorum longus (H), Peroneus brevis, longus, & tertius (I), Gastrocnemius (J), Plantaris (K), Soleus (L), Tibialis anterior (M) (Images courtesy of Mediclip, copyright 1998 Williams & Wilkins. All rights reserved).

Reference Table for Condition Assessment

This table lists a number of pathological conditions along the left-hand column. The top of the table lists common evaluation procedures. A ◆ in the box associated with a pathological condition and an evaluation procedure indicates that the procedure is commonly used to identify that pathology. A ● in the box associated with the condition and a range-of-motion or resistance test, indicates that pain is likely with that test for that pathology. Conditions are listed alphabetically.

TABLE 3 REFERENCE TABLE FOR CONDITION ASSESSMENT

	AROM	PROM	MRT	Achilles tendon pinch test	Ankle drawer test	Bone percussion	Dorsiflexion-eversion test	External rotation stress test	Interdigital squeeze test	Morton's test	Squeeze test	Talar tilt test	Thompson test	Tibialis posterior compression test	Tinel's sign
Achilles Tendon Disorder	●	●	●	◆											
Achilles Tendon Rupture	●		●										◆		
Anterior Compartment Syndrome	●	●	●												
Anterior Shin Splints	●	●	●												
Lateral Ankle Sprain	●	●	●		◆							◆			
Medial Ankle Sprain	●	●	●												
Morton's Neuroma	●	●							◆	◆					
Muscle Strains	●	●	●												
Muscular Hypertonicity	●	●													
Nerve Compression & Tension	●	●													◆
Plantar Fasciitis	●	●	●												
Posterior Shin Splints	●	●	●											◆	
Retrocalcaneal Bursitis															
Stress Fracture (Foot)						◆									
Stress Fracture (Leg)						◆									
Syndesmosis Sprain	●	●						◆			◆				
Tarsal Tunnel Syndrome	●	●					◆								◆

References

1. Clarke TE, Frederick EC, Cooper LB. Effects of shoe cushioning upon ground reaction forces in running. Int J Sports Med. Nov 1983;4(4):247-251.
2. Dixon SJ, Collop AC, Batt ME. Surface effects on ground reaction forces and lower extremity kinematics in running. Med Sci Sports Exerc. Nov 2000;32(11):1919-1926.
3. Snow RE, Williams KR. High heeled shoes: their effect on center of mass position, posture, three-dimensional kinematics, rearfoot motion, and ground reaction forces. Arch Phys Med Rehabil. 1994;75(5):568-576.
4. Hockenbury R, Sammarco G. Evaluation and treatment of ankle sprains. Physician Sportsmed. 2001;29(2).
5. Neumann DA. Kinesiology of the Musculoskeletal System. St. Louis: Mosby; 2002.
6. Stovitz SD, Coetzee C. Hyperpronation and foot pain. Physician Sportsmed. 2004;32(8).
7. Richardson J, Iglarsh ZA. Clinical Orthopaedic Physical Therapy. Philadelphia: W.B. Saunders; 1994.
8. Nordin Ma, Frankel V. Basic Biomechanics of the Musculoskeletal System. 3rd ed. Baltimore: Lippincott Williams & Wilkins; 2001.
9. Deland JT. The adult acquired flatfoot and spring ligament complex. Pathology and implications for treatment. Foot Ankle Clin. Mar 2001;6(1):129-135, vii.
10. Riddle DL. Foot and Ankle. In: Richardson JK, Iglarsh ZA, eds. Clinical Orthopaedic Physical Therapy. Philadelphia: W.B. Saunders; 1994.
11. Alexander IJ, Johnson KA. Assessment and management of pes cavus in Charcot-Marie-tooth disease. Clin Orthop Relat Res. Sep 1989(246):273-281.
12. Turner N. Pes Cavus. eMedicine. March 18. Available at: www.emedicine.com. Accessed March 23, 2005.
13. Travell J, Simons, D. Myofascial Pain and Dysfunction: The Trigger Point Manual. Vol 2. Baltimore: Williams & Wilkins; 1992.
14. Thomas S, and Barrington, R. Hallux valgus. Current Orthopedics. 2003;17:299-307.
15. Frank CJ, Robinson DE. Hallux Valgus. eMedicine. March 16. Available at: www.emedicine.com. Accessed March 25, 2005.
16. Glasoe WM, Allen MK, Saltzman CL. First ray dorsal mobility in relation to hallux valgus deformity and first intermetatarsal angle. Foot Ankle Int. Feb 2001;22(2):98-101.
17. Thomas C. Taber's Cyclopedic Medical Dictionary. 15th ed. Philadelphia: F.A. Davis Company; 1987.
18. Watson A. Hammertoe Deformity. eMedicine. April 21, 2004. Available at:www.emedicine.com.

Accessed March 21, 2005.
19. Garrick JG, Requa RK. The epidemiology of foot and ankle injuries in sports. Clin Sports Med. 1988;7(1):29-36.
20. Liu SH, Jason WJ. Lateral ankle sprains and instability problems. Clin Sports Med. 1994;13(4):793-809.
21. Thacker SB, Stroup DF, Branche CM, Gilchrist J, Goodman RA, Weitman EA. The prevention of ankle sprains in sports. A systematic review of the literature. Am J Sports Med. Nov-Dec 1999;27(6):753-760.
22. Norkin C, Levangie P. Joint Structure and Function. Philadelphia: F.A. Davis; 1983.
23. Baker CL, Brooks AA. Ankle Sprain: Operative Management. In: Torg JS, Shephard RJ, eds. Current Therapy in Sports Medicine. 3rd ed. St. Louis: Mosby; 1995:253-258.
24. Safran MR, Zachazewski JE, Benedetti RS, Bartolozzi AR, 3rd, Mandelbaum R. Lateral ankle sprains: a comprehensive review part 2: treatment and rehabilitation with an emphasis on the athlete. Med Sci Sports Exerc. Jul 1999;31(7 Suppl):S438-447.
25. Vegso JJ. Ankle Sprain: Nonoperative Management. In: Torg JS, Shephard RJ, eds. Current Therapy in Sports Medicine. 3rd ed. St. Louis: Mosby; 1995:244-248.
26. Weintraub W. Tendon and Ligament Healing. Berkeley: North Atlantic Books; 1999.
27. Smith AH, Bach BR. High ankle sprains. Physician Sportsmed. 2004;32(12).
28. Nussbaum ED, Hosea TM, Sieler SD, Incremona BR, Kessler DE. Prospective evaluation of syndesmotic ankle sprains without diastasis. Am J Sports Med. Jan-Feb 2001;29(1):31-35.
29. Teitz CC, Harrington RM. A biochemical analysis of the squeeze test for sprains of the syndesmotic ligaments of the ankle. Foot Ankle Int. Jul 1998;19(7):489-492.
30. Boytim MJ, Fischer DA, Neumann L. Syndesmotic ankle sprains. Am J Sports Med. May-Jun 1991;19(3):294-298.
31. Dawson D, Hallett M, Wilbourn A. Entrapment Neuropathies. 3rd ed. Philadelphia: Lippincott-Raven; 1999.
32. Wu KK. Morton's interdigital neuroma: a clinical review of its etiology, treatment, and results. J Foot Ankle Surg. 1996;35(2):112-119; discussion 187-118.
33. Alexander IJ, Johnson KA, Parr JW. Morton's neuroma: a review of recent concepts. Orthopedics. Jan 1987;10(1):103-106.
34. Glazer J, Bruckner P. Plantar fasciitis. Physician Sportsmed. 2004;32(11).
35. Huang CK, Kitaoka HB, An KN, Chao EY. Biomechanical evaluation of longitudinal arch

stability. Foot Ankle. Jul-Aug 1993;14(6):353-357.

36. Cavanagh PR, Lafortune MA. Ground reaction forces in distance running. J Biomech. 1980;13(5):397-406.

37. Fuller EA. The windlass mechanism of the foot. A mechanical model to explain pathology. J Am Podiatr Med Assoc. 2000;90(1):35-46.

38. Prichasuk S, Subhadrabandhu T. The relationship of pes planus and calcaneal spur to plantar heel pain. Clin Orthop Relat Res. Sep 1994(306):192-196.

39. Gill LH. Plantar Fasciitis: Diagnosis and Conservative Management. J Am Acad Orthop Surg. 1997;5(2):109-117.

40. Lemont H, Ammirati KM, Usen N. Plantar fasciitis: a degenerative process (fasciosis) without inflammation. J Am Podiatr Med Assoc. 2003;93(3):234-237.

41. Kwong PK, Kay D, Voner RT, White MW. Plantar fasciitis. Mechanics and pathomechanics of treatment. Clin Sports Med. 1988;7(1):119-126.

42. Kaufman KR, Brodine S, Shaffer R. Military training-related injuries: surveillance, research, and prevention. Am J Prev Med. 2000;18(3 Suppl):54-63.

43. Young CC. Plantar Fasciitis. eMedicine. May 6, 2002. Available at: www.emedicine.com Accessed March 28, 2005.

44. Batt ME, Tanji JL, Skattum N. Plantar fasciitis: a prospective randomized clinical trial of the tension night splint. Clin J Sport Med. 1996;6(3):158-162.

45. Wapner KL, Sharkey PF. The use of night splints for treatment of recalcitrant plantar fasciitis. Foot Ankle. 1991;12(3):135-137.

46. Brukner P, Bradshaw C, Khan KM, White S, Crossley K. Stress fractures: a review of 180 cases. Clin J Sport Med. Apr 1996;6(2):85-89.

47. Armstrong DW, 3rd, Rue JP, Wilckens JH, Frassica FJ. Stress fracture injury in young military men and women. Bone. Sep 2004;35(3):806-816.

48. Bennell KL, Malcolm SA, Thomas SA, Wark JD, Brukner PD. The incidence and distribution of stress fractures in competitive track and field athletes. A twelve-month prospective study. Am J Sports Med. Mar-Apr 1996;24(2):211-217.

49. Brukner P, Bradshaw C, Bennell K. Managing common stress fractures: let risk level guide treatment. Physician Sportsmed. 1998;26(8).

50. Cameron MH. Physical Agents in Rehabilitation. Philadelphia: W.B. Saunders; 1999.

51. DeLisa JA, Saeed MA. The tarsal tunnel syndrome. Muscle Nerve. Nov-Dec 1983;6(9):664-670.

52. Butler D. Mobilisation of the Nervous System. London: Churchill Livingstone; 1991.

53. Nagaoka M, Satou K. Tarsal tunnel syndrome caused by ganglia. J Bone Joint Surg Br. 1999;81(4):607-610.

54. Boc SF, Hatef J. Space-occupying lesions as a cause of tarsal tunnel syndrome. J Am Podiatr Med Assoc.

1995;85(11):713-715.

55. Lau JT, Daniels TR. Tarsal tunnel syndrome: a review of the literature. Foot Ankle Int. Mar 1999;20(3):201-209.

56. Jackson DL, Haglund BL. Tarsal tunnel syndrome in runners. Sports Med. 1992;13(2):146-149.

57. Upton AR, McComas AJ. The double crush in nerve entrapment syndromes. Lancet. Aug 18 1973;2(7825):359-362.

58. Walker R. Diabetes and peripheral neuropathy: keeping people on their own two feet. Br J Community Nurs. Jan 2005;10(1):33-36.

59. Kinoshita M, Okuda R, Morikawa J, Jotoku T, Abe M. The dorsiflexion-eversion test for diagnosis of tarsal tunnel syndrome. J Bone Joint Surg Am. Dec 2001;83-A(12):1835-1839.

60. Sammarco GJ. Soft Tissue Injuries. In: Torg JS, Shephard RJ, eds. Current Therapy in Sports Medicine. 3rd. ed. St. Louis: Mosby; 1995:388-398.

61. Stephens MM. Haglund's deformity and retrocalcaneal bursitis. Orthop Clin North Am. 1994;25(1):41-46.

62. Foye P, Stitik TP. Retrocalcaneal bursitis. eMedicine. July 12, 2004. Available at: www.emedicine.com. Accessed April 4, 2005.

63. Sella EJ, Caminear DS, McLarney EA. Haglund's syndrome. J Foot Ankle Surg. Mar-Apr 1998;37(2):110-114; discussion 173.

64. Haglund-Akerlind Y, Eriksson E. Range of motion, muscle torque and training habits in runners with and without Achilles tendon problems. Knee Surg Sports Traumatol Arthrosc. 1993;1(3-4):195-199.

65. McCrory JL, Martin DF, Lowery RB, et al. Etiologic factors associated with Achilles tendinitis in runners. Med Sci Sports Exerc. 1999;31(10):1374-1381.

66. Ahmed IM, Lagopoulos M, McConnell P, Soames RW, Sefton GK. Blood supply of the Achilles tendon. J Orthop Res. Sep 1998;16(5):591-596.

67. Carr AJ, Norris SH. The blood supply of the calcaneal tendon. J Bone Joint Surg Br. Jan 1989;71(1):100-101.

68. Kraushaar BS, Nirschl RP. Tendinosis of the elbow (tennis elbow). Clinical features and findings of histological, immunohistochemical, and electron microscopy studies. J Bone Joint Surg Am. 1999;81(2):259-278.

69. Almekinders LC, Temple JD. Etiology, Diagnosis, and Treatment of Tendinitis - An Analysis of the Literature. Med Sci Sport Exercise. 1998;30(8):1183-1190.

70. Khan KM, Cook JL, Bonar F, Harcourt P, Astrom M. Histopathology of common tendinopathies - Update and implications for clinical management. Sport Med. 1999;27(6):393-408.

71. Torstensen ET, Bray RC, Wiley JP. Patellar Tendinitis: A Review of Current Concepts and

Treatment. Clin J Sport Med. 1994;4(2):77-82.

72. Lin D, Marano H. Achilles tendonitis. eMedicine. July 12, 2004. Available at: www.emedicine.com. Accessed April 4, 2005.

73. Clancy WG, Jr., Neidhart D, Brand RL. Achilles tendonitis in runners: a report of five cases. Am J Sports Med. Mar-Apr 1976;4(2):46-57.

74. Khan KM, Cook JL, Taunton JE, Bonar F. Overuse tendinosis, not tendinitis - Part 1: A new paradigm for a difficult clinical problem. Physician Sportsmed. 2000;28(5):38+.

75. Corrigan B, Maitland GD. Musculoskeletal and Sports Injuries. Oxford: Butterworth Heinemann; 1994.

76. Huston KA. Achilles tendinitis and tendon rupture due to fluoroquinolone antibiotics. N Engl J Med. 1994;331(11):748.

77. Harrell RM. Fluoroquinolone-induced tendinopathy: what do we know? South Med J. 1999;92(6):622-625.

78. Williams RJ, III, Attia E, Wickiewicz TL, Hannafin JA. The effect of ciprofloxacin on tendon, paratenon, and capsular fibroblast metabolism. Am J Sports Med. May-Jun 2000;28(3):364-369.

79. Matsumoto K, Hukuda S, Nishioka J, Asajima S. Rupture of the Achilles tendon in rheumatoid arthritis with histologic evidence of enthesitis. A case report. Clin Orthop Relat Res. Jul 1992(280):235-240.

80. Lesic A, Bumbasirevic M. Disorders of the Achilles tendon. Current Orthopedics. 2004;18:63-75.

81. Clement DB, Taunton JE, Smart GW. Achilles tendinitis and peritendinitis: etiology and treatment. Am J Sports Med. 1984;12(3):179-184.

82. Shrier I, Matheson GO, Kohl HW, 3rd. Achilles tendonitis: are corticosteroid injections useful or harmful? Clin J Sport Med. 1996;6(4):245-250.

83. Lin D. Achilles tendon rupture. eMedicine. January 21, 2005. Available at: www.emedicine.com Accessed April 4, 2005.

84. Fredberg U. Local Corticosteroid Injection in Sport - Review of Literature and Guidelines for Treatment. Scand J Med Sci Sports. 1997;7(3):131-139.

85. Fadale PD, Wiggins ME. Corticosteroid Injections: Their Use and Abuse. J Am Acad Orthop Surg. 1994;2(3):133-140.

86. McGarvey WC, Singh D, Trevino SG. Partial Achilles tendon ruptures associated with fluoroquinolone antibiotics: a case report and literature review. Foot Ankle Int. 1996;17(8):496-498.

87. Korkola M. Exercise-induced leg pain. Physician Sportsmed. 2001;29(6).

88. Abdelkarim B. Compartment syndromes. eMedicine. December 22, 2003. Available at: www.emedicine.com. Accessed April 8, 2005.

89. Edwards P, Myerson MS. Exertional compartment syndrome of the leg. Physician Sportsmed. 1996;24(4).

90. Fehlandt A, Jr., Micheli L. Acute exertional anterior compartment syndrome in an adolescent female. Med Sci Sports Exerc. Jan 1995;27(1):3-7.

91. Fraipont MJ, Adamson GJ. Chronic exertional compartment syndrome. J Am Acad Orthop Surg. Jul-Aug 2003;11(4):268-276.

92. Almeida SA, Williams KM, Shaffer RA, Brodine SK. Epidemiological patterns of musculoskeletal injuries and physical training. Med Sci Sports Exerc. 1999;31(8):1176-1182.

93. Bates P. Shin splints--a literature review. Br J Sports Med. Sep 1985;19(3):132-137.

94. Couture CJ, Karlson KA. Tibial stress injuries. Physician Sportsmed. 2002;30(6).

95. Batt ME. Shin splints--a review of terminology. Clin J Sport Med. 1995;5(1):53-57.

96. Michael RH, Holder LE. The soleus syndrome. A cause of medial tibial stress (shin splints). Am J Sports Med. 1985;13(2):87-94.

97. Beck BR, Osternig LR. Medial tibial stress syndrome. The location of muscles in the leg in relation to symptoms. J Bone Joint Surg Am. 1994;76(7):1057-1061.

98. Saxena A, O'Brien T, Bunce D. Anatomic dissection of the tibialis posterior muscle and its correlation to medial tibial stress syndrome. J Foot Surg. 1990;29(2):105-108.

99. Cibulka MT, Sinacore DR, Mueller MJ. Shin splints and forefoot contact running: a case report. J Orthop Sports Phys Ther. 1994;20(2):98-102.

100. Panjabi M, White A. Biomechanics in the Musculoskeletal System. New York: Churchill Livingstone; 2001.

101. Bennell KL, Brukner PD. Epidemiology and site specificity of stress fractures. Clin Sports Med. Apr 1997;16(2):179-196.

102. Reeser JC. Stress Fracture. eMedicine. October 1, 2004. Available at: www.emedicine.com. Accessed April 9, 2005.

6 Knee and Thigh

The knee plays a critical role in shock absorption and locomotion, which requires it to withstand the strong contraction forces from the quadriceps and hamstring muscles. The knee is composed of two primary articulations: the **tibiofemoral** and the **patellofemoral** joints. An overemphasis on structural pathologies has led to a lack of attention to soft-tissue disorders of the knee, although the latter make up a significant proportion of the conditions affecting the knee.

The structure and mechanics of the tibiofemoral joint are investigated more than any other joint in the body.[1] The tibiofemoral is the largest joint in the body and is particularly susceptible to traumatic injury because it bears weight and is located at the end of two long levers.[2] The joint's rounded **femoral condyles** articulate with the relatively flat **tibial plateau** making a skeletally unstable articulation. The **lateral and medial menisci,** the multiple stabilizing ligaments, and muscles are all necessary for adequate stability in the knee. Due to the crucial role of these soft tissues, their evaluation is an important part of knee assessment.

Dysfunction in patellofemoral mechanics can also play a role in knee disorders. The patella improves the mechanical advantage of the quadriceps allowing greater force production during knee extension, which is essential during activities such as running or climbing stairs.

Pain and injury in the knee is due to a number of causes and various structural or postural problems can predispose an individual to knee pathology. It is possible for pain to be referred to the knee from conditions located in other regions. Soft-tissue pathology in the thigh or hip joint can also mimic knee pathology.[2]

Movements and Motion Testing

SINGLE-PLANE MOVEMENTS

There are two single-plane movements in the knee that are clinically measured: flexion and extension. When flexed, the knee is also capable of a small amount of medial and lateral rotation, but this movement is not measured during routine evaluation. In this text, movement past full extension or anatomical position is considered hyperextension. The associated motions, planes, axes of rotation, and range-of-motion values for the knee are listed in Table 1 at the end of the chapter.

Knee

In the knee, **flexion** and **extension** occur in the **sagittal plane** at the **tibiofemoral joint** (Figure 6.1). Flexion is the motion of bending the knee, bringing the lower leg toward the posterior thigh. Extension is the return to anatomical position; hyperextension is motion past full extension (anatomical position). Average range of motion is about 135^0 for knee flexion. Laxity of knee ligaments allows the knee to move into about 10^0 of hyperextension in some cases, which is within normal limits. Hyperextension of the knee in a standing position is called *genu recurvatum* and is discussed later in the chapter.

Capsular patterns

It is important to consider the role of the joint capsule when assessing joint function. Pathological problems in the capsule, such as fibrosis, may be visible with the joint's capsular pattern. The capsular pattern is a pattern of movement restriction that is characteristic to each individual joint. It is present in both active and passive motion. Capsular patterns are represented by a sequential listing of the movements from most likely to least likely limited. See the description of the knee's capsular pattern in Box 6.1.

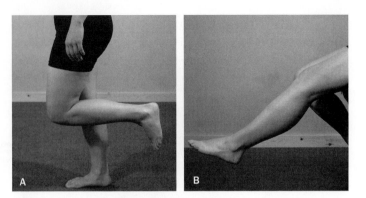

Figure 6.1 Knee flexion (A) and extension (B).

> ### Box 6.1 Capsular Pattern for the Knee
>
> Tibiofemoral (Knee) Joint
>   Flexion is more limited than extension
>   There is no limitation to rotational movements

> ### Box 6.2 Joint, Associated Motion, & End Feel
>
> Tibiofemoral (Knee) Joint
>   Flexion   Soft-tissue approximation
>   Tissue stretch
>   Extension   Tissue stretch (firm)

RANGE-OF-MOTION & RESISTIVE TESTS

Results from single-plane movement analysis form the basis for further evaluation procedures. Movement testing should be performed in a certain order, allowing for an efficient evaluation and the least amount of accumulated discomfort or pain to develop. It is also general practice to leave movements known or expected to be painful to the end of the evaluation. When possible, the pain-free side is evaluated first.

Active range-of-motion (AROM) movements are performed first to establish the client's movement abilities and pain symptoms. Passive range of motion (PROM) is performed next and manual resistive tests (MRT) follow. AROM results may make PROM assessment procedures unnecessary. If no pain occurs with active movement, pain is unlikely with passive movement. The practitioner should be familiar with the full step-by-step instructions and guidelines for how to interpret (ROM) and resistive test results explained in Chapter 3.

Active Range of Motion

Active knee flexion and extension are usually evaluated with the client in a standing position. When performing AROM evaluations, take into consideration the position of the limb to ensure the target tissues are engaged. For example, when the client actively flexes the knee by lifting the leg toward the posterior thigh, the knee flexors are engaged concentrically. When the leg returns to anatomical position it is not the knee extensors that are responsible for the action, but the knee flexors as they employ an eccentric contraction. Engaging the knee extensors requires a change in body position or in the way resistance of gravity affects the movement.

Pain with active movement indicates problems in either the contractile or inert tissues associated with that movement. Factors prematurely limiting active movement in this region include ligamentous or capsular damage, muscle contractures, pain from nerve compression or tension, tendinosis, tenosynovitis, fibrous cysts, or joint disorders such as arthritis.

Compare AROM test results with those from PROM and manual resistive tests to identify possible reasons for movement restriction. The muscles used to perform actions of the knee and thigh are listed in Box 6.3. Note that other muscles can contribute to the motion and subsequent dysfunction.

Passive Range of Motion

Passive motion is performed after active. Pain during passive movement predominantly implicates inert tissues. However, muscles and tendons that contract in the opposite direction are stretched at the end range of passive movement.

PROM testing also evaluates end feel. Box 6.2 lists the primary joint locations and their normal end feel. Review Chapter 3 for a discussion of normal and pathological end feel descriptions. Factors that could prematurely limit passive movement are the same as for active movement.

Manual Resistive Tests

A manual resistive test (MRT) produces pain when there is a mechanical disruption of tissue. Pain with an MRT indicates that one or more of the muscles and/or tendons performing that action are involved. Testing all of a muscle's actions is not necessary, as a muscle's secondary actions recruit other muscles and make the test results less accurate. Palpation elicits more information if the test alone does not produce pain or discomfort. Refer to Box 6.3 for the list of primary muscles involved with each action. Table 1 at the end of the chapter lists actions commonly used for testing muscles in the knee.

In some cases weakness is evident with MRTs. Factors that produce weakness include *lack of use, fatigue, reflex muscular inhibition*, and possibly a neurological pathology (*radiculopathy, peripheral neuropathy*, or a *systemic neurological disorder*). The nerves or nerve roots that may be involved are listed in Table 2 at the end of the chapter.

Knee

RESISTED FLEXION

The client is prone on the table with the knee flexed a little less than 90⁰. The client holds this position while the practitioner attempts to extend the knee by pressing the leg toward the table (Figure 6.2). This test can be performed in varying degrees of knee flexion, but once knee flexion is past 90⁰ there is a strong chance of producing a cramp in the hamstring muscles when resistance is engaged. It is best to perform the resistance with less than 90⁰ of knee flexion.

RESISTED EXTENSION

The client is seated on the end of the treatment table with the knee in about 45⁰ of flexion. The practitioner places a hand on the client's distal tibia. The client is instructed to hold this position as the practitioner applies pressure to the tibia, attempting to flex the client's knee (Figure 6.2).

GENERAL INSTRUCTIONS FOR ROM & RESISTIVE TESTS

Overall
- Determine motions possible at the joint to be tested.
- Select the motion to be evaluated.
- Determine the tissues involved in the motion.
- Leave motions expected to be painful to the last.
- Test the uninvolved side first.
- Ask about, note any reported pain or discomfort.

AROM
- Demonstrate the movement to be performed.
- Have the client perform the movement.

PROM
- Establish the joint's normal end feel.
- Have the client relax as much as possible.
- Use gentle and slow movements.

MRT
- Test one action at a time.
- Position should isolate the action/ muscles involved.
- If pain is suspected, start in a mid-range position.
- Client uses a strong, but appropriate amount of effort.

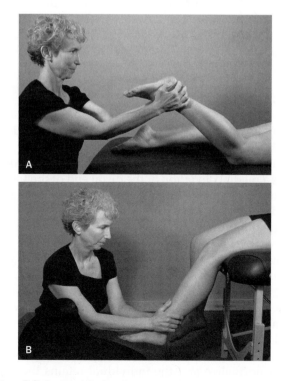

Figure 6.2 Resisted flexion (A) and extension (B).

Box 6.3 Muscle Actions of the Knee & Thigh

Knee	Flexion	Extension
	Semimembranosus	Rectus femoris
	Semitendinosus	Vastus lateralis
	Biceps femoris	Vastus intermedius
	Gracilis	Vastus medialis
	Sartorius	Tensor fasciae latae*
	Gastrocnemius	
	Plantaris	
	Tensor fasciae latae*	

*After 30^0 of knee flexion, acts through the iliotibial band

*Only near end of knee extension, acts through the iliotibial band

---

Structural and Postural Deviations

The following section covers structural or postural deviations unique to the knee and thigh. Under each condition there is a brief description of its characteristics followed by likely HOPRS findings. If applicable, orthopedic tests are included in the special tests section. If there is no special orthopedic test listed for that condition, evaluation should focus on other portions of the assessment process, such as range-of-motion testing.

GENU VALGUM

Genu valgum is also called *tibial valgus* or *knock-knees*. The condition appears concurrently with other structural dysfunctions, such as overpronation. The dysfunctional mechanics in genu valgum contribute to other pathologies, such as *patellar tracking disorders*.

Characteristics

The word *genu* means knee and the condition is named for a valgus angulation of the **tibia** in which the distal end of the tibia deviates in a lateral direction. Along with the tibial valgus, there is a corresponding *femoral varus*, which is a medial deviation of the distal end of the **femur**. **The femoral varus and tibial valgus produce the characteristic knock-knee distortion** (Figure 6.3).

Genu valgum is typical in childhood and appears as part of a normal postural growth pattern, usually normalizing with age. [3,4] In childhood an early stage of *genu varum* is followed by a later stage of genu valgum. The lower extremity eventually settles into correct postural alignment. Infants start off with physiologic bow-leg, then transition to the knock-knee posture between 2–3 years old. By the age of 5–6 years, most children's leg posture has corrected. In some cases the postural distortion does not normalize and the individual retains the genu valgum (or varum) in adolescence and adulthood. The

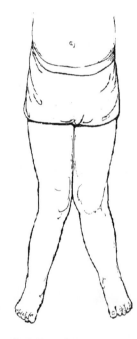

Figure 6.3 Valgus angulation of the tibia evident in genu valgum. (Mediclip image copyright, 1998 Williams & Wilkins. All rights reserved.)

posture can contribute to knee pain in adolescence, especially if the individual is engaged in vigorous activities like running or dancing.

Genu valgum is rarely an isolated problem. It routinely involves dysfunction in other parts of the lower extremity such as *hip adductor tightness* or *overpronation*. During overpronation medial rotation of the tibia is increased, which sometimes leads to genu valgum. *Coxa vara* can also cause genu valgum. This alignment problem develops when the angle between the femoral neck and shaft is less than 15^0, causing the femur to have a varus angulation and producing the corresponding tibial valgus. [5] Genu valgum could result from other disorders as well, such as *meniscal damage* or a *leg length discrepancy*. The condition can be a symptom of other pathologies such as *growth problems, trauma,* or *rickets.*[3] Presence of other conditions involving ligamentous laxity, such as *Marfan* or *Ehlers-Danlos syndromes,* makes the individual susceptible to genu valgum.

In genu valgum there is increased tensile stress on the soft tissues of the medial side of the knee. The primary tissues affected are the **medial collateral ligament, pes anserine muscle attachments**, and the **joint capsule** on the medial side. There is also compression of the lateral meniscus. The alteration in knee alignment creates dysfunctional mechanics of the **patellofemoral joint**, which can lead to *patellar dislocation* or tracking disorders such as *patellofemoral pain syndrome* or *chondromalacia patellae.*[6] Pathology sometimes results from compressive stress patterns on the ends of the **femur** and **tibia**.[3]

History
The client may report knee pain, but not necessarily. The condition might have developed in childhood or be an acquired condition, such as one resulting from overpronation. Ask about other conditions that could be related to the problem.

Observation
Visual inspection is the primary means of evaluating genu valgum. The client has clearly observable tibial valgus and femoral varus when viewed from the front or back. The medial side of the knees generally touch each other when the client is standing with the feet slightly apart.

Palpation
There are no specific findings with palpation.

Range-of-Motion and Resistance Testing
AROM: Active range of motion is not impaired.
PROM: There are no restrictions to passive movement.
MRT: No unusual findings with manual resistive tests.

Suggestions for Treatment
Correcting a postural distortion such as genu valgum involves retraining the neuromuscular patterns that created the problem. Structural bodywork or massage could be helpful in some cases, especially in conjunction with postural approaches. It is not an easy process for the client and requires their constant attention to posture and movement patterns. In more advanced cases that lead to continual knee problems, surgical intervention is periodically chosen.

GENU VARUM

Genu varum is named for the **varus angulation of the tibia** and is also called *tibial varus.* The common name for this postural distortion is *bow-leg.* While not as prevalent as valgus angulations of the tibia, genu varum can lead to a number of pathological conditions of the knee.

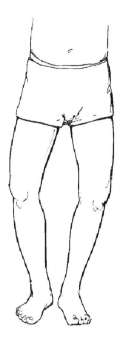

Figure 6.4 The common bow-leg deformity appearance of genu varum. (Mediclip image copyright, 1998 Williams & Wilkins. All rights reserved.)

Characteristics
In this condition, *tibial varus* and *femoral valgus* **cause the characteristic bow-legged appearance** (Figure 6.4). A varus angulation is one in which the distal end of a bony segment deviates in a **medial** direction. Like genu valgum, genu varum is typical in childhood and appears as part of a normal postural growth pattern, usually normalizing with age.[4] The early stage of genu varum is followed by a later stage of genu valgum before the lower extremity eventually settles into correct postural alignment. Infants start off with physiologic bow-leg, then transition to knock-knee posture between 2–3 years old. By the age of 5–6 most children's leg posture has corrected. In some cases the postural distortion does not normalize and the individual retains the genu varum (or valgum) in adolescence and adulthood.

Genu varum can develop in childhood from pathological biomechanics, as well such as systemic conditions such as *rickets* or *Blount's disease.*[7] Genu varum also occurs later in life as an acquired postural compensation where it affects other regions of the body. The postural distortion usually involves dysfunction in other parts of the kinetic chain, such as *hip abductor tightness* or *excessive supination* of the foot.

The condition can develop after childhood from *osteoarthritis* or other pathological conditions involving *internal joint damage* or instability, such as loss of a **medial meniscus**. Prolonged postural stresses to the knee, such as those caused by horseback riding, sometimes produce genu varum. As with genu valgum, presence of systemic conditions involving *ligamentous laxity* such as

Marfan or *Ehlers-Danlos syndromes* predispose the individual to the condition.

Genu varum causes increased tensile stress on lateral knee tissues, such as the **iliotibial band**, **lateral collateral ligament**, and **joint capsule of the knee**. There is compressive stress on the **medial meniscus**. Dysfunctional stress on the knee from genu varum can lead to numerous soft-tissue disorders such as *meniscal injury, patellar tracking problems, ligament sprains, osteoarthritis,* or *iliotibial band friction syndrome.*[8]

History

Identify any factors of prolonged postural stress, such as long periods of horseback riding. Inquire about other conditions in the client's history, such as the disorders mentioned above. The condition could develop in childhood or be an acquired disorder, resulting from pathological mechanics such as excessive supination.

Observation

Genu varum is easily identifiable with visual examination. The client has tibial varus and femoral valgus when viewed from the front or back. The individual also appears to stand on the lateral edge of the foot.

Palpation

There are no specific findings with palpation.

Range-of-Motion and Resistance Testing

AROM: Active range of motion is not impaired.
PROM: No significant restrictions to passive movement.
MRT: No unusual findings exist with MRT.

Suggestions for Treatment

Soft-tissue treatments help reduce muscular hypertonicity, but the overall joint mechanics and postural movement patterns must be addressed with postural and neuromuscular re-education. Orthotics are helpful in some cases. If the condition continues to be problematic, surgical correction may be necessary.

GENU RECURVATUM

Hyperextension in the knee is called *genu recurvatum.* The disorder is a structural deviation that can be inherited, produced by other postural dysfunctions, or caused by systemic conditions. Knee hyperextension impairs proper posture and can lead to other structural conditions.

Characteristics

Laxity in the internal ligaments of the knee **causes the knee to bow in a posterior direction at the end of extension**. Hyperextension of the knee is limited by tautness in both the **anterior** and **posterior cruciate ligaments**, as well as the **posterior joint capsule**.[9] Some hyperextension when standing is desirable as it prevents the quadriceps from constantly contracting to maintain the standing

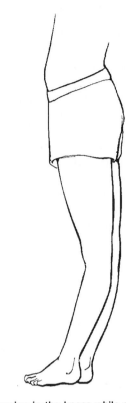

Figure 6.5 Hyperextension in the knees while standing produces genu recurvatum. (Mediclip image copyright, 1998 Williams & Wilkins. All rights reserved.)

posture. It is normal for there to be about 5^0–10^0 of hyperextension in the knee, but more than 10^0 of extension is considered a structural deviation (Figure 6.5).[5]

In addition to ligament laxity, genu recurvatum is caused by *poor neuromuscular control* of the knee extensor muscles which eventually overwhelm the posterior capsule and internal ligaments of the knee.[10] Strong contractions of the quadriceps near the end of extension can repeatedly stress the restraining ligaments and joint capsule enough to cause the condition. The condition can also occur as a result of an injury that forces the knee into hyperextension and permanently stretches the ligaments and posterior capsule. *Systemic disorders* involving *ligament weakness* or developmental neuromuscular disorders of impaired proprioception or coordination, such as *multiple sclerosis, cerebral palsy,* or *polio* also produce the condition.[11]

Genu recurvatum causes other structural disorders throughout the kinetic chain. As the knee moves farther into hyperextension, the line of gravity moves anterior to the knee's axis of rotation. The resultant shift in weight-bearing leads to numerous structural compensations such as *anterior pelvic tilt, increased lumbar lordosis,* and *overuse of the plantar flexor muscles.*

History

Ask the client about previous or existing neuromuscular disorders, such as multiple sclerosis, cerebral palsy, or polio. Identify conditions or injuries that cause laxity or weakness in connective tissues, especially ligaments and joint capsule.

Observation

Visual inspection is the primary means of evaluating this problem. It is best viewed from a lateral direction in relation to a vertical reference, such as a plumb line. There will be visible posterior bowing of the lower extremity. Measurement with a goniometer helps determine the degree of hyperextension.

Palpation

There are no specific findings with palpation.

Range-of-Motion and Resistance Testing

AROM: Active range of motion is not impaired. The additional degree of knee extension is visible during active extension, if it is performed with the client in a seated position with the legs fully stretched out in front. With the knees extended, the client is asked to tighten the quadriceps. If genu recurvatum exists the client's heel(s) will rise several inches.

PROM: No restrictions to full range in passive movement exist. If genu recurvatum is present a greater degree of hyperextension is visible with passive extension of the knee.

MRT: There are no unusual findings with MRT.

Suggestions for Treatment

If the primary cause of the problem is neuromuscular control, proprioceptive training or bracing can be used to improve muscular coordination and prevent excessive hyperextension. Little can be done for ligamentous laxity, so improving neuromuscular control is important. It is important to address the corresponding postural compensations that occur simultaneously, such as anterior pelvic tilting and exaggerated lumbar lordosis.

EXCESSIVE Q ANGLE

The Q angle illustrates aspects of patellofemoral biomechanics, particularly related to patellar tracking during knee extension. An *excessive Q angle* can cause dysfunctional biomechanics and lead to knee disorders.

Characteristics

The **Q (or quadriceps) angle** is determined by measuring the angle between two imaginary lines on the anterior thigh. The first line connects the **tibial tuberosity** with the **midpoint of the patella** and continues in a superior direction. The second line connects the **midpoint of the patella** with the **anterior superior iliac spine (ASIS)**. The angle created between these lines is the Q angle and

defines the quadriceps' angle of pull (Figure 6.6).

Three of the four quadriceps muscles attach to the femur proximally and the tibia distally. Because the patella is embedded in their distal tendon, its mechanics are influenced by these muscles' angle of pull. Due to the normal **varus angulation** of the femur, the quadriceps group pulls the patella in a superior and lateral direction. **In an excessive Q angle, the lateral pull is greater than it should be.**

An excessive Q angle is usually caused by postural relationships that are genetically determined. *Genu valgum* can increase the Q angle and women have a larger Q angle than men due to the wider pelvis. An excessive Q angle is associated with various knee pathologies such as *patellofemoral tracking disorders, patellar subluxation or dislocation, anterior knee pain, chondromalacia patellae,* and *anterior cruciate ligament injuries.*[12-16] Controversy exists in the literature about what constitutes an excessive Q angle and the lack of a consistent standard is problematic.[17] Some sources cite problems with values as low as 10^0, while others say the Q angle is not a concern until it exceeds 20^0.[5] Without established standards for what constitutes a pathological Q angle, it is best not to place too much emphasis on the angle, unless it is extreme. A large

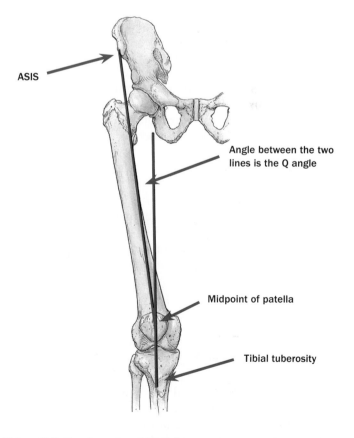

ASIS

Angle between the two lines is the Q angle

Midpoint of patella

Tibial tuberosity

Figure 6.6 The Q angle, which influences lateral patellar tracking. (Mediclip image copyright, 1998 Williams & Wilkins. All rights reserved.)

Q angle may not cause adverse symptoms until the client starts activities that intensify knee extension.

History

Ask the client about activities such as running or jumping, which indicate repetitive use of the quadriceps group. The client may indicate anterior knee pain associated with these activities, which could result from an excessive Q angle.

Observation

Several factors help identify a Q angle. A broad pelvis naturally causes the distal femur to angle medially, and increases the size of the Q angle. Genu valgum also increases the size of the Q angle. Accurate measurement of the Q angle is difficult, but can be performed with a goniometer. The large fluctuation in what is considered excessive for the Q angle makes the value of measurements questionable. Practitioners often use visual approximation to determine the existence of an excessive Q angle.

Palpation

There are no specific findings with palpation, but the soft tissues around the knee could be tender if there is a corresponding patellar tracking disorder.

Range-of-Motion and Resistance Testing

AROM: Active range of motion is not impaired.
PROM: There are no restrictions to passive movement.
MRT: There are no unusual findings with MRT.

Suggestions for Treatment

An excessive Q angle is typically determined by genetic factors beyond the individual's control (like a broad pelvis) and manual treatment does little to correct it. In some cases postural retraining and lower extremity biomechanical interventions, such as orthotics, are helpful.

SQUINTING PATELLA

Dysfunctional patellofemoral biomechanics can result from a structural problem in the femur, causing a disorder called the *squinting patella*. Individuals are born with this deviation and it can create pain and dysfunction.

Characteristics

During flexion and extension, the patella moves superiorly and inferiorly in a groove between the **femoral condyles**. In anatomical position both femoral condyles should point straight forward, with the anterior surface or *face* of the patella pointing forward. **A squinting patella develops when the femoral condyles are turned slightly toward the midline of the body, causing the face of each patella to angle toward the midline** (Figure 6.7). It is not medial rotation of the hip that produces the deviation. Rather, the primary cause is a dysfunctional twist within

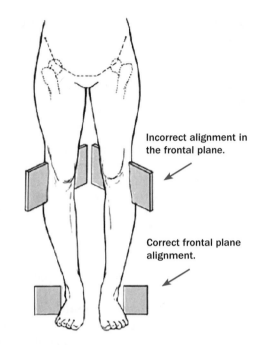

Incorrect alignment in the frontal plane.

Correct frontal plane alignment.

Figure 6.7 Femoral anteversion creates the inward pointing knees of squinting patella. (Mediclip image copyright, 1998 Williams & Wilkins. All rights reserved.)

the femoral shaft called *femoral anteversion* that forces the distal portion of the femur to face more medially than the proximal portion.

There is a natural degree of lateral pull on the patella. When a squinting patella is present, the lateral tensile force on the patella pulls the structure against the lateral condyle of the femur during knee extension. In more severe cases there are episodes of *patellar subluxation* or dislocation. *Anterior knee pain* and *joint dysfunction* can result due to excessive friction between the patella and lateral femoral condyle.

History

The client may complain of anterior knee pain, but the condition does not always produce pain. Identifying femoral anteversion requires an x-ray. Ask if the client has previously dislocated or subluxed the patella.

Observation

This postural distortion is best viewed from an anterior direction. The patella will angle in a medial direction instead of facing anteriorly.

Palpation

There are no specific findings with palpation.

Range-of-Motion and Resistance Testing

AROM: Active range of motion is generally not impaired, but there might be pain near the end of knee extension with actions that produce more resistance, such as standing from a squatting position.
PROM: Passive motion is not impaired.

MRT: In some cases there is anterior knee pain with resisted knee extension that results from a patellar tracking disorder.

Suggestions for Treatment

A squinting patella cannot be corrected with manual therapy. Subsequent problems that arise from the condition, such as patellar tracking disorders, can be addressed with soft-tissue treatment and are discussed later in the chapter.

Common Injury Conditions

ANTERIOR CRUCIATE LIGAMENT SPRAIN

Damage to the primary ligaments of the knee is common. The **anterior cruciate ligament (ACL)** is the most frequently injured.[18,19] Third degree sprains are more common than second or first degree, and some estimates suggest that as many as 85% of *ACL sprains* involve a complete rupture.[20] The majority of ACL injuries result from sporting activities, particularly those that involve deceleration, twisting, rapidly changing direction or jumping.

Characteristics

The ACL attaches to the **anterior tibia** and the **posterior femur** (Figure 6.8). Inside the knee the ACL forms a cross with the **posterior cruciate ligament** (PCL) in order to provide dynamic stability in the sagittal plane. The ACL's primary function is to prevent anterior translation of the **tibia** in relation to the femur. It also assists in preventing rotation at the knee.[9]

The ACL passes between the **femoral condyles** in a passage called the **intercondylar notch**. The notch plays a role in the onset of ACL injury because if the notch is narrow, the ACL can rub against the medial side of the **lateral femoral condyle**. This is particularly true in conditions of genu valgum. How much the friction contributes to ACL injury is debated.[21]

Mechanical overload is the primary cause of ACL injury and is common in sporting activities. For example, when an individual is running and suddenly changes direction on a planted foot, the rotational stress to the knee can produce ACL injury. Another mechanism of injury involves suddenly stopping in the midst of running. To quickly slow the body's momentum, the quadriceps engage intense contractions as the foot is planted. The attachment site of the quadriceps is on the **anterior tibia**, so the contraction pulls the tibia in an anterior direction stressing the ACL. The abrupt load on the ACL can cause a ligament tear. Another cause of ACL sprain is an **extreme hyperextension** injury to the knee, such as a direct blow to an extended knee or from landing improperly from a jump with the knee hyperextended.

Women sustain ACL injuries at a higher rate than men. There are several possible explanations for this increased risk. Hormone concentrations cause some degree of *ligamentous weakness*. In addition, the **larger Q angle** in women causes vulnerability to ACL injury, as the ACL is more likely to rub against the side of the femoral condyles in the intercondylar notch making it increasingly vulnerable to tensile stress injury.[22] Strength imbalances between the quadriceps and hamstrings is another factor. There are also indications that men are more dependent on muscle development for knee stability, while women are more dependent on ligamentous support.[23]

ACL injuries rarely happen alone. Instead, they coincide with damage to other ligaments such as the **medial collateral (MCL)** or **posterior cruciate ligaments (PCL)**. It is common to have ACL injury in addition to *meniscal damage*. The term *unhappy triad* is used to describe concurrent damage to the ACL, MCL, and **medial meniscus**. Recent reports indicate that the **lateral meniscus** is involved in some cases.[24]

Despite the fact that the ACL is not palpable due to its location within the knee joint, ACL injury is routinely evaluated with physical examination. One author suggests that 90% of ACL sprains can be identified with physical examination and an accurate history.[25] The excessive hypermobility of the knee makes third degree sprains relatively easy to identify. In fact, first or second degree sprains are harder to detect than third degree.

History

The client describes a sudden motion or activity that caused immediate knee pain. Encourage the client to elaborate on the mechanics of the incident to determine whether the ACL was exposed to a sudden high tensile load. The client might describe a loud pop or snap at the onset of injury. The client commonly experiences weakness in the knee immediately after the injury and reports the knee *giving way*.

Sharp pain is felt at the time of injury and can persist due to swelling or partially torn ligament fibers. Pain may

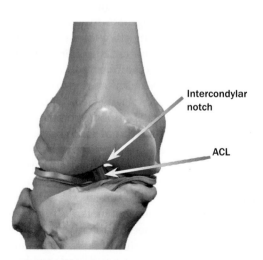

Figure 6.8 Anterior view of the right knee with patella removed. The ACL is visible deep within the joint. (3-D anatomy image courtesy of Primal Pictures Ltd. www.primalpictures.com.)

be worse if the ligament is only partially torn. If the fibers are completely disrupted (third degree sprain) there is pain at the initial point of injury but less or no pain and increased hypermobility once swelling has subsided because of complete disruption of the ligament fibers.

Swelling is generally reported at the time of the injury or shortly thereafter. Swelling produces pain as the fluid presses on many free nerve endings in the joint. The client could report stiffness around the knee due to muscle splinting.

Observation

Ligament damage produces swelling with some ACL injuries, but it is generally contained within the capsule and not visible. Alterations in gait are probable, due to instability in the knee and pain. If there is excessive hyper-mobility of the knee, there is an increased prominence of the anterior margin of the **tibial plateau** compared to the unaffected side in certain positions.

Palpation

Swelling may or may not be evident with palpation. Because the ligaments are too deep to be palpated, tenderness from ligament damage is not felt with palpation. Tensile stress must be applied to the ligament in order to reproduce symptoms.

Range-of-Motion and Resistance Testing

AROM: In some cases AROM is impaired due to protective muscle spasm, especially if the spasm involves the hamstrings. In this case active motion in knee extension is somewhat restricted.

PROM: Passive motion could be restricted by pain at the end range of knee extension as the damaged ligament is stretched. Passive knee flexion generally does not produce pain.

MRT: Some pain and forward movement of the tibia during resisted knee extension could be due to the quadriceps pulling the proximal tibia in an anterior direction. Pain is not typical with other MRTs. Pain can cause reflex muscular inhibition, particularly in the quadriceps, making the muscles appear weak during MRTs.

Special Tests

Anterior Drawer Test

The client is supine on the table with the hip flexed to 45^0, the knee flexed at 90^0, and the client's foot flat on the table. The client's foot is stabilized by anchoring the toes beneath the practitioner's thigh (Figure 6.9). The practitioner places both hands around the posterior side of the proximal tibia and gives a firm anterior pull on the tibia. A positive test results with a mushy end feel, pain, and/or anterior movement of the tibia. Anterior translation of the tibia may be visible. Evaluate this movement by watching the anterior edge of the tibial plateau during the test.

Explanation: The primary role of the ACL is to restrain anterior movement of the tibia in relation to the femur.

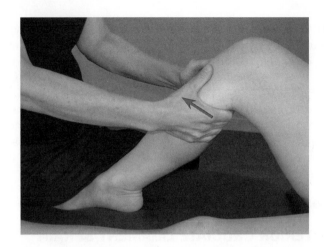

Figure 6.9 Anterior drawer test. The arrow indicates the direction of the practitioner's force.

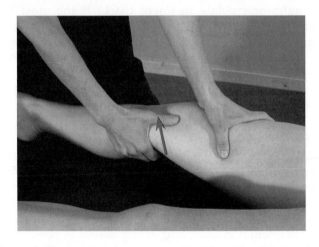

Figure 6.10 Lachman test. The arrow indicates the direction of the practitioner's force. Emphasis is on the force applied to the tibia.

By pulling the tibia in an anterior direction, direct tensile stress is applied to the ACL. False negatives are not unusual with this test due the angle of the knee during the test, which is why it is not as accurate as the Lachman test. If the hamstrings are in spasm, they prevent anterior movement of the tibia as their line of pull is in the same direction as the practitioner's pulling force on the tibia. A spasm in the hamstrings can prevent the forward shifting of the proximal tibia, even with a severe cruciate ligament injury, which gives the appearance of stability although there is an injury present (false negative). If the ligament is completely ruptured considerable movement is observed, but there is generally no pain during the test because the two ends of the ligament are separated.

Lachman Test

The client is supine on the table. This test can be performed with the knee in straight extension or in partial flexion. The client's anterior distal femur is stabilized with one hand and the other hand is placed behind the proximal tibia (Figure 6.10). A firm anterior pull is applied to the tibia. If there is movement, pain, or a mushy end feel,

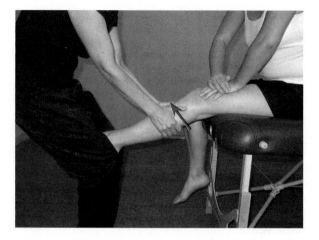

Figure 6.11 Lachman test variation. The arrow indicates the direction of the practitioner's force.

damage to the ACL is probable.

Explanation: The mechanics of the Lachman test are the same as the anterior drawer in that an anterior force is being applied to the proximal tibia and pulls on the ACL. However without significant knee flexion, the hamstrings' angle of pull is unlikely to give false negatives as it does with the anterior drawer test. Practitioners with small hands may have trouble with the traditional Lachman test position and therefore the variation listed next is effective. A complete ligament rupture allows considerable movement, but no pain because the fibers are disconnected.

Lachman Test Variation
The client is seated on the end of the table with the legs hanging down. The client presses down on the distal femur to stabilize it during the test. The client's foot is held between the practitioner's legs so the knee is in partial flexion (Figure 6.11). At the same time the practitioner grasps the posterior proximal tibia with both hands and gives a firm anterior pull on the tibia. Pain, mushy end feel, or anterior translation of the proximal tibia is indicative of ACL injury.

Explanation: The mechanics of this test are the same as the standard Lachman test. The client's assistance with stabilization and the practitioner's use of both hands to pull the proximal tibia forward make this test easier to perform than the traditional Lachman's position.

Differential Evaluation
MCL or PCL sprain, meniscal injury, tibial fracture, patellar tendon avulsion, osteoarthritis, osteochondritis dissecans.

Suggestions for Treatment
The ACL is inaccessible to palpation, and massage is not able to address the actual ligament tear. If the tear is minor, a physician may recommend no treatment. In other cases, surgery is advised. Advances in arthroscopic

surgery have improved the techniques used to repair the ligament and dramatically shortened recovery time.

Massage is helpful for returning normal biomechanical balance to surrounding muscles that are in protective spasm. Strength training of the quadriceps and hamstrings is used to encourage proper muscular coordination around the knee.

POSTERIOR CRUCIATE LIGAMENT SPRAIN

The **posterior cruciate ligament (PCL)** is one of the primary stabilizers of the knee. Injuries to the PCL are not as common because this ligament is broader and stronger than the ACL. *PCL sprains* do not produce as much functional disability as ACL sprains. These sprains appear with the greatest frequency in athletes, but result from falls or automobile accidents as well.

Characteristics
The PCL attaches to the **posterior tibia** and the **anterior femur** (Figure 6.12). The ligament's primary function is to prevent posterior movement of the tibia in relation to the femur, which occurs with either posterior movement of the tibia or anterior movement of the femur. The PCL also functions to resist lateral rotation of the tibia.[9] **The majority of injuries result from the tibia being thrust in a posterior direction.**

PCL injuries happen in athletic situations where there is a direct blow to the proximal tibia while the knee is hyperextended. More often they result from anterior impacts on the tibia with the knee in a flexed position. The PCL becomes taut at the end of knee flexion making it particularly vulnerable to sprain. For example, this type of PCL injury results from head-on automobile accidents when the flexed knee hits the dashboard and the tibia is thrust posteriorly. Another mechanism of injury is cre-

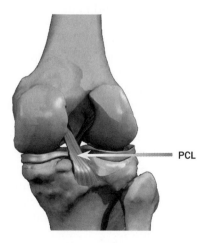

Figure 6.12 Posterior view of the right knee showing the PCL and its attachment to the posterior tibia. (3-D anatomy image courtesy of Primal Pictures Ltd. www.primalpictures.com.)

ated when the individual falls on the knee with the foot plantar flexed, so the proximal tibia hits the ground first. If the client has a prominent tibial tuberosity, such as that resulting from *Osgood-Schlatter disease*, the force driving the tibia posterior will be exaggerated.[26]

The PCL is usually injured in conjunction with other structures of the knee. It is estimated that half of all PCL injuries involve damage to other knee structures, such as the **ACL** or **joint capsule**.[5] Evidence shows that many PCL injuries go undetected, which means it is likely that there are more PCL injuries than are reported.[27] PCL injuries alter **patellofemoral mechanics** and can produce *anterior knee pain* following the injury.[26]

Sharp pain is felt at the time of injury and can persist due to swelling or damaged ligament fibers. Pain may be worse if the ligament is only partially torn. If the fibers are completely disrupted (third degree sprain), pain might be felt at the initial point of injury, but subside once the swelling goes down because the ligament is completely torn, even though there is considerably hypermobility.

History

The client describes a sudden motion or activity performed which immediately causes pain. Identify the mechanics of the injury, such as an automobile accident or fall, to determine if a tensile stress injury to the PCL is likely. The client may describe hearing a loud pop or snap at the onset of injury. Ask the client about weakness in the knee immediately after the injury. Muscle splinting, swelling, and difficulty with locomotion are reported.

Observation

Although the PCL is deep in the knee, it lies outside the margins of the joint capsule. Consequently, swelling resulting from ligament damage is typically more evident with PCL sprains than with ACL. Swelling can be prominent on the posterior side of the knee. A contusion might be visible on the anterior proximal tibia, if there was a direct blow. Alterations in gait are probable, due to instability in the knee and pain.

Palpation

Swelling could be evident with palpation, particularly if other structures are damaged along with the PCL. Local tenderness is typical and results from swelling or other damaged structures. The ligament itself is not palpable.

Range-of-Motion and Resistance Testing

AROM: In some cases AROM is impaired due to protective muscle spasm or movement pain. Active movement without resistance is generally not painful unless the ligament is severely damaged. In some cases, knee extension is painful if the injury caused alterations to proper patellofemoral mechanics.

PROM: Pain is not usually felt with passive flexion or extension short of the end range. However, the PCL becomes increasingly taut during flexion of the knee, so pain might be elicited near the end of full flexion as the ligament fibers are stretched. The PCL is also stretched if posterior pressure is added to the anterior proximal tibia at the end range of hyperextension.

MRT: Pain is sometimes felt with posterior movement of the tibia during resisted knee flexion. Pain results from the hamstrings pulling the proximal tibia in a posterior direction, which stretches the injured ligament. The special orthopedic tests outlined below are particularly effective at stretching the PCL. In some cases ligament pain causes reflex muscular inhibition of other knee muscles, causing them to appear weak during MRTs.

Special Tests
Posterior Drawer Test

The client is supine on the table with the hip flexed to 45^0, the knee flexed at 90^0, and the client's foot flat on the table (Figure 6.13). The client's foot is stabilized by anchoring the toes beneath the practitioner's thigh. The practitioner places both hands around the proximal tibia and gives a firm posterior push on the tibia. A positive result is pain, a mushy end feel, or posterior movement of the tibia. Posterior translation of the tibia may be visible. To evaluate this movement watch the anterior edge of the tibial plateau during the test to see if it moves posteriorly.

Explanation: The primary role of the PCL is to prevent posterior movement of the tibia. Pushing the tibia farther in this direction helps detect damage to the ligament. When performing the posterior drawer test, it is helpful to do the Sag Sign or Gravity Drawer tests first in order to determine if there is posterior sagging of the proximal tibia. If the tibia is sagging in a posterior direction due to gravity, posterior movement may not be apparent. In this situation, pull the tibia forward into a neutral position and redo the test. Laxity is evident if the test is positive. If the ligament is completely ruptured considerable movement is usually observed, but there may be no pain during the test because the ligament ends are separated.

Sag Sign or Gravity Drawer

The client is in a similar starting position to the anterior and posterior drawer tests: supine on the table but with the hip flexed to 45^0, knee flexed at 90^0, and foot flat on the table (Figure 6.14). The practitioner views the tibial tuberosity to see if it drops posteriorly.

Another variation on this position is called the Godfrey test (Figure 6.14). In this test the client's hip is flexed to 90^0, the knee is also flexed to 90^0, and the practitioner holds the client's foot. The practitioner examines the level of the tibial tuberosity to determine if there is a posterior drop or sag in the proximal tibia. The sag can be accentuated by pressing down on the proximal tibia or by having the client attempt resisted knee flexion while resistance is offered under the distal tibia or posterior heel. If the client attempts a quadriceps contraction from the test position, anterior movement of the tibia is likely to be visible as it is brought back to a neutral position.

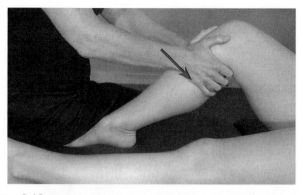

Figure 6.13 Posterior drawer test. The arrow indicates the direction of the practitioner's force.

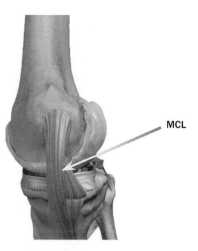

Figure 6.15 Medial view of the right knee showing the MCL and its attachment to the tibia. (3-D anatomy image courtesy of Primal Pictures Ltd. www.primalpictures.com.)

Suggestions for Treatment

Because the PCL is deep inside the joint and inaccessible to palpation, massage can not be used to address the ligament tear. If the tear is minor, physicians occasionally recommend no treatment. In other cases, surgery is suggested. PCL tears are ordinarily treated conservatively with physical therapy prior to, or instead of, surgery. Massage is beneficial for reducing spasm in surrounding muscles.

MEDIAL COLLATERAL LIGAMENT SPRAIN

The **medial collateral ligament (MCL)** is the largest stabilizing ligament of the knee. *MCL sprains* are relatively common and can coincide with other structural pathologies in the knee. Tears in the MCL are more likely when there are other structural problems, such as *genu valgum* or *overpronation*, which make the MCL more susceptible to tensile stress damage.

Characteristics

The MCL is also called the **tibial collateral ligament** due to its distal attachment to the **tibia** (Figure 6.15). This ligament is the larger of the two collateral ligaments and has a fibrous attachment to the **medial meniscus**. As a result, tensile stress injuries to the MCL often cause tearing of the outer edge of the medial meniscus. The MCL is connected with the **joint capsule**, making MCL sprains particularly painful due to the rich innervation of the capsule.

The primary function of the MCL is to prevent valgus stress to the knee; **sprains can result when the knee is forced toward the position of genu valgum.** Valgus stress is frequent in contact sports where the knee receives a blow to its lateral side, but it may also happen without direct impact. For example, MCL injuries occur in snow skiing when a skier catches an edge of a ski and the lower extremity is pulled laterally. As the individual falls, there

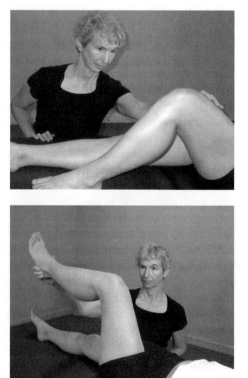

Figure 6.14 Evaluating posterior drop of the tibia with the gravity drawer test (A) and Godfrey test (B).

Explanation: If the PCL is damaged, the ligament cannot resist the pull of gravity and a posterior movement of the proximal tibia results. Visual examination alone is generally not accurate enough to identify a PCL injury, but is helpful when used in conjunction with other procedures. Do not confuse a prominent tibial tuberosity, which may be a result of having *Osgood-Schlatter disease* as a child, with a posterior drop of the tibia.

Differential Evaluation

ACL, MCL, or LCL sprain, meniscal injury, tibial fracture, posterolateral capsule damage.

is a strong valgus load on the knee that may cause a tear in the MCL.[28]

In addition to valgus force, the MCL has a fundamental role in stabilizing the knee against rotational stress. In particular the MCL resists medial rotation of the **femur** on the tibia. **Rotational stress injuries** to the ligament are common in running activities that require the individual to plant a foot and abruptly turn the body to the opposite side.

Injuries that damage the MCL can damage other knee structures as well. ACL sprains are concurrent with those of the MCL in many cases. Simultaneous ACL and MCL sprains cause **multi-directional instability** in the knee. The knee may then need supportive bracing to prevent further injury during stressful activities.

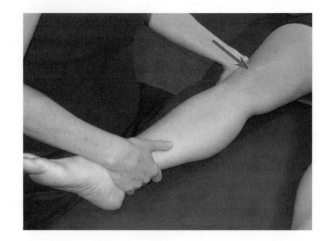

Figure 6.16 Valgus stress test. The arrow indicates the direction of the practitioner's force applied to the lateral joint line.

History

The client reports a sudden injury that involves a valgus or rotary stress to the knee. Ask the client about a recent blow to the outside of the knee or injury from a non-contact valgus force, such as slipping on the ice. A loud pop might have been heard at the time of injury. The client experiences weakness in the knee immediately after the injury, often reported as the knee giving way. Muscle splinting, swelling, and difficulty with locomotion are reported.

An MCL sprain causes sharp pain on the medial side of the knee. As a result of the ligament being superficial, the client is usually able to reproduce the pain by pressing on the site of injury. If the fibers are completely disrupted (third degree sprain), there is pain at the initial point of injury but less or no pain once swelling has subsided. Complete disruption of the ligament may not produce further pain as the tissues are no longer stressed. In the third degree sprain, there is considerable hypermobility of the joint.

Observation

Swelling is ordinarily evident due to the superficial nature of this ligament. Damage to other structures, such as the joint capsule or muscle, also produces swelling. Alterations in gait are probable, due to instability in the knee and pain. *Ecchymosis* arises if other richly vascular tissues like muscles are torn.

Palpation

The usual site of injury is directly over the joint line (the articulation between the tibia and femur) in the middle of the ligament's length. Palpation of the area usually produces pain. Disruption of the continuity of ligament fibers may also be palpable. Edema is evident on the medial side of the knee.

Range-of-Motion and Resistance Testing

AROM: Active motion may not be limited, but pain or discomfort can be reported as the knee moves through flexion and extension. If pain is severe, limitation in active

movement is observed. Movement restriction is generally due to pain avoidance, not from tissue restriction.

PROM: The same principles apply as for active movement.

MRT: There are no major restrictions with MRTs. In some cases there is pain from tensile stress on the ligament during resisted adduction of the thigh, if the hand offering resistance is distal to the knee. This position creates valgus stress to the knee.

Special Test
Valgus Stress Test

The client is supine on the table. The practitioner stabilizes the distal medial tibia with one hand, while applying valgus force to the lateral knee with the other hand (Figure 6.16). The amount of valgus force to apply will vary, but is best described as moderate. Make sure the middle of the hand applying the valgus force is placed directly over the joint line and not superior or inferior. If the hands are not in the right position, the practitioner cannot adequately feel movement in the joint. Pain or a mushy end feel indicates damage to the MCL. A small amount of gapping over the medial joint line may be visible as the valgus force is applied.

The accuracy of the test is increased by placing the knee in approximately 15^0–20^0 of flexion. In the standard position of full extension, the ACL opposes some valgus stress to the knee and if the ACL is intact, the MCL can appear to not have laxity although it is injured. When the knee is slightly flexed, the ACL does not offer the same degree of resistance to valgus force and the test's accuracy improves.

Explanation: By applying valgus force, the practitioner stresses the MCL's primary function. Although muscles and tendons cross the region, they do not offer much support against valgus stress. If the ligament is completely ruptured movement is often visible, but pain is not always present because the ligament ends are separated.

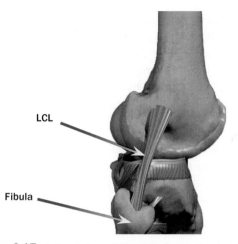

Figure 6.17 Lateral view of the right knee showing the LCL and its attachment to the fibula. (3-D anatomy image courtesy of Primal Pictures Ltd. www.primalpictures.com.)

Differential Evaluation

ACL sprain, meniscal injury, distal adductor strain, pes anserine bursitis, tibial plateau fracture, patellofemoral pain syndrome, arthritis.

Suggestions for Treatment

If the ligament damage is not severe, the primary focus of treatment is to encourage the development of healthy scar tissue in the ligament. It is important to prevent the scar tissue from adhering the ligament to underlying bone. An effective way to accomplish these goals is with deep transverse friction massage applied directly to the injured ligament. Addressing muscular hypertonicity around the knee joint is important. Consult with the physician or other health care providers to make sure massage treatment goals and methods are complementary to other rehabilitative techniques being employed.

LATERAL COLLATERAL LIGAMENT SPRAIN

The **lateral collateral ligament (LCL)** is the least frequently injured of the four primary stabilizing ligaments of the knee. Due to its smaller size, LCL injuries are also less severe. The most common cause of LCL sprain is a direct blow to the inside of the knee, which can occur in contact sports like rugby or football.

Characteristics

The lateral collateral ligament is also called the **fibular collateral ligament** due to its distal attachment to the **fibular head**. It runs between the **lateral epicondyle of the femur** and the **head of the fibula** (Figure 6.17). The tendon of the **biceps femoris** muscle lies directly over it. As a result, tendon pathology of the biceps femoris can be mistaken for LCL injury. Unlike the MCL, the LCL has no fibrous connection to the meniscus or joint capsule.

The primary function of this ligament is to resist varus forces to the knee, where the knee is forced further toward the position of *genu varum*. Varus force usually results from a blow to the medial knee that pushes the knee laterally.

One reason for reduced injury in the LCL is that the ligament is protected by other structures. For example, if an individual is hit from the right side, the right knee takes a valgus impact and protects the left knee from excessive varus force. An ankle sprain is more likely to result than an LCL sprain when a laterally directed force hits the medial side of the knee. The lateral ankle ligaments are a weaker point in the kinetic chain and are therefore more susceptible to injury.

The LCL also resists internal rotation of the **tibia** the ligament becomes taut when the knee is extended and loosens when flexed. Sprains can occur when the knee is exposed to rotational stress while extended, such as when planting the foot and twisting the body. Overlying structures, such as the **biceps femoris tendon** or the **iliotibial band**, could also produce lateral knee pain.

History

The client reports a sudden injury that involves a varus and/or rotary stress to the knee. Pain from an LCL sprain is felt on the lateral side of the knee and is pronounced at the time of the injury. A loud pop might have been heard at the time of injury. Ask the client about weakness in the knee immediately after the injury. Muscle splinting, swelling, and difficulty with locomotion are reported.

The client is usually able to reproduce the pain by pressing on the site of injury. If the fibers are completely disrupted (third degree sprain), there is pain at the initial point of injury but less or no pain once swelling has subsided. In the third degree sprain, there is considerable hypermobility of the joint.

Observation

Swelling is prevalent in the area following the injury, but is not always visible. Bruising results if other vascular tissues in the area are damaged. The client may demonstrate visible knee stiffness and walk with a limp due to motion restriction.

Palpation

There is tenderness over the lateral collateral ligament. The site of injury could vary along the length of the ligament, but usually lies over the joint line. The LCL is easy to palpate as the ligament's attachment sites are obvious landmarks. If the injury is severe there is palpable disruption in the continuity of ligament fibers. Some swelling is evident with palpation, even when not visible. Local tenderness with palpation can be due to concurrent injury of the biceps femoris tendon, iliotibial band, or posterolateral joint capsule.

Range-of-Motion and Resistance Testing

AROM: Active movement is not generally limited. Because the LCL is not contiguous with the joint capsule,

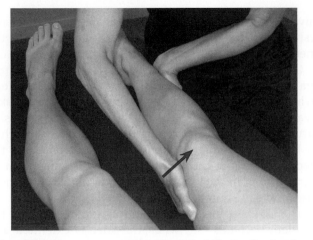

Figure 6.18 The varus stress test. The arrow indicates the direction of the practitioner's force applied to the medial joint line.

flexion and extension are not as likely to cause pain as occurs with an MCL injury. However, friction against the overlying iliotibial band may cause discomfort during these motions.

PROM: The same principles apply as for AROM.

MRT: No restrictions are evident with MRTs. If the hand offering resistance is distal to the knee, there may be pain from tensile stress on the ligament during resisted abduction of the thigh, which produces varus stress.

Special Test
Varus Stress Test
The client is supine on the table. The practitioner stabilizes the lateral distal tibia with one hand, while applying varus force to the lateral knee with the other (Figure 6.18). The amount of force will vary, but is best described as moderate. Ensure the middle of the hand applying the force is placed immediately over the joint line, not superior or inferior. If the hand is not in the right position the practitioner cannot adequately feel movement in the joint. Pain or a mushy end feel indicates damage to the LCL. A small amount of gapping over the lateral joint line may be visible as the varus force is applied.

The accuracy of the test is increased by placing the knee in approximately 15⁰–20⁰ of flexion. In the standard position of full extension, the ACL can oppose some varus stress to the knee and if the ACL is intact, the LCL can appear to not have laxity although it is injured. When the knee is slightly flexed, the ACL cannot offer the same degree of resistance and the test's accuracy is improved.

Explanation: By applying a varus force, the integrity of the LCL is tested. Damage to the ligament is evident if there is pain and/or excess motion. If the ligament is ruptured, movement is likely to be visible but pain is not always present because the ligament ends are separated.

Differential Evaluation
Meniscal injury, iliotibial band friction syndrome, biceps femoris tendon avulsion, tibial plateau fracture.

Suggestions for Treatment
Similar to the MCL, the LCL has a superficial location and is therefore accessible for treatment with massage. Treatment goals are the same as those for MCL sprain. These include developing a healthy functional scar and preventing unwanted adhesions with adjacent tissues. Because the LCL does not have fibrous continuity with the joint capsule as the MCL does, there is less chance of adverse adhesions developing at the capsule.

LCL sprains are treated with surgery less often than MCL injuries. Whether surgery is performed or not, massage plays a valuable role in speeding recovery. Deep transverse friction massage can be applied directly to the injured ligament. Addressing muscular hypertonicity around the knee joint is important. Consult with the physician to develop an appropriate focus for massage treatment in the post-surgical stage.

PATELLOFEMORAL PAIN SYNDROME

Patellofemoral pain syndrome (PFPS) is anterior knee pain of variable origin primarily caused by a patellar tracking disorder. While the anterior knee pain of the syndrome is widespread and recognizable, an adequate understanding of the cause has yet to be developed. The condition is moderately frequent, particularly in the athletic population.

Characteristics
PFPS is a disorder of the **extensor mechanism** of the knee, which includes the **quadriceps** group, **patellar tendon**, **femur**, **tibia**, **patella**, **quadriceps retinaculum,** and **fascia**.[29, 30] Reviewing the structure and function of the patellofemoral articulation aids in understanding this condition. A ridge on the underside of the patella fits in a groove between the **femoral condyles** helping it track correctly (Figure 6.19). The patella is imbedded within the **patellar (quadriceps) tendon** and is tethered on the medial and lateral sides by fibers of the **quadriceps retinaculum**. There is fibrous continuity of the retinaculum with numerous restraining ligaments around the knee as well. All of these tissues are involved in movements of the **patellofemoral joint**.[31]

As the knee moves in flexion and extension, the patella glides in a superior and inferior direction over the top of the femoral condyles. The soft tissues that tether the patella from different directions keep it tracking correctly between the condyles. **Patellar tracking disorders result when there is an imbalance of forces pulling on the patella** or some other structural disorder and the patella does not glide evenly. Tracking disorders are a cause of PFPS.

Several structural and functional factors are implicated in patellar tracking disorders. Due to the natural varus angulation of the femur, there is a greater tendency for the patella to be pulled in a lateral direction. Lateral tracking disorders are more common in a person with a

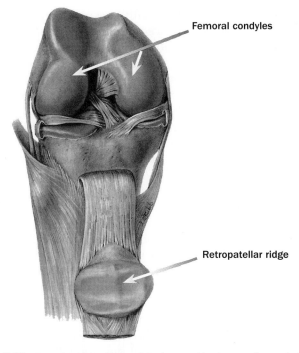

Femoral condyles

Retropatellar ridge

Figure 6.19 Anterior view of the right knee with the patella peeled back to show the ridge on the underside that fits between the femoral condyles. (Mediclip image copyright, 1998 Williams & Wilkins. All rights reserved.)

large Q angle due to the increased *femoral varus. Genu valgum* or *femoral anteversion* and a *squinting patella* can also produce a *lateral tracking disorder*.

Muscle imbalances are another factor thought to contribute to lateral tracking problems. The most distal portion of the vastus medialis muscle is called the **vastus medialis obliquus**, or **VMO**, because its fibers angle toward the patella at an oblique angle. The angle allows it to counteract the lateral pull of the vastus lateralis on the opposite side of the patella. It is suggested that *vastus lateralis tightness* combined with **VMO weakness** could lead to lateral tracking disorders.[32]

While the anatomical structures around the knee are well studied, the actual source of pain in PFPS remains a mystery. The **quadriceps retinaculum**, particularly on the medial side, is often implicated.[33] Due to the tracking disorder, *hyaline cartilage degeneration* develops on the underside of the patella and is sometimes described as the source of pain in PFPS. However, hyaline cartilage has little innervation making it an unlikely cause. Irritation and degeneration of the richly innervated **subchondral bone** is a more reasonable cause of knee pain.[6] This theory is still controversial and other anatomical structures in the area, such as the **infrapatellar fat pad**, **quadriceps muscles, tibiofemoral joint capsule, patellar tendon**, and **synovium,** produce similar pain.[29]

PFPS usually develops as a chronic condition, especially after activities involving repetitive knee flexion and extension such as running, jumping, hiking, or dancing. The condition is particularly prevalent in the athletic pop-

ulation and frequently results from sudden increases in activity levels, such as beginning a new training program or engaging in athletic activities without prior conditioning. In some cases weakness or buckling of the knees is felt with PFPS, especially during forceful extension like climbing stairs, due to reflex muscular inhibition from pain.[34]

PFPS is generally considered an early warning sign of *chondromalacia patellae*, which may develop if the dysfunctional biomechanics of PFPS are not corrected. Chondromalacia literally means softening of the cartilage and the term is sometimes used to refer to anterior knee pain. But because there is little innervation in the cartilage, it is unlikely that cartilage degeneration is producing the knee pain.[35] The term chondromalacia is best reserved for degenerative conditions in the cartilage and not for patellofemoral tracking disorder pain.

History

The client describes anterior knee pain associated with activities emphasizing knee flexion and extension, such as running, jumping, climbing or descending stairs, hiking, and squatting. Activities that engage more resistance are likely to create more pain. Ask about sudden changes in activity level. Holding the knee in a flexed position for long periods, such as sitting in a movie theater, tends to aggravate symptoms. The pain subsides when the knee is extended or the person begins to move around again. This pain pattern associated with long periods of knee flexion is known as a **positive movie sign** or **theater sign**.

Clients routinely describe the pain as coming from under the kneecap (retropatellar), but are unable to identify a specific site. The tissues under the patella are not necessarily the cause of pain as other tissues could refer pain to the region. Pain is customary in the midst of activity, but can develop with delayed onset—coming on even a full day after activity. Pain can be sharp at times, but is generally a non-specific aching that improves with rest and is aggravated with activity. Grinding or grating sensations during knee extension might be reported.

Observation

There are no visible signs specifically for PFPS, although certain biomechanical or postural distortions can play a role in the condition, . Especially important is the presence of genu valgum, squinting patella, or a large Q angle.

As a result of pain and reflex muscular inhibition, some muscles atrophy rapidly. In particular, anti-gravity muscles such as the quadriceps atrophy faster than other muscles.[36] Visual evaluation of extensor muscle dysfunction can be accomplished by measuring the circumference of the distal quadriceps with a flexible tape measure and comparing it to the opposite side. If there is a discrepancy, muscle atrophy is probable on the smaller side. While this measurement does not specifically identify PFPS, it does indicate a problem that is causing the quadriceps to atrophy and PFPS may play a role in the condition.

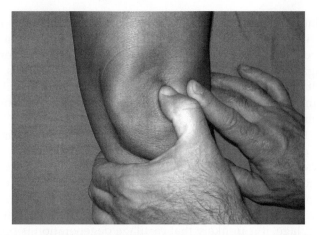

Figure 6.20 Patellar mobility test applied to the left knee. More than adequate mobility is demonstrated in this individual.

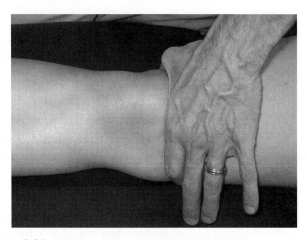

Figure 6.21 Clarke's sign for patellofemoral dysfunction.

Palpation

In some cases it is difficult to reproduce the pain of PFPS with palpation, while in other cases it is easy. For example, if the pain is due to irritation of the sub-chondral bone on the underside of the patella, light or moderate palpation anywhere around the knee does not always produce discomfort. If the patella is pressed against the femoral condyles, pain could be elicited by placing pressure upon the patella.

If the superficial tissues around the knee such as the quadriceps retinaculum are involved, palpation reproduces the client's pain. If the knee is in flexion, pain will be exaggerated as the tissues are stretched.

Range-of-Motion and Resistance Testing

AROM: Pain is possible during active knee flexion or extension. Pain is greater if these movements are performed in a weight-bearing position, such as squatting. Crepitus during flexion or extension with either weight-bearing or non-weight-bearing positions is typical.

PROM: Pain is unusual with passive movement unless the condition is advanced. Crepitus might be evident with flexion or extension. Pain is sometimes felt at full knee flexion as anterior knee tissues, such as the patellar tendon and the extensor retinaculum, are stretched.

MRT: Pain is possible with resisted knee extension. Pain is more probable as the patella moves during active resisted extension and not during an isometric contraction. Reflex muscular inhibition can cause a quadriceps contraction to appear weak as the muscles decrease contraction strength in response to pain.

Special Tests

Patellar Mobility Test

The client is seated or supine on the table with the knees extended and relaxed. The practitioner pushes the edge of the patella, attempting to move it medially and laterally (Figure 6.20). If the patella moves less than one quarter of the patella's width in a medial direction, there may be restriction to proper tracking.

Explanation: The patella should be able to move about half its width from a neutral position either medially or laterally. If the patella is unable to move medially, it indicates tightness in the lateral soft-tissue restraints, such as the lateral retinaculum or vastus lateralis. When these tissues are tight they pull the patella laterally during extension causing the lateral tracking disorder.

Clarke's Sign

The client is supine on the table with the knee fully extended. The practitioner places one hand over the distal end of the suprapatellar tendon, just above the superior margin of the patella. The webbing between the practitioner's thumb and hand should be pressing straight down (toward the table) into the suprapatellar tendon and quadriceps retinaculum (Figure 6.21). The client slowly contracts the quadriceps until a full contraction is achieved. Pain is a positive result for patellofemoral dysfunction.

If the client has an advanced case of PFPS, this test can be very painful. The client should contract the quadriceps slowly to reduce pain intensity. One way to determine if a genuine problem exists is to repeat the test several times using different pressure levels each time. The practitioner should begin the testing process with light pressure, gradually increasing pressure each time. If the condition is unilateral, compare the results on the affected side with those of the unaffected side to determine problem severity.

Explanation: As the quadriceps contract, the patella is pulled in a superior direction. Because the knee is already in a position of extension at the start of the test, the greatest degree of superior patella movement is allowed. During the contraction, pressure on the patella pulls on the soft-tissue restraints, such as the retinaculum. This pressure magnifies the effect of the stress caused by the tracking disorder and reproduces the client's pain.

Differential Evaluation

Chondromalacia patellae, meniscal damage, osteochondritis dissecans, complex regional pain syndrome, patellar tendinosis, synovial plica, loose body in the joint.

Suggestions for Treatment

A primary concern in PFPS is improper tracking of the patella due to vastus lateralis tightness. Massage is effective in reducing hypertonicity and helping to achieve a balanced pull on the patella. Techniques such as deep longitudinal stripping, sweeping superficial cross fiber methods, broadening techniques, or active engagement help accomplish this goal.

In addition, strengthening the VMO is an important aspect of treatment. The VMO is most active in the last 15^0–20^0 of extension, and strengthening activities are best performed in this final stage of extension. A combined approach of soft-tissue treatment and strengthening is more effective than either alone.

ILIOTIBIAL BAND FRICTION SYNDROME

Iliotibial band (ITB) friction syndrome is an overuse condition and results from repetitive flexion and extension of the knee in activities such as running, where it is the primary cause of lateral knee pain.[37] Several factors contribute to the problem, including structural deviations in the hip or knee, tightness of the hip muscles, or lack of proper conditioning.

Characteristics

ITB friction syndrome is an overuse condition caused by friction of the ITB over the lateral epicondyle of the femur (Figure 6.22). The iliotibial band is a thickened band of the **fasciae latae**, which is a cylindrical tube of connective tissue encompassing the thigh.[38] The ITB covers the lateral thigh and functions as a long, flat tendon for the distal attachments of the **tensor fasciae latae** and **gluteus maximus muscles**. At its distal end, the band passes over the epicondyle of the femur on the lateral side of the knee.

There is evidence of a **small bursa** between the **ITB** and the **lateral epicondyle** of the femur in some people.[39] Researchers sometimes describe this structure as a separate bursa or in some cases an extension of the knee's joint capsule.[40] Inflammatory activity in the lateral knee is present with ITB friction syndrome and could result from soft-tissue inflammation, but not necessarily an inflamed bursa.[41]

When the knee is in extension, the band lies **anterior** to the **lateral epicondyle** of the femur. At approximately 30^0 of flexion the ITB begins to move across the lateral epicondyle.[42] The **posterior fibers** of the ITB are the first to contact the bony prominence. Thickening of the posterior fibers of the ITB has been observed in some patients.[39] It is not clear if the thickened edge of the band is a cause of the excess friction or a result of it.

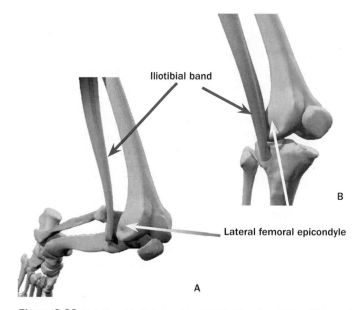

Figure 6.22 Relationship between the iliotibial band and lateral femoral epicondyle with the right knee in flexion (A) and close to full extension (B). (3-D anatomy images courtesy of Primal Pictures Ltd. www.primal-pictures.com).

Several biomechanical factors contribute to ITB friction syndrome. The condition appears in runners, with distance runners particularly affected due to stride mechanics. Sprinters continue to accelerate during their entire running time, while distance runners spend greater time in the weight-bearing phases of the running gait. It is the weight-bearing phase that stresses the ITB.

Excess tension in the ITB is a primary cause of ITB friction syndrome. The ITB is not a contractile tissue and tension in the structure differs from that of muscles. Excess tension in the ITB is due to *hypertonicity* of the **tensor fasciae latae** and **gluteus maximus muscles** that pull on the band. The ITB is under its greatest tension during the first third of the stance phase in running or walking.[43] There is increased tension on the ITB when decelerating the body's momentum, such as walking or running downhill. With greater tension on the ITB, the band is pulled more firmly against the epicondyle.

Genu varum or a **prominent lateral epicondyle** of the femur increase the risk of ITB friction syndrome as the band is pulled taut over the protruding knee structures. The condition develops frequently when a person is running on a sloped surface, such as a beach or the side of the road. The leg that is on the downhill side has a greater varus stress at the knee, increasing ITB friction.

An interesting biomechanical method can be used to confirm ITB irritation. In those with ITB friction syndrome lateral knee pain can be drastically reduced or even eliminated when they walk backwards down the stairs or a steep slope. The quadriceps take the primary role in decelerating motion and even though the knee is moving in flexion and extension the pain will be reduced.

History

The client describes aching pain on the lateral aspect of the knee that increases with activity. Onset is gradual and associated with repetitive flexion and extension of the knee, such as running or cycling. Ask the client about sudden increases in activity prior to symptom onset. If running or walking precipitated the symptoms, determine if there are other risk factors such as running on a sloped surface or excessive distances going downhill. In some cases, there is an audible popping or snapping sensation associated with the pain.

Observation

There are rarely visible signs of ITB friction syndrome. Other biomechanical factors increase the likelihood of developing the problem, such as genu varum.

Palpation

The ITB is tender with palpation near the lateral epicondyle of the femur. The posterior edge of the band may be more painful, as this is the section that first rubs across the bony prominence. Palpate the band with the knee in several positions. In full extension, the band does not lie directly over the epicondyle and is likely to be less tender. Once the knee is past 30^0 of flexion, there is a greater chance of tenderness when the band is palpated (see the Noble compression test below).

Range-of-Motion and Resistance Testing

AROM: Pain is routinely felt with active knee flexion and extension, particularly when the knee is flexed past 30^0. In many cases, pain only presents if active motion is performed while bearing weight.

PROM: Unless the condition is inflamed or severe, pain is not felt with passive motion. If the condition is severe, pain is felt during flexion and extension as the band is rubbed across the lateral epicondyle of the femur.

MRT: MRTs do not tend to aggravate ITB pain, as pain is produced primarily during motion.

Special Tests

Modified Ober Test

The client is side-lying on the treatment table and positioned diagonally so the leg and thigh of the upper side can drop off the back edge of the table. The practitioner brings the client's leg into abduction and hyperextension, then slowly lowers it as far as it will go (Figure 6.23). Make sure the pelvis stays vertically aligned as the leg is dropped or proper tension will not be placed on the ITB. If the leg drops below horizontal, it is considered within normal limits for ITB flexibility. If the leg does not drop below horizontal, then excess tension is evident in the ITB (from gluteus maximus and tensor fasciae latae).

Explanation: While this procedure is not specific for ITB friction syndrome, muscle tightness in the muscles and the associated ITB can be a prominent factor in the condition. In some cases the leg drops only slightly below

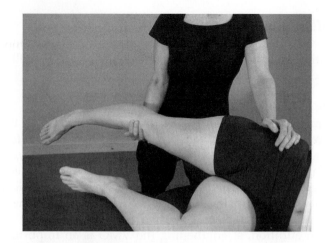

Figure 6.23 Modified Ober test.

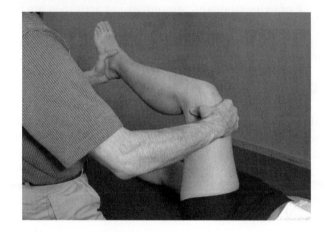

Figure 6.24 Noble compression test.

horizontal, but remains within normal parameters. This mild limitation may still indicate restriction in the ITB and could contribute to the syndrome.

The original Ober test is performed with the knee in 90^0 of flexion rather than full extension. The modified Ober position (pictured) allows greater hip adduction than the original test.[44, 45] An inability to drop the leg below horizontal is more indicative of restriction with the modified version. Because additional hip adduction is possible with the modified Ober position, practitioners should not use the tests interchangeably.

Noble Compression Test

The client is supine with the hip flexed and knee extended (Figure 6.24). The practitioner applies moderate pressure to the ITB just proximal to the lateral epicondyle of the femur with one or both thumbs. Once pressure is applied, the client or the practitioner flexes the client's knee. If pain is felt around 30^0 of flexion there is a good likelihood of ITB friction syndrome.

Explanation: By holding the ITB close to the epicondyle during flexion and extension, the irritated fibers are further compressed, reproducing the client's pain.

Differential Evaluation

Meniscal injury, biceps femoris strain or tendinosis, synovial plica, osteoarthritis, lateral collateral ligament injury, myofascial trigger point pain.

Suggestions for Treatment

Treatment of ITB friction syndrome should focus on reducing the mechanical cause of irritation. In some cases activity modification is sufficient. For example, changing from running on a sloped surface, like the side of the road, to flat ground could reduce symptoms. Massage is beneficial for reducing tightness in the tensor fasciae latae and gluteal muscles that attach to the ITB, and freeing any adhesions between the band and the vastus lateralis.

Some practitioners attempt to address the fiber degeneration in the ITB itself with friction treatments to the primary site of pain and injury near the lateral knee. If this treatment option is chosen, the friction may inflame the synovial pouch directly under the ITB. Further aggravation of this injury can be reduced by maintaining the knee in at least 90⁰ of flexion while friction treatment is performed (notice in Figure 6.22 how the ITB is not directly over the epicondyle when the knee is in flexion). In this way, the underlying bursa or synovial tissue is not pinched against the lateral epicondyle of the femur during treatment.

MENISCAL DAMAGE

Meniscal dysfunction can contribute to various knee pathologies. Due to a poor understanding of their function, it used to be general practice to remove the menisci if there was evidence of damage or degeneration. Now, however, the biomechanical importance of the menisci is well understood and a serious effort is made to preserve proper function of the structure.

Characteristics

Inside the knee there is a **lateral** and **medial meniscus** (plural **menisci**). These fibrocartilage structures disburse weight loads from the **femur** to the **tibia**, as well as provide shock absorbency. The menisci sit directly on top of the **tibial plateau** (Figure 6.25). The medial meniscus is larger and somewhat C-shaped, while the lateral meniscus is the shape of a nearly closed circle. Each meniscus is thicker on its outer edge and increasingly thins toward the middle. Their shape provides a greater area of contact surface for the femoral condyles, increases joint lubrication, reduces friction, and helps guide correct knee mechanics.[46] There is limited blood supply to the menisci, but it is greatest in the peripheral border of each meniscus and poorest toward the center.[5]

The menisci are attached primarily to the tibia by means of several ligaments. The **coronary ligaments** that connect the outer edge of the meniscus to the **tibial plateau** provide the main connection (Figure 6.26). The **medial meniscus** has a fibrous connection to the **medial**

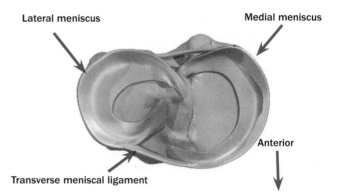

Figure 6.25 Medial and lateral menisci on top of the tibial plateau. (3-D anatomy image courtesy of Primal Pictures Ltd. www.primalpictures.com.)

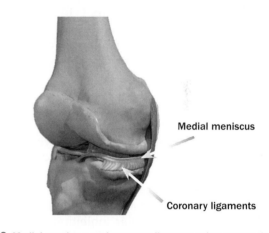

Figure 6.26 Medial meniscus and coronary ligaments that secure the meniscus to the tibia. (3-D anatomy image courtesy of Primal Pictures Ltd. www.primalpictures.com.)

collateral ligament. There is no such connection between the **lateral collateral ligament** and the **lateral meniscus**. There are also attachments between the lateral and medial meniscus, such as the **transverse meniscal ligament** (Figure 6.25). Some muscles play a role in translation of the meniscus during knee motions through indirect attachments.[46, 47]

Meniscal damage is generally caused by excessive compressive loads. Compressive forces in the knee reach 2–3 times body weight during walking and are much greater during running.[5] The importance of the meniscus in shock absorption is illustrated with biomechanical studies that show that loss of the lateral meniscus increases forces on the tibial plateau over 300%.[48]

Due to a heavy load, the meniscus may crack, chip, or tear. In some cases tensile stress on a meniscal attachment, such as that between the MCL and the medial meniscus, will cause the tear. Meniscal damage is usually an acute injury, associated with twisting the knee during a weight-bearing activity such as planting the foot and twisting the body while running.[49] Valgus or varus stresses to the knee that accompany twisting may also cause meniscal damage. Tearing or cracking of the meniscus can cause a loose chunk of cartilage to become dislodged into the joint cavity. The chunk, sometimes referred to as a *joint mouse*, can impair movement by floating around in the joint space and intermittently becoming lodged between the two bones.

History
The client typically reports a sudden movement or activity that caused a sharp pain in the knee. The primary location of pain is generally near the joint line (the articulation between the tibia and femur). A loud pop or click at the moment of injury might have been heard as well. Identify the injury's biomechanical forces to determine what kind of stress (e.g. medial rotation, valgus, etc.) the knee was exposed to at injury. Swelling immediately and for several hours after the injury is likely. The client routinely describes a sensation of locking or buckling in the knee, especially with extension movements, which can be indicative of a loose body of cartilage (joint mouse) in the joint.

Observation
There is little visible evidence of meniscal injury. While swelling accompanies the injury for several hours afterward, it is usually not visible as it is contained within the capsule. Bruising can develop if ligaments or other superficial tissues were torn during the incident, but it is not always visible. If a long-standing meniscal injury has caused reflex muscular inhibition, atrophy may be visible in the quadriceps muscles, particularly the vastus medialis.

Palpation
Meniscal damage ordinarily occurs near the periphery of the meniscus and pain may be elicited by placing pressure on the lateral or medial joint line near the site of the meniscus tear. Sometimes there is tenderness in other muscles of the region due to hypertonicity and reflexive muscle spasm.

Range-of-Motion and Resistance Testing
AROM: Pain is typical during knee flexion or extension. Pain is more common if active motion is performed with resistance and with the individual bearing weight or in a closed-chain position (the distal extremity fixed during motion). If the individual is not weight-bearing or is in an open-chain position during movement, pain is not likely. PROM: Pain is possible during passive motion, but not as prevalent as pain with active weight-bearing movement. It is possible for a loose body of cartilage to move around within the joint capsule and cause a springy block end feel at the end of knee extension or flexion. When performing the evaluation, the end feel may be apparent one moment, and then not when the motion is repeated because the cartilage fragment moved into another position.

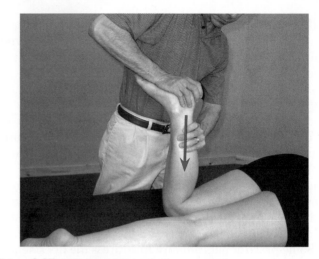
Figure 6.27 Apley compression test.

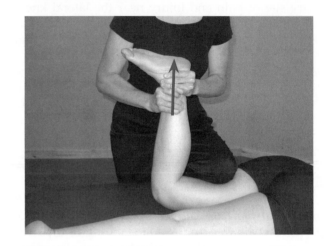
Figure 6.28 Apley distraction test.

MRT: There are no specific findings with MRTs for meniscal damage.

Special Tests
Apley Compression and Distraction Tests
These tests compare pain symptoms produced with compression and distraction. The two procedures place selective stress on different structures. The tests are primarily designed to differentiate between ligamentous damage and meniscal damage. There are two parts: the compression test and the distraction test.

Compression Test
The client is in a prone position on the table with the knee flexed to 90°. The practitioner grasps the client's ankle with one hand and uses the other hand to press down (toward the table) on the heel so the tibia is pressed against the femoral condyles (Figure 6.27). With the knee flexed, there is some rotational capability due to slackening of the ligaments in this position. Once pressure is placed on the tibia, the practitioner gently rotates the tibia through

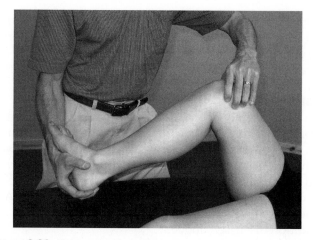

Figure 6.29 McMurray test. In this picture the knee is being extended after having been initially rotated.

its full range of motion both medially and laterally. Make sure the rotational force is directed toward the knee and not toward the foot/ankle complex. Note whether this motion causes pain or discomfort and then proceed to the distraction test.

Distraction Test

The client is in the same starting position as for the compression test. The practitioner places a knee on the client's posterior thigh to stabilize it against the table, then uses both hands to pull the client's leg so that it is distracted (lifted) from the femoral condyles (Figure 6.28). Once the distraction force is applied, the practitioner gently rotates the tibia through its full range of motion both medially and laterally. Make sure the rotational force is directed to the knee and does not twist the foot/ankle region. Note whether this motion causes pain or discomfort.

Explanation: Pain in the compression test means either ligamentous or meniscal damage, as the ligaments are being twisted and the menisci compressed. If there is pain with the compression test, but no pain with the distraction test, meniscal tissues are likely the source of pain because the ligaments are being twisted in both tests, but the menisci are not compressed in the distraction test. If there is pain with both the compression and distraction tests, and the pain is similar in each test, it is expected that the ligaments are at fault because they are the only tissues stressed in both cases.

McMurray Test

The McMurray test also tests the medial and lateral meniscus and has several variations. The following is one of the most common variations and is easier to perform than the others. The test has two maneuvers. The first tests the lateral meniscus; the second, tests the medial meniscus.

The client is supine on the table with the knee fully flexed so the heel comes as close to the buttock as possible. The practitioner has one hand cupping the client's heel and the other hand grasping the medial and lateral

joint line of the knee. The tibia is medially rotated as far as possible (Figure 6.29). A slight degree of valgus stress is sometimes added to this position.

Once in full medial rotation the client's knee is extended until it is completely straight either actively by the client or passively by the practitioner. If pain, popping, or snapping sensations occur during this motion, it is likely that there is a problem with the meniscus. When the leg is medially rotated, particularly with additional valgus stress, problems with the lateral meniscus are more evident.

To test the medial meniscus, the same starting position is used. The knee is fully flexed and then laterally rotated. A slight degree of varus stress is sometimes added to this position. Once the knee is laterally rotated, fully extend the knee to evaluate pain, popping, or snapping symptoms.

Explanation: In this procedure the tibia is rotated against the femoral condyles in order to evaluate the edge of the meniscus for a torn piece of cartilage. When the femoral condyles rub over the torn or chipped cartilage it often produces a snapping sensation and may produce pain. By fully rotating the tibia (both medially and laterally) and then extending the leg, pressure is applied against much of the outer rim of the menisci where tears develop with the greatest frequency.

Differential Evaluation

Sprain to the ACL, PCL, or MCL, patellar tendinosis, synovial plica, osteoarthritis, myofascial trigger point pain, osteochondritis dissecans, loose fragments in knee.

Suggestions for Treatment

Meniscal damage sometimes resolves on its own, depending on what region of the meniscus is damaged. Massage therapy is not indicated as a direct treatment for meniscal damage; no techniques enhance the healing of damaged cartilage tissue. Soft-tissue therapy can be used as an adjunct treatment for the resultant muscle spasm and biomechanical dysfunction that develop along with other pathologies in the region.

PATELLAR TENDINOSIS

Most overuse tendon disorders result from collagen degeneration in the tendon and are not inflammatory conditions.[50-53] *Tendinosis* is the term used to describe these conditions. *Patellar tendinosis*, also called *jumper's knee*, is a prevalent injury in the athletic population, particularly with those engaged in vigorous running or jumping activities. The strong eccentric load placed on the quadriceps tendon during landing from a jump often causes this condition and is the reason it is known as *jumper's knee*.

Characteristics

The **patellar tendon** is the distal attachment tendon for the **quadriceps femoris** group. The patella is imbedded

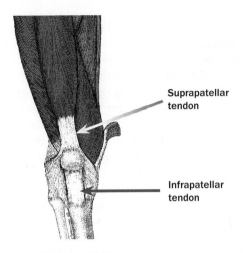

Figure 6.30 Anterior view of the knee showing the supra- and infrapatellar portions of the patellar tendon. (Mediclip image copyright, 1998 Williams & Wilkins. All rights reserved.).

within the patellar tendon dividing the tendon into an upper and lower section (Figure 6.30). The upper section is called the **suprapatellar tendon** and the lower section, the **infrapatellar tendon**. The lower section is sometimes erroneously identified as the **patellar ligament** because the fibers pass from the patella to the tibia, connecting bone to bone. The patella is imbedded within the tendon, making it structurally, functionally, and physiologically tendon tissue.

Tendinosis occurs in either the suprapatellar or infrapatellar tendon. The condition appears in order of frequency at the infrapatellar tendon's insertion into the patella (65% of cases), the attachment of the suprapatellar tendon into the patella (25% of cases), and the patellar tendon insertion into the tibial tuberosity (10% of cases).[54,55] Dysfunction with the infrapatellar portion of the tendon accounts for 75% of all cases. If the tendinosis is not properly managed, a complete rupture of the tendon can result.[56]

The primary function of the patella is to improve the quadriceps' angle of pull on the tibia. As a result, the tendon transmits high force loads to the tibia. **When these loads are applied repetitively, collagen degeneration within the tendon can result.**[57]

Tendinosis is more likely to develop if the tendon is already under some degree of stress. Long periods of activity stress the tendon and fatigue eventually leads to collagen breakdown. Collagen degeneration develops with sudden bouts of activity for which the individual did not properly train. Certain biomechanical factors such as *genu valgum* or *varum, abnormal Q angle,* or *patellar instability* can contribute to the condition.[53] The degree of severity of the condition is determined by the quality of pain. Pain arises in distinct stages, progressing from least to most problematic. First, pain is felt only after activity. Next, pain starts at the beginning of activity, dissipates after warm-up, and recurs with fatigue. As the condition

worsens, pain becomes prolonged and takes place during and after activity, with increasing difficulty in performing at a satisfactory level. Finally, complete rupture of the infrapatellar tendon occurs, requiring surgical repair.[56]

History
The client usually describes a repetitive activity involving strong quadriceps contractions, such as running or jumping, prior to the onset of symptoms. Anterior knee pain is the primary symptom. Because both the suprapatellar and infrapatellar portions of the tendon are superficial, the client can generally locate the specific site of pain. Ask about pain levels in regard to the stages of pain and the condition discussed above.

Observation
Tendinosis is not an inflammatory problem and there are no visible signs of the condition. If the condition is chronic, it is possible that quadriceps atrophy might result from reflex muscular inhibition.

Palpation
Pain and tenderness exist with palpation throughout the entire tendon, but are exaggerated near the inferior pole of the patella where the infrapatellar tendon fibers meet the border of the patella. Palpation can cause referred pain sensations deeper in the knee as well.

Range-of-Motion and Resistance Testing
AROM: Pain is felt near the end range of knee flexion as the involved tendon is stretched. There may be pain with extension, if the load placed on the tendon during the evaluation is severe enough. For example, if the tendinosis is mild and active extension is performed in a non-weight-bearing position, it rarely causes pain. If the tendinosis is advanced and active movement is performed against greater resistance, pain is customary.
PROM: Pain is felt near the end range of knee flexion as the involved tendon is stretched. Pain is proportional to the severity of the condition. Knee extension does not cause discomfort as tensile stress is taken off the tendon during passive extension.
MRT: Resisted knee extension elicits the client's pain.

Differential Evaluation
ACL or PCL sprain, osteochondritis dissecans, meniscal injuries, Osgood-Schlatter disease, patellar injury or dislocation, synovial plica, osteoarthritis, myofascial trigger point pain, loose fragments in the knee, PFPS, pes anserine bursitis, irritation of infrapatellar fat pad.

Suggestions for Treatment
Rest from offending activities is a crucial treatment for tendinosis. Because rebuilding the damaged collagen fibers can take a long time, it is important to keep stress off the tendon for some time after it is no longer symptomatic. It is valuable to reduce tightness in the quadriceps

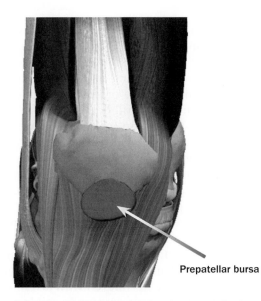

Prepatellar bursa

Figure 6.31 Anterior view of the knee showing the prepatellar bursa. (3-D anatomy image courtesy of Primal Pictures Ltd. www.primalpictures. com.)

group with massage and stretching. Using deep friction massage to stimulate fibroblast activity is important to help rebuild collagen. In some cases, ice applications are used in conjunction with massage to reduce pain associated with the condition or with treatment.

PREPATELLAR BURSITIS

Prepatellar bursitis **is usually caused by direct compression of the bursa, but other systemic conditions can cause an inflammatory reaction in the bursa.** This is a moderately widespread occupational injury, especially for those who spend long periods working on their knees. Due to its occurrence in people who do a great deal of cleaning activities, the condition is also known as *housemaid's knee.*

Characteristics
The body has more than 150 bursae designed to reduce friction between adjacent structures. One of the most superficial and prominent of these is the **prepatellar bursa,** lying just underneath the skin and directly on top of the **patella** (Figure 6.31). There are numerous bursae in and around the knee joint. Irritation and inflammation to any of these bursae constitutes bursitis of the knee, but prepatellar bursitis is the most common.[58]

There are three basic types of bursitis, each of which can affect the prepatellar bursa: **acute, chronic non-septic,** and **chronic infected.** The most common is the chronic non-septic variation. Acute prepatellar bursitis results from a direct blow to the knee causing inflammation, which gradually subsides with time. This is the least problematic form of bursitis as it is tied to one particular event. With no further aggravation, the inflamed bursa recovers on its own.

Chronic non-septic bursitis also develops from mechanical compression, although not from a single incident but from frequent compression. This form of bursitis affects individuals who perform occupational activities requiring long periods of work on their knees. For example, it is prevalent among carpet layers, airline luggage handlers, and gardeners. The bursa is irritated by repeated mechanical compression, but avoiding the activities that cause compression may not be easy. The severity of the condition progresses in this case.

Chronic infection of the bursa can also cause prepatellar bursitis. The bursa becomes inflamed and swollen, but the infection usually arises in the absence of trauma. Previous trauma can precede the infectious variation in some cases. Infections develop in the bursa from a number of systemic disorders or from cuts in the skin where the bursa gets exposed to outside infectious agents.[59, 60] Chronic infectious bursitis might develop from crystal deposits due to *gout* or *rheumatoid arthritis.*[58]

History
The client reports pain and other signs of inflammation in the anterior knee region such as redness, swelling, puffiness, difficulty in walking, or increased local heat. Ask questions in the interview process that establish whether the onset is acute or chronic. Ask about the client's occupation or activities where there are long periods of compression on the knee, such as roofing, plumbing, carpet laying, or house cleaning. If there is no mechanical trauma to the area, ask the client if a physician has been consulted to evaluate the presence of an infectious agent.

Observation
There is a prominent visible enlargement under the skin, directly over the patella. The size of the bump is dependent on the extent of the bursitis. The more inflamed the bursa, the larger the bump on the patella. Swelling in the area can produce a bump the size of a golf ball.

BOX 6.4 CLINICAL NOTES

Swelling in the knee

Prepatellar bursitis and Baker's cysts are inflammatory conditions that produce swelling around the knee. However, there are other causes of knee joint inflammation. It is important to consider other possible causes of swelling when making a thorough examination.

In some injuries, such as cruciate ligament sprains, swelling may be within the joint capsule and harder to detect in physical examination. Other injuries such as external ligament sprains, meniscal damage, gout, infection, patellar dislocation, or a host of systemic disorders can produce swelling around the knee that is more easily palpable.

Palpation

Because the inflamed bursa lies directly under the skin and is richly innervated, pressure is painful. Tenderness varies with an individual's pain tolerance or the severity of the bursitis, but the anterior knee is generally very tender when palpated. Excess fluid accumulation in the region is also palpable. Heat is usually felt when the hand is placed close to or on the knee. Crepitation might be palpated during range-of-motion evaluation.

Range-of-Motion and Resistance Testing

AROM: Pain may be felt during knee flexion as the skin over the bursa is pulled taut, increasing compression on the inflamed bursa.
PROM: The same principles apply as for passive motion.
MRT: Pain with MRTs is unlikely as no muscles place pressure on the bursa during isometric contraction.

Differential Evaluation

Sprain to the ACL or PCL, osteochondritis dissecans, meniscal injuries, osteoarthritis, pes anserine bursitis, quadriceps rupture, rheumatoid arthritis.

Suggestions for Treatment

Anti-inflammatory medications are usually prescribed for the inflamed bursa, particularly if the primary cause is mechanical compression. Antibiotic agents are used to treat infectious varieties. In chronic non-septic variations, the best treatment is to remove or reduce the aggravating compressive loads. For example, if there is an occupational activity that is causing pressure on the bursa, limiting (or eliminating) the time the client is on the knees is essential. Massage should not be applied directly to the inflamed bursa as there is no benefit and it is detrimental.

BAKER'S CYST

The majority of *Baker's (popliteal) Cysts* are benign, but can cause pain and are frequently an indication of other pathologies. These fluid-filled cysts cause pain and discomfort in the posterior knee region.

Characteristics

The Baker's cyst is the most common mass to develop in the **popliteal** region.[61] **The cyst appears as a small pouch or cyst on the posterior side of the joint capsule that collects excess fluid** (Figure 6.32). The sac is located directly behind the **medial femoral condyle,** between the medial head of the **gastrocnemius muscle** and the **semimembranosus tendon**. A one-way valve at the opening allows fluid to pass from the knee joint into the cyst.

The assumed function of the valve is that it allows fluid to escape the knee joint in order to minimize pressure on sensitive structures within the joint.[61, 62] As fluid accumulates, the cyst can press on nerves or vascular tissues in the popliteal region and produce pain. For example, the cyst could compress the **sciatic nerve** and cause neurological symptoms in the leg. The cyst may press on the **popliteal artery** and **vein** and produce vascular symptoms in the lower leg such as coldness in the feet, discoloration, or problems with swelling in the foot or leg due to poor venous return. Presence of the cyst can also prevent or cause discomfort with full flexion or possibly extension.

Baker's cysts develop for a number of reasons, but a clear cause is not always evident. They can result from conditions such as *rheumatoid arthritis, gout, meniscal tears, cruciate ligament tears,* or *osteochondritis dissecans,* with *osteoarthritis* producing the largest majority of cysts.[63] The probability of a Baker's cyst developing is increased as the number and extent of damaged tissues increases.[64]

Baker's cysts are more prevalent in older people due to the increased incidence of osteoarthritis. An exception is Baker's cysts in children with juvenile rheumatoid arthritis. When the cysts develop in children, they resolve faster than those in their adult counterparts.

Complications can develop with the cysts, such as rupture and fluid leakage into the posterior calf; other complications include *deep vein thrombosis, pulmonary embolism, infection, posterior compartment syndrome,* and *trapped calcified bodies.* [61]

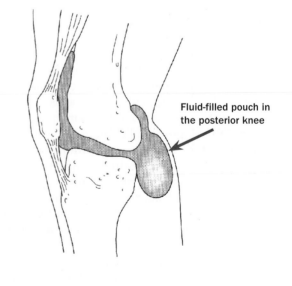

Fluid-filled pouch in the posterior knee

Figure 6.32 Medial view of the knee showing a Baker's cyst in the posterior knee region. (Used with permission from Magee D. Orthopedic Physical Assessment. 3rd ed. Philadelphia: W.B. Saunders; 1997.)

History

The client usually describes a feeling of fullness in the popliteal region and may report catching, popping, or locking of the knee. A recent knee trauma or inflammatory condition, such as arthritis, is sometimes reported. Inquire about symptoms such as paresthesia, numbness, coldness, or sensations of swelling that indicate pressure on neurovascular structures. The client reports the greatest discomfort when flexing the knee.

Observation

A Baker's cyst produces a large mass on the posterior medial aspect of the knee. A lump may be evident just below the skin. The cyst may not be large enough to be visible, but other symptoms could indicate its presence. It is important to have a physician confirm the cyst with a high-tech diagnostic procedure, such as MRI, ultrasound, or arthrography.

Palpation

The Baker's cyst is a palpable nodule or mass on the posterior-medial aspect of the knee. The client may feel pain when the mass is palpated, but not always. The cyst is filled with fluid and is likely to have a puffy feeling. Use caution when palpating the cyst. Pressing too firmly may cause damage as the one-way valve at the connection with the joint capsule does not permit fluid to flow back into the joint capsule. Too much pressure could also cause the cyst to rupture.

Range-of-Motion and Resistance Testing

AROM: Pain in the posterior knee can be felt with active motion, especially in flexion. The cyst is further compressed when the knee moves into flexion. In some cases pain does not present, but the client perceives an obstruction to movement. There may be limitation in extension of the knee, but this is not common.
PROM: The same principles apply as for passive motion.
MRT: No pain results from an MRT because further pressure or irritation is not placed on the cyst from resisted isometric contractions.

Differential Evaluation

Deep vein thrombosis, popliteal artery aneurysm, soft-tissue tumors, septic arthritis, hemorrhage, tear of distal hamstrings or proximal gastrocnemius attachments, meniscal injury, ACL or PCL sprain.

Suggestions for Treatment

Baker's cysts are usually treated with cold applications and anti-inflammatory medications. If the underlying pathology is addressed, the cyst generally resolves on its own. Needle aspiration can be attempted, but the fluid within the cyst is often too thick to be aspirated. Massage is contraindicated for this problem as further compression of the cyst aggravates the situation. Lymphatic drainage approaches can be helpful as the cyst begins to subside.

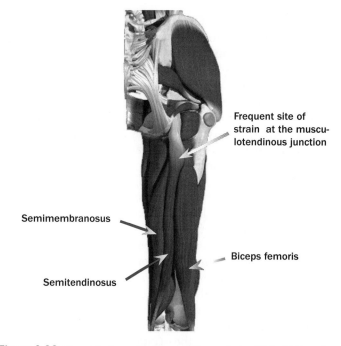

Figure 6.33 Hamstring muscle group on the posterior thigh. (3-D anatomy image courtesy of Primal Pictures Ltd. www.primalpictures.com.)

HAMSTRING STRAIN

Muscle strains can develop in several muscles around the knee, but are particularly common in the hamstrings. The hamstrings are a powerful muscle group that plays fundamental roles in locomotion and maintaining static postures, making them more vulnerable to *hamstring strains*.

Characteristics

A hamstring strain, also called a *pulled hamstring*, **involves a tear in the muscle-tendon unit of any of the three hamstring muscles** and are predominantly an acute injury. The hamstrings are composed of the **semimembranosus, semitendinosus**, and **biceps femoris muscles** on the posterior thigh (Figure 6.33). With the exception of the short head of the biceps femoris, the proximal attachments are on the **ischial tuberosity**. The concentrated tensile stress at the conjoined tendon makes the musculotendinous junction of these muscles the primary site for injury.

The structural and biomechanical demands placed on the hamstrings are one reason strains develop in this muscle group with greater frequency than strains to other lower extremity muscles. With the exception of the short head of the biceps femoris, the hamstrings are **multiarticulate muscles** (meaning they cross more than one joint), making them susceptible to muscle strain. Other factors contribute to strains as well, including lack of flexibility, muscle fatigue, insufficient warm-up, and strength imbalances between the hamstrings and quadriceps.[67, 68] Once a hamstring strain has occurred, the individual is prone to re-injury. Chronic shortening from previous injuries makes future strains more likely.[65, 66]

The **biceps femoris** is the muscle most often injured, although one of its heads is not multi-articulate.[69] A possible reason for frequent biceps femoris injuries may be the muscle's **dual innervation**.[70] The muscle's long and short heads eventually blend together at their distal attachment. Yet the long head is innervated by the **tibial division** of the sciatic nerve and the short head by the **peroneal division**. The different innervation signals sometimes cause impairments to proper neurological coordination and lead to strain. In addition, because the biceps femoris is a shorter muscle, its limited flexibility could cause it to sustain strain injuries first.

Adverse neural tension in the sciatic nerve also plays a part in the onset of hamstring strains.[71] Increases in neural tension cause elevated levels of sympathetic nervous system activity, which produces greater muscle tonus and can lead to further injury. Fibrous adhesions or scar tissue in the hamstring muscles from a previous strain can restrict mobility of the sciatic nerve and increase its irritation. A vicious cycle of neural tension and hamstring strain then develops.[72]

Hamstring strains are routine in runners, dancers, or others performing lower extremity activities requiring long strides. Due to the multi-articulate nature of the hamstrings, they are under high eccentric load at the very end of the **swing-through phase** of gait. It is at this point that hamstring strains can occur. In some cases, the strain results from high tensile loads during maximal contraction, which is the type of force experienced during sprinting.[73] In other cases, even if performed slowly a maximal stretch can produce a tear.

History

The client reports sudden pain associated with an activity that overwhelmed the hamstrings. A loud popping or snapping sound might be heard at the point of injury. Mild to severe pain is reported with the injury, with pain decreasing after the initial trauma. Have the client describe the mechanics of the activity as clearly as possible. Ask the client about previous strains, as recurrent hamstring strains are common. Ask about sensations of tightness or restriction in the posterior thigh muscles.

Observation

Depending on the severity of the injury, the client may be limping or walking with some degree of impairment. If the strain is in a highly vascularized region of the muscle, bruising is to be expected and can appear worse several days after the initial injury. Disrupted capillaries leak blood into the interstitial spaces. Gravity eventually pulls that blood toward the feet and the bruised area increases in size and appears to run down the posterior thigh. In some cases swelling from the injury site is visible, but generally not. If there is a severe hamstring injury, a defect in the continuity of the muscle may be visible.

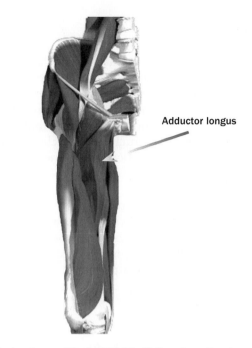

Adductor longus

Figure 6.34 Adductor group of the inner thigh. (3-D anatomy image courtesy of Primal Pictures Ltd. www.primalpictures.com.)

Palpation

The hamstrings are likely to be hypertonic due to reflexive muscle spasm, with exaggerated tenderness near the site of the tissue tearing. Depending on injury severity, there may be a palpable defect in the muscle that feels like an indentation or disruption in the continuity of the fibers.

Range-of-Motion and Resistance Testing

AROM: Active motion is limited in hip flexion with knee extension, as the damaged fibers are stretched. Tensile stress on the site of the injury causes pain and typically produces a reflexive tightening of the muscle as well. There may be pain with active flexion depending on the amount of resistance. For example in a mild strain, the active motion of lifting the leg off the floor by flexing the knee from a standing position may not require enough resistance to cause pain.

PROM: As with active motion, pain results from stretching the hamstrings in hip flexion and knee extension. Pain is possible with passive knee flexion, but not generally expected.

MRT: Pain is felt with resisted knee flexion as it recruits the hamstrings in active contraction. The severity of the pain is proportional to the injury. Weakness compared to the other side during the MRT is expected because the muscle is functionally impaired. Palpating the site of injury during the MRT elicits greater tenderness.

Differential Evaluation

Lumbar radiculopathy, myofascial trigger point pain, tensile stress injury to sciatic nerve, tendon avulsion (especially at ischial tuberosity), piriformis syndrome.

Box 6.5 Clinical Notes

What about quadriceps strains?

The quadriceps are a powerful muscle group on the anterior thigh. In the process of locomotion they produce strong contractile forces to extend the knee, allowing us to jump, walk, run and stand up from a deep-knee position.

Despite the high force loads on the muscle group, strains to the quadriceps are not as common as those to the hamstrings. Quadriceps strains are less common because the quadriceps are much stronger than the hamstrings, giving them a greater resistance to the tensile overload that produces a strain. The quadriceps (with the exception of rectus femoris) also cross only one joint, whereas the hamstrings cross two. Crossing multipe joints makes a muscle more susceptible to strain. When quadriceps strains do occur, they are most common in the rectus femoris, the one quadriceps muscle that crosses two joints.

Suggestions for Treatment

There are two major goals for treating hamstring strains. It is important to address the hypertonicity in the hamstring muscle group with general relaxation massage techniques. Proper tone must return to the muscle for adequate healing. The damaged tissue site should also be treated. Deep friction massage to the injury site is the best strategy for developing a healthy and functional scar. This treatment can only be performed after the initial inflammatory stage has subsided. Stretching methods integrated with massage will assist in preventing future strains.

ADDUCTOR STRAINS

Although the adductors act primarily on the hip joint, *adductor strains* are addressed in this chapter because the adductors are considered thigh muscles. Adductor strains are relatively common in the athletic community and are called *groin pulls*. Due to their proximity to the genital area, respect for the individual's privacy during assessment and treatment is essential. The practitioner is advised to use extra caution and very clear communication about therapeutic intentions, so the client feels comfortable with the evaluation and treatment process. Proper draping methods are imperative.

Characteristics

There are five primary adductor muscles: **adductor magnus, brevis,** and **longus, and the pectineus** and **gracilis**. The muscles originate from the **pubis** and insert on the **femur**, with the exception of gracilis which inserts on the medial tibia. Their primary action is to pull the femur into adduction. The majority of adductor strains occur at the proximal musculotendinous junction near the pubis, with very few involving the muscle belly or distal musculotendinous junctions. Of the five adductors, the **adductor longus** is the most frequently strained (Figure 6.34).[74] The region of adductor attachments on the pubis has a poor blood supply as well as rich innervation. This may explain in part the slower healing time and strong pain sensations associated with adductor strains.[75]

Similar to other muscle strains, adductor strains are caused by strong eccentric forces on the muscle. For example, these injuries are common in soccer when one player is running to kick the ball with the instep of the foot and another player blocks the kick. The momentum of the first player's body and the blocked leg causes a sudden eccentric load on the adductors. Sudden changes in direction while running can put high tensile loads on the adductor muscles. Adductor strains also result from sudden resistance to abduction, such as slipping on the ice with the legs going in separate directions. Some of the primary factors that lead to muscle strains are lack of flexibility, poor conditioning, inadequate warm-up, and fatigue.[76] In particular, improper flexibility is a primary factor because the adductors aren't emphasized as much as other major muscles of the lower extremity such as the hamstrings and quadriceps during regular stretching activities.

The largest number of strains are acute injuries and are directly attributable to a single incident of over stressing the muscle. However, high force loads are not always required to produce the injury. Strains can develop from low level tensile stress to a fatigued muscle. In addition, muscles that have been previously injured are limited in their pliability, making them increasingly susceptible to future strain injury. Chronic strains are familiar in the adductor group.

History

The client reports an instance of sudden overload on the adductor muscles, which is accompanied by sharp pain at the site of the muscle tear. The large majority of strains appear at the musculotendinous junction and the client typically reports the primary region of pain near the groin as opposed to farther down the medial thigh. Pain ranges from mild to severe depending on the extent of the injury. If the strain is chronic as opposed to acute, pain may be described as a dull ache rather than a sharp pain.

Observation

Gait disturbances may be evident depending on the severity of the strain. Alterations in gait are evident during the swing-through phase because the adductors are most active during this period. Turning and pivoting on a weight-bearing leg can cause irritation of the torn adductor fibers and therefore produce a visible compensation pattern. In some cases swelling or bruising is visible, but generally not.

Palpation

Use clear communication and the cautions advised in the introduction prior to palpating this area. Hypertonicity in the adductors is usually palpable. The proximal tendons are short and therefore pain is felt when the muscle is palpated near the attachments on the pubis. Depending on the severity of the injury, there may be a palpable defect in the muscle that feels like an indentation or disruption in the continuity of the fibers. The defect is more characteristic when the tear is located in the fibers of the muscle belly, rather than in the musculotendinous junction.

Range-of-Motion and Resistance Testing

AROM: Pain is felt near the end of abduction as the damaged fibers are stretched. In some cases there is pain with active adduction, if performed against resistance. For example if the client lies on the affected side and attempts to adduct the leg, the resistance of gravity is such that pain can be felt with active motion even with a mild strain. Due to accessory actions of the adductors, some pain is generally felt with hip flexion.

PROM: Pain develops with passive abduction near the end range as the damaged fibers are stretched. Some pain periodically occurs at the end range of hip extension.

MRT: Pain that reproduces the primary complaint is felt with resisted adduction.

Differential Evaluation

Hernia, iliopsoas or rectus femoris strain, iliopsoas bursitis, stress fractures, avulsion fractures, femoral nerve compression, snapping hip syndrome, chronic prostatitis, osteitis pubis, urological disorders, sacroiliac dysfunction, gastrointestinal disorders.

Suggestions for Treatment

See the treatment description for hamstring strains and apply these principles to the adductor group. Attention is focused on reducing hypertonicity in the muscle group and addressing torn fibers at the site of the injury. Use clear communication, proper draping, and the cautions advised in the introduction prior to treating this area.

GENERAL NEUROMUSCULAR DISORDERS

In many cases, soft-tissue dysfunctions are not given a specific name. Adequate assessment is required to determine the tissues most likely involved and to take into account pathologies that may or may not have specific titles. Chapter 4 provides a discussion of the pathological processes of hypertonicity, myofascial trigger points, muscle strains, nerve compression and tension, tendinosis, tenosynovitis, ligament sprains, and osteoarthritis in any region of the body. Chapter 4 also includes the history, observation, palpation, relevant tests, and treatment suggestions sections for these conditions. The principles are the same for these conditions wherever they occur in the body.

Included in this section are specific tables and graphics for the knee and thigh, including dermatomes, cutaneous innervation, trigger point referral patterns, and findings for MRTs. Nerve compression or tension pathologies

produce symptoms in the knee and thigh from either a lumbar radiculopathy (spinal nerve root compression) or a peripheral neuropathy (peripheral lower extremity nerve injury). There are only a few locations in the proximal lower extremity where peripheral neuropathies develop. Other regions where nerve compression occurs near the knee and thigh are listed in Box 6.6.

Sensory symptoms from a lumbar radiculopathy may be felt in the proximal or distal lower extremity and are experienced within the dermatome associated with that nerve root (Figure 6.35). Sensory symptoms of peripheral neuropathy are felt in the region of cutaneous innervation for the nerve affected (Figure 6.36). Radiculopathies or peripheral neuropathies can cause motor dysfunction and produce weakness in the muscles innervated by the affected nerve (Box 6.7).

Muscular hypertonicity develops in the proximal lower extremity as a result of repetitive stress. As a result of chronic muscular tension, myofascial trigger points can develop in the affected muscle(s). Myofascial trigger points refer pain or characteristic neurological sensations to various regions of the knee and thigh. Common myofascial trigger point referral patterns for the major muscles in this region are shown in Figure 6.37.

Box: 6.6 REGIONS OF POSSIBLE NERVE ENTRAPMENT

Peroneal nerve
Near the fibular head

Sciatic nerve
Adjacent to the piriformis muscle

Femoral nerve
Underneath the inguinal ligament

Lateral femoral cutaneous nerve
Underneath the inguinal ligament

Posterior femoral cutaneous nerve
Adjacent to the piriformis muscle

Superior gluteal nerve
Adjacent to the piriformis muscle

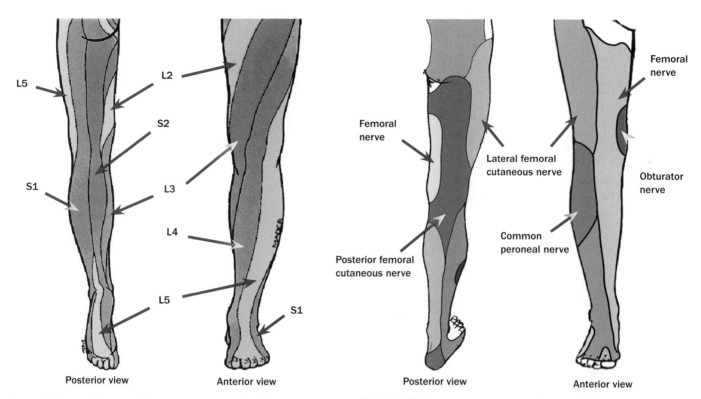

Figure 6.35 Dermatomes of the lower extremity (Mediclip image copyright, 1998 Williams & Wilkins. All rights reserved).

Figure 6.36 Cutaneous innervation of the proximal lower extremity.

Box: 6.7 Innervation of Distal Lower Extremity Muscles

Femoral Nerve
- Rectus femoris
- Vastus lateralis
- Vastus medialis
- Vastus intermedius
- Pectineus

Sciatic Nerve (Tibial Division)
- Biceps femoris (long head)
- Semimembranosus
- Semitendinosus
- Adductor magnus (inferior fibers)

Sciatic Nerve (Peroneal Division)
- Biceps femoris (short head)

Obturator Nerve
- Adductor longus
- Adductor brevis
- Gracilis
- Adductor magnus (superior, middle fibers)
- Obturator externus

Table 1 Joints, Associated Motions, Planes of Motion in Anatomical Position, Axis of Rotation, and Average ROM

Joint	Motion	Plane of Motion	Axis of Rotation	Avg. ROM (degrees)
Knee	Flexion	Sagittal	Medial-Lateral	135
	Extension	Sagittal	Medial-Lateral	0-10

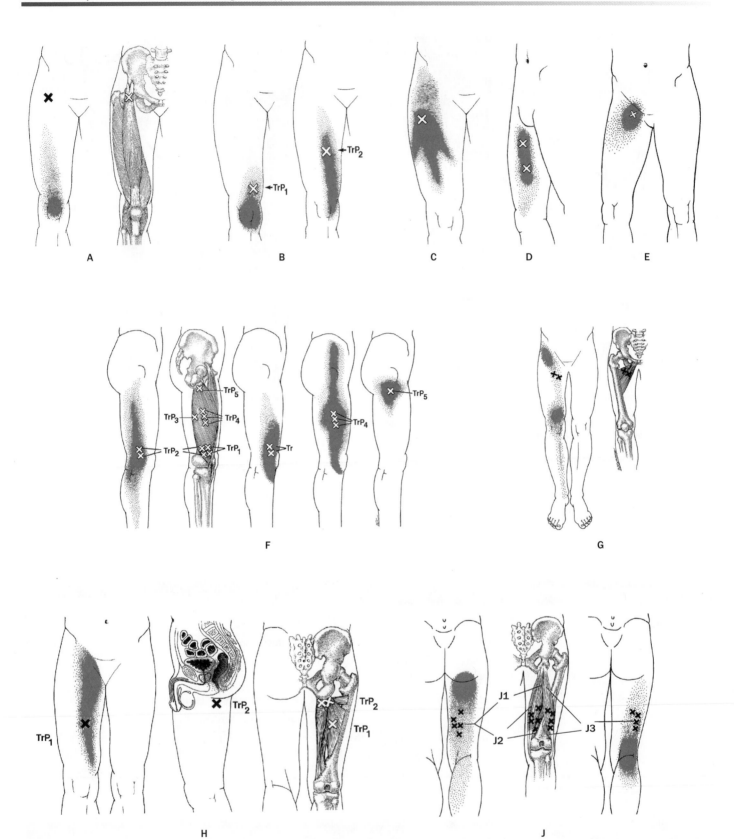

Figure 6.37 Myofascial trigger point referral patterns: Rectus Femoris (A), Vastus medialis (B), Vastus intermedius (C), Gracilis (D), Pectineus (E), Vastus lateralis (F), Adductor longus and brevis (G), Adductor magnus (H), Semitendinosus (J1), Semimembranosus (J2), Biceps femoris (J3). (Images courtesy of Mediclip, copyright 1998 Williams & Wilkins. All rights reserved).

TABLE 2 WEAKNESS WITH MANUAL RESISTIVE TEST AND POSSIBLE NERVE INVOLVEMENT

Muscle	Resisted Action	Possible Nerve Involvement if Action Weak
Semimembranosus	Knee flexion	Tibial division of sciatic nerve (L5 - S2)
Semitendinosus	Knee flexion	Tibial division of sciatic nerve (L5 - S2)
Biceps femoris (long head)	Knee flexion	Tibial division of sciatic nerve (L5 - S2)
Biceps femoris (short head)	Knee flexion	Peroneal division of sciatic nerve (L5 - S2)
Rectus femoris	Knee extension	Femoral nerve (L2 - L4)
Vastus intermedius	Knee extension	Femoral nerve (L2 - L4)
Vastus lateralis	Knee extension	Femoral nerve (L2 - L4)
Vastus medialis	Knee extension	Femoral nerve (L2 - L4)

Reference Table for Condition Assessment

This table lists a number of pathological conditions along the left-hand column. The top of the table lists common evaluation procedures. A ◆ in the box associated with a pathological condition and an evaluation procedure indicates the procedure is commonly used to identify that pathology. A ● in the box associated with the condition and a range-of-motion or resistance test, indicates pain is likely with that test for that pathology. Conditions are listed alphabetically.

TABLE 3 REFERENCE TABLE FOR CONDITION ASSESSMENT

	AROM	PROM	MRT	Anterior drawer test	Apley compression test	Apley's distraction test	Clarke's sign	Gravity drawer test	Lachman test	McMurray test	Noble compression test	Ober (modified) test	Patellar mobility test	Posterior drawer test	Valgus stress test	Varus stress test
ACL Sprain	●			◆					◆							
Adductor Strain	●	●	●													
Baker's Cyst	●	●														
Hamstring Strain	●	●	●													
ITB Friction Syndrome	●										◆	◆				
LCL Sprain	●															◆
MCL Sprain	●														◆	
Meniscal Damage	●				◆	◆				◆						
Muscular Hypertonicity	●	●														
Nerve Compression & Tension	●	●														
Patellar Tendinosis		●	●													
PCL Sprain	●							◆						◆		
PFPS	●						◆						◆			
Prepatellar Bursitis																

References

1. Soderberg G. Kinesiology: Application to Pathological Motion. Baltimore: Williams & Wilkins; 1986.
2. Magee D. Orthopedic Physical Assessment. 3rd ed. Philadelphia: W.B. Saunders; 1997.
3. Stevens PM, Holmstrom MC. Genu Valgum, Pediatrics. eMedicine. March 16, 2005. Available at: www.emedicine.com. Accessed April 24, 2005.
4. Zayer M. Long-term results after physiological genu varum. J Pediatr Orthop B. Oct 2000;9(4):271-277.
5. Neumann DA. Kinesiology of the Musculoskeletal System. St. Louis: Mosby; 2002.
6. Fulkerson JP. Diagnosis and treatment of patients with patellofemoral pain. Am J Sports Med. May-Jun 2002;30(3):447-456.
7. DeOrio M, DeOrio J. Blount Disease. eMedicine. March 15, 2005. Available at: www.emedicine.com. Accessed September 19, 2005.
8. Hinterwimmer S, von Eisenhart-Rothe R, Siebert M, Welsch F, Vogl T, Graichen H. Patella kinematics and patello-femoral contact areas in patients with genu varum and mild osteoarthritis. Clin Biomech (Bristol, Avon). Aug 2004;19(7):704-710.
9. Kapandji IA. The Physiology of the Joints: Volume 2- Lower Limb. Vol 2. 5th ed. Edinburgh: Churchill Livingstone; 1987.
10. Loudon JK, Goist HL, Loudon KL. Genu recurvatum syndrome. J Orthop Sports Phys Ther. May 1998;27(5):361-367.
11. Isakov E, Mizrahi J, Onna I, Susak Z. The control of genu recurvatum by combining the Swedish knee-cage and an ankle-foot brace. Disabil Rehabil. Oct-Dec 1992;14(4):187-191.
12. Caylor D, Fites R, Worrell TW. The relationship between quadriceps angle and anterior knee pain syndrome. J Orthop Sports Phys Ther. Jan 1993;17(1):11-16.
13. Hvid I, Andersen LI, Schmidt H. Chondromalacia patellae. The relation to abnormal patellofemoral joint mechanics. Acta Orthop Scand. Dec 1981;52(6):661-666.
14. Papagelopoulos PJ, Sim FH. Patellofemoral pain syndrome: diagnosis and management. Orthopedics. Feb 1997;20(2):148-157; quiz 158-149.
15. Zimbler S, Smith J, Scheller A, Banks HH. Recurrent subluxation and dislocation of the patella in association with athletic injuries. Orthop Clin North Am. Oct 1980;11(4):755-770.
16. Huston LJ, Greenfield ML, Wojtys EM. Anterior cruciate ligament injuries in the female athlete. Potential risk factors. Clin Orthop Relat Res. Mar 2000(372):50-63.
17. Horton MG, Hall TL. Quadriceps femoris muscle angle: normal values and relationships with gender and selected skeletal measures. Phys Ther. Nov 1989;69(11):897-901.
18. Swenson TM, Harner CD. Knee ligament and meniscal injuries. Current concepts. Orthop Clin North Am. Jul 1995;26(3):529-546.
19. Arnold T, Shelbourne KD. A perioperative rehabilitation program for anterior cruciate igament surgery. Physician Sportsmed. 2000;28(1).
20. Evans NA, Chew HF, Stanish WD. The natural history and tailored treatment of ACL injury. Physician Sportsmed. 2001;29(9).
21. Harner CD, Paulos LE, Greenwald AE, Rosenberg TD, Cooley VC. Detailed analysis of patients with bilateral anterior cruciate ligament injuries. Am J Sports Med. 1994;22(1):37-43.
22. Arendt E, Dick R. Knee injury patterns among men and women in collegiate basketball and soccer. NCAA data and review of literature. Am J Sports Med. 1995;23(6):694-701.
23. Cabaud HE, Rodkey WG. Philosophy and rationale for the management of anterior cruciate injuries and the resultant deficiencies. Clin Sports Med. Apr 1985;4(2):313-324.
24. Shelbourne KD, Nitz PA. The O'Donoghue triad revisited. Combined knee injuries involving anterior cruciate and medial collateral ligament tears. Am J Sports Med. 1991;19(5):474-477.
25. Johnson DL, Warner JJ. Diagnosis for anterior cruciate ligament surgery. Clin Sports Med. Oct 1993;12(4):671-684.
26. Morgan EA, Wroble RR. Diagnosing posterior cruciate ligament injuries. Physician Sportsmed. 1997;25(11).
27. Parolie JM, Bergfeld JA. Long-term results of nonoperative treatment of isolated posterior cruciate ligament injuries in the athlete. Am J Sports Med. 1986;14(1):35-38.
28. Paletta GA, Warren RF. Knee injuries and Alpine skiing. Treatment and rehabilitation. Sports Med. Jun 1994;17(6):411-423.
29. Crossley K, Bennell K, Green S, McConnell J. A systematic review of physical interventions for patellofemoral pain syndrome. Clin J Sport Med. 2001;11(2):103-110.
30. Thomee R, Augustsson J, Karlsson J. Patellofemoral pain syndrome: a review of current issues. Sports Med. 1999;28(4):245-262.
31. Desio SM, Burks RT, Bachus KN. Soft tissue restraints to lateral patellar translation in the human knee. Am J Sports Med. 1998;26(1):59-65.
32. Sakai N, Luo ZP, Rand JA, An KN. The influence of weakness in the vastus medialis oblique muscle on the patellofemoral joint: an in vitro biomechanical study. Clin Biomech (Bristol, Avon). Jun 2000;15(5):335-339.
33. Biedert RM, Sanchis-Alfonso V. Sources of anterior

knee pain. Clin Sports Med. Jul 2002;21(3):335-347, vii.

34. LaBotz M. Patellofemoral syndrome. Physician Sportsmed. 2004;32(7).

35. Post WR. Patellofemoral pain: Let the physical exam define treatment. Physician Sportsmed. 1998;26(1).

36. Liebenson Ce. Rehabilitation of the Spine. Baltimore: Williams & Wilkins; 1996.

37. Barber FA, Sutker AN. Iliotibial band syndrome. Sports Med. 1992;14(2):144-148.

38. Moore K, Dalley A. Clinically Oriented Anatomy. 4th ed. Philadelphia: Lippincott Williams & Wilkins; 1999.

39. Ekman EF, Pope T, Martin DF, Curl WW. Magnetic resonance imaging of iliotibial band syndrome. Am J Sports Med. 1994;22(6):851-854.

40. Nemeth WC, Sanders BL. The lateral synovial recess of the knee: anatomy and role in chronic Iliotibial band friction syndrome. Arthroscopy. 1996;12(5):574-580.

41. Nishimura G, Yamato M, Tamai K, Takahashi J, Uetani M. MR findings in iliotibial band syndrome. Skeletal Radiol. 1997;26(9):533-537.

42. Martens M. Iliotibial Band Friction Syndrome. In: Torg JS, Shephard RJ, eds. Current Therapy in Sports Medicine. St. Louis: Mosby; 1995:322-324.

43. Martinez J, Honsik K. Iliotibial Band Syndrome. eMedicine. April 8, 2005. Available at: www.emedicine.com. Accessed May 1, 2005.

44. Gajdosik RL, Sandler MM, Marr HL. Influence of knee positions and gender on the Ober test for length of the iliotibial band. Clin Biomech (Bristol, Avon). Jan 2003;18(1):77-79.

45. Reese NB, Bandy WD. Use of an inclinometer to measure flexibility of the iliotibial band using the Ober test and the modified Ober test: differences in magnitude and reliability of measurements. J Orthop Sports Phys Ther. Jun 2003;33(6):326-330.

46. Malone T, McPoil T, Nitz A. Orthopedic and Sports Physical Therapy. 3rd ed. St. Louis: Mosby; 1997.

47. Kim YC, Yoo WK, Chung IH, Seo JS, Tanaka S. Tendinous insertion of semimembranosus muscle into the lateral meniscus. Surg Radiol Anat. 1997;19(6):365-369.

48. Paletta GA, Jr., Manning T, Snell E, Parker R, Bergfeld J. The effect of allograft meniscal replacement on intraarticular contact area and pressures in the human knee. A biomechanical study. Am J Sports Med. Sep-Oct 1997;25(5):692-698.

49. Silbey MB, Fu FH. Knee Injuries. In: Fu FH, Stone D, eds. Sports Injuries. Baltimore: Williams & Wilkins; 1994.

50. Kraushaar BS, Nirschl RP. Tendinosis of the elbow (tennis elbow). Clinical features and findings of histological, immunohistochemical, and electron microscopy studies. J Bone Joint Surg Am. 1999;81(2):259-278.

51. Almekinders LC, Temple JD. Etiology, Diagnosis, and Treatment of Tendinitis - An Analysis of the Literature. Med Sci Sport Exercise. 1998;30(8):1183-1190.

52. Khan KM, Cook JL, Bonar F, Harcourt P, Astrom M. Histopathology of common tendinopathies - Update and implications for clinical management. Sport Med. 1999;27(6):393-408.

53. Torstensen ET, Bray RC, Wiley JP. Patellar Tendinitis: A Review of Current Concepts and Treatment. Clin J Sport Med. 1994;4(2):77-82.

54. Fredberg U, Bolvig L. Jumper's knee. Review of the literature. Scand J Med Sci Sports. Apr 1999;9(2):66-73.

55. Ferretti A. Epidemiology of jumper's knee. Sports Med. Jul-Aug 1986;3(4):289-295.

56. Depalma MJ, Perkins RH. Patellar tendinosis. Physician Sportsmed. 2004;32(5).

57. Khan KM, Bonar F, Desmond PM, et al. Patellar Tendinosis (Jumpers Knee) - Findings at Histopathologic Examination, Us, and MR-Imaging. Radiology. 1996;200(3):821-827.

58. Albright J, Foster D. Prepatellar Bursitis. In: Torg JS, Shephard RJ, eds. Current Therapy in Sports Medicine. St. Louis: Mosby; 1995:316-322.

59. Ho G, Jr., Tice AD, Kaplan SR. Septic bursitis in the prepatellar and olecranon bursae: an analysis of 25 cases. Ann Intern Med. Jul 1978;89(1):21-27.

60. Wilson-MacDonald J. Management and outcome of infective prepatellar bursitis. Postgrad Med J. Oct 1987;63(744):851-853.

61. Bui-Mansfield L, Youngberg R. Baker Cyst. eMedicine. May 3, 2004. Available at: www.emedicine.com. Accessed May 2, 2005.

62. Lindgren G, Rauschning W. Clinical and arthrographic studies on the valve mechanism in communicating popliteal cysts. Arch Orthop Trauma Surg. 1979;95(4):245-250.

63. Fam AG, Wilson SR, Holmberg S. Ultrasound evaluation of popliteal cysts on osteoarthritis of the knee. J Rheumatol. May-Jun 1982;9(3):428-434.

64. Miller TT, Staron RB, Koenigsberg T, Levin TL, Feldman F. MR imaging of Baker cysts: association with internal derangement, effusion, and degenerative arthropathy. Radiology. Oct 1996;201(1):247-250.

65. Brockett CL, Morgan DL, Proske U. Predicting hamstring strain injury in elite athletes. Med Sci Sports Exerc. Mar 2004;36(3):379-387.

66. Croisier JL. Factors associated with recurrent hamstring injuries. Sports Med. 2004;34(10):681-695.

67. Worrell TW. Factors associated with hamstring injuries. An approach to treatment and preventative measures. Sports Med. 1994;17(5):338-345.

68. Kujala UM, Orava S, Jarvinen M. Hamstring injuries. Current trends in treatment and prevention. Sports Med. 1997;23(6):397-404.

69. Garrett WE, Jr., Rich FR, Nikolaou PK, Vogler JB, 3rd. Computed tomography of hamstring muscle strains. Med Sci Sports Exerc. 1989;21(5):506-514.

70. Best TM, Garrett WE. Hamstring strains. Physician Sportsmed. 1996;24(8).

71. Kornberg CaL, P. The Effect of Stretching Neural Structures on Grade One Hamstring Injuries. Journal of Orthopaedic and Sports Physical Therapy. 1989;June:481-487.

72. Turl SE, and George, K. P. Adverse Neural Tension - A Factor in Repetitive Hamstring Strain. J Orthop Sport Phys Therapy. 1998;27(1):16-21.

73. Askling C, Tengvar M, Saartok T, Thorstensson A. Sports related hamstring strains--two cases with different etiologies and injury sites. Scand J Med Sci Sports. 2000;10(5):304-307.

74. Karlsson J, Sward L, Kalebo P, Thomee R. Chronic groin injuries in athletes. Recommendations for treatment and rehabilitation. Sports Med. Feb 1994;17(2):141-148.

75. Fry B, Brunner R. Adductor Strain. eMedicine. April 8, 2005. Available at: www.emedicine.com. Accessed May 3, 2005.

76. Garrett WE. Muscle strain injuries. Am J Sports Med. 1996;24(6 Suppl):S2-8.

7 Hip & Pelvis

The hip and pelvis's biomechanical function is complex and has profound impacts on the overall function of the body. This region makes up the structural core of the body and contains its center of gravity. The hip and pelvis have two major articulations on each side of the body: the sacroiliac (SI) joint and the iliofemoral (hip) joint. Iliofemoral and sacroiliac joint mechanics are closely related and understanding the numerous pathologies in this region requires familiarity with both joints.

Motion at the SI joint is controlled by ligaments and numerous muscles, some of which cross the joint and others that do not. Unlike most joints in the body, no muscles directly connect the two adjacent bones of the joint. While there are muscles that cross the SI joint, there are none that attach to the sacrum and the ilium, specifically controlling the joint. Due to the functional relationship between the SI region and the lumbar spine, a thorough evaluation of mechanical dysfunction in the lumbar spine must include consideration of SI joint mechanics.[1, 2]

The iliofemoral, or hip, joint is a large ball-and-socket articulation that permits movement in several planes. Its structure provides stability and transmits weight to the lower extremity, which results in fewer injuries compared to similarly designed joints such as the shoulder. While muscles acting across the hip joint can generate large force loads, hip joint pathologies generally result from chronic compressive stress.

Movements and Motion Testing

SINGLE-PLANE MOVEMENTS

There are six primary movements in the iliofemoral joint: flexion, extension, abduction, adduction, medial rotation, and lateral rotation. There are two motions at the SI joint: nutation and counternutation. The SI joint is usually not included in general range-of-motion evaluations because its range of motion is only a few degrees and is difficult to measure. However, SI joint mechanics are evaluated with a number of the special orthopedic tests included in this chapter. The associated motions, planes, axes of rotation, and range-of-motion values for the hip and pelvis are listed in Table 1 at the end of the chapter.

Hip (iliofemoral) joint

Flexion and **extension** occur in the **sagittal plane** (Figure 7.1). In flexion the thigh is brought toward the anterior surface of the torso. Extension is the return to anatomical position from any flexed position, with motion past anatomical position considered hyperextension. Average range of motion is 120^0 for flexion and 30^0 for extension.

Abduction and **adduction** occur in the **frontal plane** (Figure 7.2). During abduction the thigh is brought away from the midline of the body. Adduction is the return to anatomical position from an abducted position, as well as movement across the body toward the midline. Average range of motion is 45^0 for abduction and 30^0 for adduction, noting that adduction is measured only from anatomical position moving toward the opposite side.

Medial and **lateral rotations** occur in the **transverse plane** (Figure 7.3). Rotational movements are easier to evaluate when the knee is flexed. Medial rotation is rotary movement of the anterior thigh toward the midline of the body. Lateral rotation is rotary movement of the anterior thigh away from the midline of the body. Average range of motion in medial or lateral rotation is 45^0.

Sacroiliac joint

Nutation and **counternutation** are movements in the **sagittal plane** (Figure 7.4). Nutation is the anterior tipping of the upper portion of the sacrum relative to the innominate. This movement can occur with the sacrum rotating anteriorly or the innominate (ilium, ischium, and pubis) rotating posteriorly. Counternutation is the posterior tipping of the sacrum and results from the sacrum rotating posteriorly or the innominate rotating anteriorly.

Capsular patterns

It is important to consider the role of the joint capsule when assessing joint function. Pathological problems in the capsule, such as *fibrosis*, may be evident from the joint's **capsular pattern**. The capsular pattern is a pattern of movement restriction that is characteristic to each individual joint. It is present in both active and passive motion. Capsular patterns are represented by a sequential listing of the movements from most likely to least likely limited. See the capsular pattern for this region in Box 7.1.

RANGE-OF-MOTION & RESISTIVE TESTS

Results from single-plane movement analysis form the basis for further evaluation procedures. Movement testing should be performed in a certain order, allowing for an efficient evaluation and the least amount of accumulated discomfort or pain to develop. It is also general practice to leave movements known or expected to be painful to the end of the evaluation. When possible, the pain-free side is

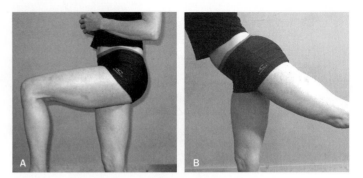

Figure 7.1 Hip flexion (A) and extension (B).

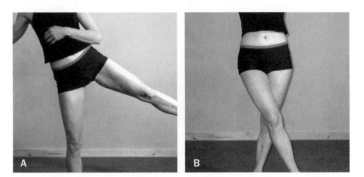

Figure 7.2 Hip abduction (A) and adduction (B).

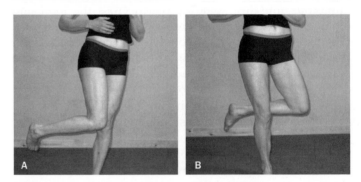

Figure 7.3 Hip medial rotation (A) and lateral rotation (B).

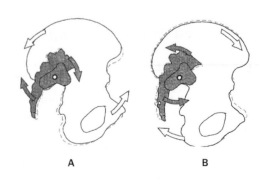

Figure 7.4 Sacral nutation (A) and counternutation (B). (Mediclip image copyright, 1998 Williams & Wilkins. All rights reserved.)

BOX 7.1 CAPSULAR PATTERN FOR THE HIP

Iliofemoral (Hip) Joint
- Medial rotation is most restricted
- Flexion and abduction are limited
- Extension may be slightly limited
- Adduction is not likely limited
- Lateral rotation is not likely limited

BOX 7.2 JOINT, ASSOCIATED MOTION, & END FEEL

Iliofemoral Joint		
	Flexion	Tissue stretch
	Extension	Tissue stretch
	Abduction	Tissue stretch (soft)
	Adduction	Soft-tissue approximation
	Medial rotation	Tissue stretch
	Lateral rotation	Tissue stretch

---

evaluated first.

Active range-of-motion (AROM) movements are performed first to establish the client's movement abilities and pain symptoms. Passive range of motion (PROM) is performed next and manual resistive tests (MRT) follow. AROM results may make PROM assessment procedures unnecessary. If no pain occurs with active movement, pain is unlikely with passive movement. The practitioner should be familiar with the full step-by-step instructions and guidelines for how to interpret ROM and resistive test results as explained in Chapter 3.

Active Range of Motion

Active hip motions are usually evaluated with the client in a standing position. When performing AROM evaluations, take into consideration the position of the body to ensure the target tissues are engaged. For example, when the client actively flexes the hip by lifting the leg toward the torso, the hip flexors are engaged concentrically. When the leg returns to anatomical position it is not the hip extensors that are responsible for the action, but the hip flexors as they employ an eccentric contraction. Engaging the hip extensors requires a change in body position or the way resistance to the movement is offered.

Pain with active movement indicates problems in either the contractile or inert tissues associated with that movement. Factors prematurely limiting active movement in this region include *ligamentous or capsular damage*, *muscle contractures*, pain from *nerve compression or tension*, *tendinosis*, *fibrous cysts*, or *joint disorders* such as *arthritis*. Compare AROM test results with those from PROM and manual resistive tests to identify possible reasons for movement restriction. The muscles used to perform actions of the hip and pelvis are listed in Box 7.3. Note that other muscles can contribute to the motion and subsequent dysfunction.

Passive Range of Motion

Passive motion is performed after active. Pain during passive movement predominantly implicates inert tissues. However, muscles and tendons that contract in the opposite direction are stretched at the end range of passive movement.

PROM testing also evaluates end feel. Box 7.2 lists the primary joint locations and their normal end feel. Review Chapter 3 for a discussion of normal and pathological end feel descriptions. Factors that could prematurely limit passive movement are the same as for active movement.

Manual Resistive Tests

The MRT produces pain when there is a mechanical disruption of tissue. Pain with an MRT indicates that one or more of the muscles and/or tendons performing that action are involved. Testing all of a muscle's actions is not necessary, as a muscle's secondary actions recruit other muscles and make the test results less accurate. Palpation during manual resistance elicits more information if the test alone does not produce pain or discomfort. Refer to Box 7.3 for the list of primary muscles involved with each action. Table 2 at the end of the chapter lists actions commonly used for testing muscles in the hip and pelvis.

GENERAL INSTRUCTIONS FOR ROM & RESISTIVE TESTS

Overall
- Determine motions possible at the joint to be tested.
- Select the motion to be evaluated.
- Determine the tissues involved in the motion.
- Leave motions expected to be painful to the last.
- Test the uninvolved side first.
- Ask about, note any reported pain or discomfort.

AROM
- Demonstrate the movement to be performed.
- Have the client perform the movement.

PROM
- Establish the joint's normal end feel.
- Have the client relax as much as possible.
- Use gentle and slow movements.

MRT
- Test one action at a time.
- Position should isolate the action/muscles involved.
- If pain is suspected, start in a mid-range position.
- Client uses a strong, but appropriate amount of effort.

BOX 7.3 MUSCLE ACTIONS OF THE HIP

Hip	**Flexion**	**Extension**

Flexion

- Iliopsoas
- Rectus femoris
- Sartorius
- Pectineus
- Adductor longus
- Adductor magnus (superior portion)
- Tensor fasciae latae
- Gluteus medius (anterior portion)

Extension

- Gluteus maximus
- Biceps femoris
- Semitendinosus
- Semimembranosus
- Adductor magnus (inferior portion)
- Gluteus medius (posterior portion)

Abduction

- Gluteus medius
- Gluteus minimus
- Tensor fasciae latae
- Sartorius
- Piriformis (w/flexed hip)
- Gemellus superior (w/flexed hip)
- Gemellus inferior (w/flexed hip)
- Obturator internus (w/flexed hip)

Adduction

- Adductor magnus
- Adductor longus
- Adductor brevis
- Pectineus
- Gracilis

Medial rotation

- Gluteus medius (anterior portion)
- Gluteus minimus
- Tensor fasciae latae
- Semimembranosus
- Semitendinosus
- Adductor magnus
- Adductor longus

Lateral rotation

- Gluteus maximus
- Piriformis
- Gemellus superior
- Obturator internus
- Gemellus inferior
- Obturator externus
- Quadratus femoris
- Sartorius
- Biceps femoris (long head)
- Gluteus medius (posterior portion)
- Iliopsoas

In some cases weakness is evident with MRTs. Factors that produce weakness include *lack of use, fatigue, reflex muscular inhibition*, and possibly a neurological pathology (*radiculopathy, peripheral neuropathy,* or a *systemic neurological disorder*). The nerves or nerve roots that may be involved are listed in Table 3, which occurs at the end of the chapter.

Hip
RESISTED FLEXION AND EXTENSION
To test flexion the client is seated on the treatment table. The practitioner places a hand on the client's distal thigh while the client attempts to lift the thigh against the practitioner's resistance (Figure 7.5).

To test extension the client is prone on the treatment table with the knee flexed to 90⁰. The practitioner offers resistance with a hand placed near the distal portion of the client's thigh as the client attempts to lift the thigh against the practitioner's resistance (Figure 7.5).

RESISTED ABDUCTION AND ADDUCTION
To test abduction the client is supine on the treatment table with the thigh partially abducted. The client may hold on to the sides of the table to stabilize the torso if desired.

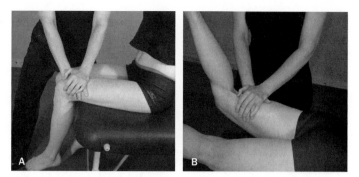

Figure 7.5 Resisted hip flexion (A) and extension (B).

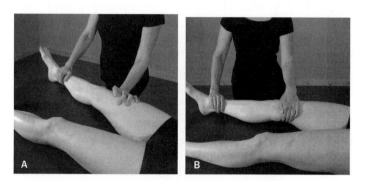

Figure 7.6 Resisted hip abduction (A) and adduction (B).

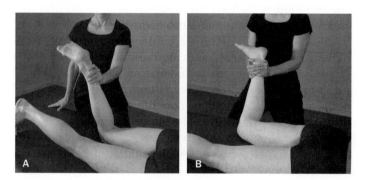

Figure 7.7 Resisted hip medial rotation (A) and lateral rotation (B).

The practitioner places one hand at the lateral aspect of the distal thigh and the other hand against the lower leg, to stabilize the lower extremity. The client holds this position as the practitioner attempts to move the thigh back to anatomical position (Figure 7.6). The practitioner's hand at the distal thigh offers resistance.

To test adduction the client is supine with the thigh partially abducted. The practitioner places one hand on the medial aspect of the distal thigh and the other hand on the medial aspect of the leg for stabilization. The client holds this position as the practitioner attempts to pull the thigh into further abduction (Figure 7.6).

RESISTED MEDIAL AND LATERAL ROTATION

To test medial rotation the client is prone on the treatment table with the knee flexed to 90⁰. The practitioner places a hand on the lateral aspect of the client's distal leg near the ankle. The client holds this position as the practitioner attempts to push the leg in a medial direction (Figure 7.7). This position uses the leg as a lever to achieve motion in the hip. For most people this will not be a problem, but this position should not be used if there is a knee pathology that could be aggravated by the force on the lower leg. It may seem backward to push the client's leg in a medial direction to achieve a resisted medial rotation, but with the client prone and the knee flexed, the lower leg moves laterally during medial rotation. The client attempts to medially rotate the hip to resist the practitioner's pressure.

To test lateral rotation the client is in the same starting position as for medial rotation. The practitioner places a hand on the medial aspect of the client's distal leg. The client holds this position as the practitioner attempts to pull the client's leg in a lateral direction (Figure 7.7). As with medial rotation, this position should not be used if there is a knee pathology involving joint instability.

Structural and Postural Deviations

The following section covers structural or postural deviations unique to the hip and pelvis. Under each condition there is a brief description of the condition's characteristics followed by likely HOPRS findings. If applicable, orthopedic tests are included in the special tests section. If there is no special orthopedic test listed for that condition, evaluation should focus on other portions of the assessment process, such as range-of-motion testing.

There are important considerations for some of the special tests included in this chapter. While the majority of special tests in other chapters have a relatively high degree of specificity and sensitivity, some tests in the hip and pelvis region are under scrutiny due to poor test reliability.[3-5] Issues that affect accuracy include difficulty in identifying anatomical landmarks, inability to perceive motion correctly, and failure to establish a causal relationship between motion disturbance and a specific pathology. However, that doesn't mean that the tests are not of clinical importance. They still provide beneficial information for evaluating disorders in the region.

Instead of focusing on individual tests, a broader clinical picture including a variety of testing methods and information from other portions of your assessment should be considered The multiple factors that make up a comprehensive physical examination must be investigated for a complete and accurate picture of the condition.[6-8] Special tests are only part of a broader evaluation. In addition, postural deviations in the hip and pelvis routinely exist along with conditions in other regions of the body. These other conditions should also be investigated.

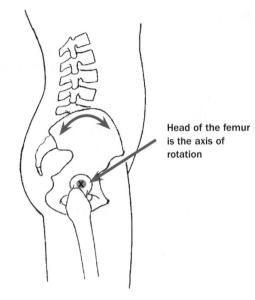

Head of the femur is the axis of rotation

Figure 7.8 Axis for anterior or posterior innominate rotation. (Mediclip image copyright, 1998 Williams & Wilkins. All rights reserved.)

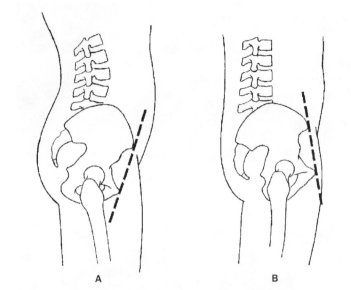

A   B

Figure 7.9 Anterior (A) and posterior (B) innominate rotations. (Mediclip image copyright, 1998 Williams & Wilkins. All rights reserved.)

ANTERIOR OR POSTERIOR INNOMINATE/ PELVIC ROTATION

Anterior innominate or pelvic rotation is a common postural distortion and occurs in conjunction with an *exaggerated lumbar lordosis. Posterior innominate rotation* reduces the lumbar lordosis. Both conditions are typically produced by muscular imbalance. Pain is not always felt from these disorders, but when present appears in the lumbar or sacral regions.

Anterior innominate rotation can increase compressive load on the spinal facet joints and alter other factors of lumbo-sacral mechanics.

Characteristics

Three bones compose each half of the pelvis, the **ilium, ischium** and **pubis,** and are referred to as the **left** or **right innominates**. The **sacrum** and the innominates make up the pelvic girdle. The axis for innominate rotation is through the **iliofemoral (hip) joint** and around the head of the **femur** (Figure 7.8).[9] The slight degree of motion at the **sacroiliac (SI) joint** makes only a minimal contribution to innominate rotation. Innominate rotation is necessary for normal movement, such as flexion and extension in the lumbar spine and hips. Each innominate is able to move to a very slight degree independently of the other, as would occur in walking.

When there is pathological rotation, the left and right innominate generally rotate in the same direction, either anteriorly or posteriorly (Figure 7.9). Posterior rotations are not as common as anterior rotations. Because the innominates can move independently, it is possible to have one anteriorly rotated and the other not, or rotated posteriorly. When this occurs, the condition is called a *left*

or *right anteriorly* or *posteriorly rotated innominate.*

Anterior innominate rotation is sometimes described as causing a *functionally longer leg* (with the long leg being on the side of the anteriorly rotated innominate). The hip joint is the axis for innominate rotation and the innominate rotates around the head of the femur. As a result, the innominate cannot force the lower extremity in an inferior direction. A functional leg length discrepancy results from a tight **quadratus lumborum** on the apparent short side (see *Lateral Pelvic Tilt*). A tight quadratus lumborum or hip flexors could contribute to an exaggerated lumbar lordosis and anterior innominate rotation.

Rotational distortions of the innominate generally develop as acquired *postural disorders.* Anterior innominate rotation is primarily caused by *hypertonicity* in the **lumbar extensors** and the **hip flexors** (iliopsoas and rectus femoris). These muscles can work together to produce a *force couple* that produces the rotational distortion (Figure 7.10). Clients may experience no detrimental symptoms or pathology, but the condition can contribute to biomechanical problems, especially in the low back.

Anterior innominate rotations increase *lumbar lordosis.* As a result, other conditions such as *facet joint pathology, increased weight-bearing by the posterior vertebral structures,* and *SI joint pathology* can develop or be exacerbated.[2, 10-12] Individuals with anterior innominate rotations may also experience an increase in *hamstring strains.* As the innominate rotates anteriorly, the hamstrings are lengthened and become susceptible to strain.

Habitual postural patterns that stem from poor sitting posture are the primary instigators of posterior innominate rotation.[9] **Hypertonicity** in the **hamstrings** and **abdominals** can also produce the force couple that creates posterior rotations (Figure 7.11). There is a loss of lordo-

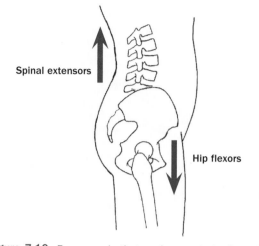

Figure 7.10 Force couple that produces anterior innominate rotation. (Mediclip image copyright, 1998 Williams & Wilkins. All rights reserved.)

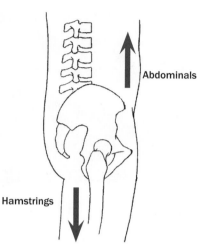

Figure 7.11 Force couple that produces posterior innominate rotation. (Mediclip image copyright, 1998 Williams & Wilkins. All rights reserved.)

sis in this condition, particularly when both innominates rotate in the same direction. When the lumbar lordosis is decreased, there is a measurable increase in the compressive load on the intervertebral discs, which can lead to *degeneration* and eventual *herniation* in some cases. Muscular hypertonicity and adopted neuromuscular patterns can create a vicious cycle that is difficult to change without constant attention to postural correction.

Innominate rotation is evaluated in a standing position. The degree of innominate rotation should not be overly emphasized as a pathological factor. What is more important than the static position, is the way in which the innominates interact with the spine and lower extremity during movement. The body is capable of compensating for postural distortions and some pelvic rotations can be overcome without pathology.

Evaluating the degree of innominate rotation is challenging. Assessment methods rely on visual analysis of bony landmarks or estimation with a goniometer.[13] It is difficult to make accurate measurements and determine the clinical significance of those measurements. Philip Greenman argues that to accurately identify pelvic positional dysfunctions, problems must be evident in asymmetry, range of motion, and tissue texture.[14]

History

It is common for the client to experience no major symptoms. With either anterior or posterior rotation, the client may report some degree of discomfort in the low back region. In anterior innominate rotation clients might complain of pain from muscular hypertonicity or facet joint compression. The client with posterior rotation may report hamstring tightness. Inquire about poor sitting postures or any prolonged positions that may exaggerate the posterior innominate rotation. In-depth questioning is sometimes necessary, as the client may not recognize a connection between the alignment problem and their symptoms. Ask about previous or existing injuries and

determine what effect innominate rotation could have on those conditions as either a cause or effect.

Observation

A person with an anteriorly rotated innominate appears to have an *exaggerated lumbar lordosis* and prominent gluteal region. An anterior rotation is more evident with higher heeled shoes. With a posterior rotation, the lumbar region appears flat with no lordotic curvature and the gluteal region appears tucked under or flattened. Posterior innominate rotation is often observed in conjunction with an *upper thoracic kyphosis*.

Palpation

In an anterior rotation, hypertonicity is typically evident in the spinal extensors, quadratus lumborum, rectus femoris, and the iliopsoas. With a posterior rotation, muscular hypertonicity is sometimes evident in the hamstrings or abdominal muscles .

Range-of-Motion and Resistance Testing

AROM: In anterior innominate rotation, trunk flexion is generally restricted due to tightness in the spinal extensors. Limitations in hip extension are expected due to hypertonicity in the iliopsoas muscle, which is best identified with a muscle length test such as the modified Thomas test described below. There are no specific findings with active motion for posterior innominate rotation. Pain is unlikely although there may be some reduced hip flexion due to hamstring tightness.
PROM: The same principles apply as for active motion.
MRT: No unusual findings exist with MRTs

Special Tests
Anterior and Posterior Innominate Rotation Test
This test is designed to evaluate the degree of anterior or posterior innominate rotation. For effective evaluation, anatomical landmarks must be accurately palpated, but

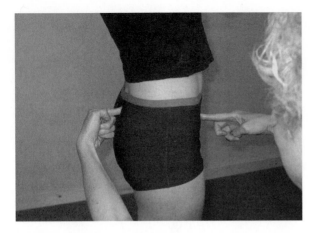

Figure 7.12 Anterior and posterior innominate rotation test.

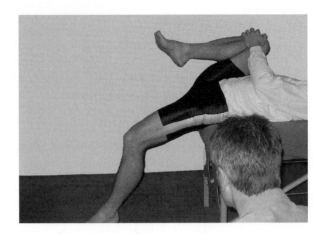

Figure 7.13 Modified Thomas test.

finding these may be difficult. The client stands barefoot with feet shoulder width apart. The practitioner kneels at the client's side so the client's pelvis is at eye level. The practitioner places one finger on the client's **posterior superior iliac spine (PSIS)** and another finger on the client's **anterior superior iliac spine (ASIS)** and evaluates the level of the fingers (Figure 7.12).

If the innominate is in a normal position, the ASIS and PSIS are level or the ASIS is slightly lower. If the ASIS is more than a half-inch lower, an anterior innominate rotation is indicated. Due to shape differences in the female pelvis, a little more than the half-inch difference may be considered normal for women. If the PSIS is lower than the ASIS, a posterior innominate rotation is indicated. It is important to check both innominates, as they may have different degrees or directions of rotational distortion.

Explanation: The relationship between the relative height of the ASIS and PSIS changes when the innominate is rotated. Due to anatomical variations or areas of adipose tissue, the practitioner may find it difficult to accurately locate the PSIS and ASIS bony landmarks, which makes test accuracy questionable.

Modified Thomas Test

This test is for a hypertonic iliopsoas. The client leans on the edge of the treatment table without fully sitting on the table. The client brings the knee that is not being tested to the chest. Once the knee is drawn to the chest, the practitioner assists the client in rolling back onto the treatment table. The thigh being held to the chest should be at about a 45⁰ angle to the table. The practitioner observes the client's extended thigh from a lateral view (Figure 7.13). If the thigh is at horizontal or above, hypertonicity in the iliopsoas is indicated. If the thigh drops below horizontal, the iliopsoas is considered within normal parameters for flexibility. If the rectus femoris is at normal length, the lower leg should drop toward the floor at a vertical angle. If the lower leg is not vertical some hypertonicity in the rectus femoris is evident.

Safety note: If you are performing this procedure on a portable treatment table that folds in the middle, take extra caution. When the client sits on the edge of the table, it may start to fold up in the middle, causing the table to collapse and the client to fall. The table's middle should be stabilized with the practitioner applying weight directly over the middle of the table. The practitioner should also use caution when helping the client out of the position and off the treatment table at the conclusion of the test.

Explanation: Hypertonicity, particularly in the iliopsoas, plays a fundamental role in most anterior innominate rotations. The modified Thomas test evaluates the level of hypertonicity in the iliopsoas and rectus femoris muscles by measuring their length. Holding the knee to the chest on the side opposite that being tested prevents excessive anterior innominate rotation. With the innominates in a normal degree of rotation, tightness in the iliopsoas is evident because it pulls the thigh of the test side toward the chest and lifts it above horizontal.

The original version of this test was performed with the client supine on the treatment table. While the iliopsoas can be tested in this position because the extended thigh can lift off the table, the rectus femoris cannot be tested due to hip hyperextension and knee flexion are blocked by the table. It is important to evaluate the contribution of rectus femoris to innominate rotation, so the modified Thomas test is the preferred method.

Suggestions for Treatment

Reducing tension in the iliopsoas or lumbar extensor muscles is paramount for decreasing anterior rotation. Reducing tightness in the hamstring and abdominal muscles may assist the innominate in regaining its proper alignment in a posterior rotation. Massage, stretching, and other neuromuscular methods, such as muscle energy technique, reduce hypertonicity in the affected muscles. Despite the benefits of soft-tissue treatment, postural retraining is imperative in order to change the dysfunctional motor patterns which perpetuate these conditions.

LATERAL PELVIC TILT

Lateral pelvic tilts result from either structural (skeletal) or functional (muscular) disorders. It is crucial to identify what is producing the tilt for the most appropriate treatment. Treating for a structural leg length discrepancy, for example, when the condition derives from muscular hypertonicity can perpetuate and even exacerbate the client's condition.

Characteristics

In addition to rotating in the **sagittal plane**, the pelvis can tilt from side to side in the **coronal plane**. An individual can have either a left or right *lateral pelvic tilt*. If the left side is higher, the pelvis tilts down to the right and it is considered a *right* lateral pelvic tilt; if the pelvis tilts down to the left, it is a *left* lateral tilt. The analogy of the pelvis as a bowl of water is often used to illustrate the posture. With a right tilt, the water pours out the right side and vice versa. Lateral pelvic tilting can alter the position of the **S-I joint** and affect motion in the **lumbar spine**. There is not a clear axis of rotation in the pelvis, which makes biomechanical analysis difficult.

Skeletal sources of lateral pelvic tilt include *structural leg-length discrepancies, small innominate (hemi-pelvis)* and *congenital scoliosis*. Leg-length inequality is relatively common, but is not necessarily pathological. When the bones of one leg are longer than the other, the **innominate** is pushed superiorly on the side of the longer leg (Figure 7.14). For example, if the right leg is longer, the right innominate will be raised, causing a left lateral pelvic tilt. How much leg-length difference is pathological has not been determined because the body is capable of significant compensation for leg length differences.[8,15] However, pathological problems are possible even with small variations in leg lengths that are considered normal.[16]

Lateral pelvic tilts are also caused by muscular *hypertonicity* and can produce a *functional leg-length discrepancy*. Tightness in the **quadratus lumborum** can lift the ipsilateral innominate superiorly, causing a lateral tilt to the opposite side. A functional scoliosis and leg-length discrepancy can result. Functional disorders are far more common than structural and can develop from a number of causes. Acute muscle spasm from a low back injury, sitting on a large wallet, or improper and/or prolonged postures can all produce tightness in the quadratus lumborum.

Lateral pelvic tilts are often only evaluated in a supine position by making a leg-length comparison, which does not determine the cause of the discrepancy (Figure 7.15). Additional assessment must be performed. If not sufficiently evaluated, a functional disorder could be mistaken for a structural distortion. Such an error in evaluation could lead to poor treatment. Mistaking a hypertonic quadratus lumborum for a true leg-length discrepancy could lead to the improper use of heel lifts and exacerbate the problem.

History

The client with a lateral pelvic tilt may complain of low back or SI joint pain, especially after long periods of sitting or standing. Ask the client if they have been diagnosed with congenital scoliosis or have had a low back injury. Inquire about unequal forces on the pelvis, such as sitting on a large wallet.

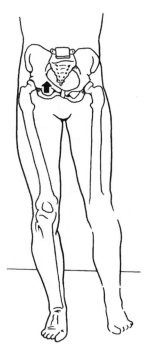

Figure 7.14 A structurally longer right leg causes the right side of the pelvis to appear higher, producing a left lateral tilt. (Mediclip image copyright, 1998 Williams & Wilkins. All rights reserved.)

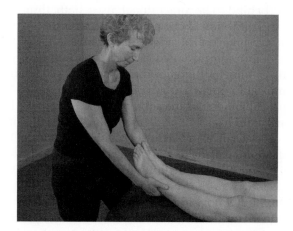

Figure 7.15 Supine position leg-length comparison.

Observation

When viewed in a standing position from an anterior or posterior direction, the client appears to have one hip raised in relation to the other. If the condition is severe, there may be alterations in gait. Compensations are typically visible farther up the postural chain. For example, the shoulders may be tilted to the opposite side of the pelvic tilt in an effort to compensate.

Palpation

Hypertonicity is generally evident in the lumbar muscles on the high side, especially if the problem is functional. Tissues can also feel tight on the low side due to overstretching and tautness. Tenderness and myofascial trigger points are likely in the low back muscles on the side of the elevated innominate.

Range-of-Motion and Resistance Testing

AROM: If hypertonicity in the quadratus lumborum produced the pelvic tilt, low back pain and restricted motion are felt when laterally flexing the torso toward the low side of the pelvic tilt. For example, a client with a left lateral tilt may have pain on the right side when laterally flexing to the left. Pain and restriction result from tightness in the right quadratus lumborum. Pain or discomfort in the SI joint region could be felt during active lateral flexion to either side.

PROM: Passive motion evaluation is challenging due to the weight of the torso, but can be performed with the client in a supine position with feet together. The practitioner grasps the client's ankles and pulls both lower extremities to the side. Results should be similar to those in active motion.

MRT: MRTs are rarely painful. In some cases, attempting to engage the quadratus lumborum in an MRT on the side of the elevated innominate may activate myofascial trigger points and produce local or referred pain.

Special Tests

Lateral Pelvic Tilt Test

The client stands barefoot and the practitioner kneels directly behind. The practitioner uses both thumbs to find the high point of the iliac crest on each side. Evaluate the relative height of each iliac crest (Figure 7.16). This test can also be performed with the practitioner facing the front of the client and using each ASIS as the landmark for comparison.

Explanation: This test evaluates lateral pelvic tilt by measuring the height of one ilium in relation to the other, but it does not determine the reason for the tilt. Other procedures discussed below will help determine whether the height difference is structural or functional.

Leg Length Measurement

The client is supine on the treatment table. The practitioner uses a tape measure to compare the lengths of each lower extremity. One end of the tape measure is placed

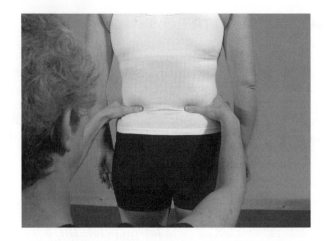

Figure 7.16 Lateral pelvic tilt test.

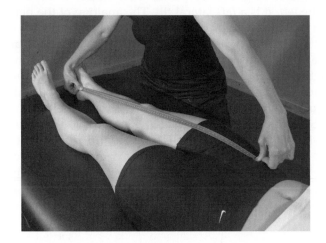

Figure 7.17 Leg length measurement.

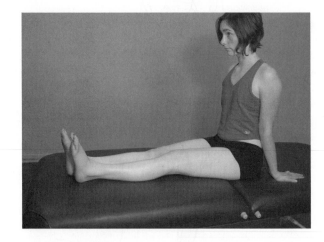

Figure 7.18 Supine-to-sit test with a tight left quadratus lumborum.

at the inferior lip of the ASIS and the other end is placed on the underside of the medial malleolus (Figure 7.17). The length of each side should be the same, but a difference of 1–1.5 cm is considered within normal limits. Even though it is within normal limits this difference could still produce pathological symptoms.

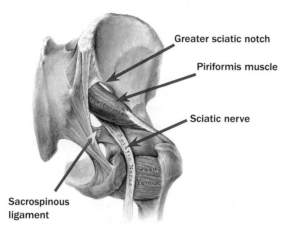

Figure 7.19 Normal path of the sciatic nerve in relation to the piriformis muscle and other nearby structures. (Mediclip image copyright, 1998 Williams & Wilkins. All rights reserved.)

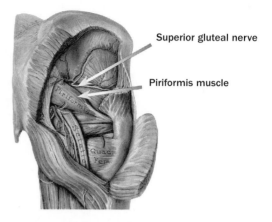

Figure 7.20 Susceptibility of the superior gluteal nerve to compression by the piriformis muscle. (Mediclip image copyright, 1998 Williams & Wilkins. All rights reserved.)

Explanation: The leg-length measurement evaluates the femur and tibia because they are the primary weight-bearing bones in the lower extremity so they are the ones that create the length difference. The ASIS is used because it has a more prominent location than any point on the femur and a better measurement can be made. Take into consideration any degree of innominate rotation that might throw off the measurement on either side.

The medial malleolus is used as the distal measurement point because it is located on the weight-bearing tibia. Differences in muscle bulk in the quadriceps could alter accuracy of the measurement as the tape measure must cross the quadriceps. The lateral malleolus of the fibula could be used as the inferior landmark to cross reference and validate findings with the medial malleolus.

Supine-to-Sit Test
The client is supine on the treatment table. The practitioner grasps the client's ankles and provides a slight degree of traction on both legs to make sure they are fully extended. The practitioner then examines the position of each medial malleolus in relation to the other. The client is then instructed to sit upright. As the client sits up, the practitioner watches the medial malleolus on each leg (Figure 7.18). If one malleolus moves more superior than the other, it is an indication that a functional disorder is contributing to the lateral pelvic tilt.

Explanation: As the client sits upright the low back muscles are pulled taut. If the quadratus lumborum is hypertonic, it pulls the ilium and the lower extremity on that side in a superior direction. The practitioner will see the lower limb glide superiorly at the ankle relative to the non-moving side.

Suggestions for Treatment
If the lateral tilt is created by muscle hypertonicity, massage and stretching methods to the quadratus lumborum are effective for restoring proper alignment. If the cause is a structural leg-length discrepancy, a heel lift can be placed in the shoe on the short side. The lift helps compensate for the length difference and allows the pelvis to return to a neutral position. Other structural disorders such as scoliosis may be addressed through functional braces or in severe conditions through implanted postural correction devices.

Common Injury Conditions

PIRIFORMIS SYNDROME

Radiating neurological pain that courses down the back of the leg is often diagnosed as originating from disc herniations in the lumbar spine. However, nerve compression at other sites can produce similar symptoms. One of the most common compression sites is in the gluteal region where **nerves are compressed by the piriformis muscle, creating a condition known as** *piriformis syndrome.* In the medical literature, nerve compression syndromes in this region are controversial because of the difficulty in establishing a definitive diagnosis.[17-19]

Characteristics
The primary nerve compressed in piriformis syndrome is the **sciatic.** The sciatic nerve derives from the **L4-S2 nerve roots** and courses anterior to the **sacrum,** before passing inferior to the **piriformis muscle** (Figure 7.19). The nerve can be compressed by tendinous bands within the muscle. It can also be compressed between the **piriformis muscle** and the **sacrospinous ligament,** a dense and unyielding connective tissue. Even a low level of pressure applied to the nerve for a long period of time can create symptoms.[17] Neurological symptoms include pain, paresthesia, numbness, or muscle weakness in the gluteal region or posterior lower extremity.

Others nerves may be compressed in this region. The definition of piriformis syndrome is sometimes expanded

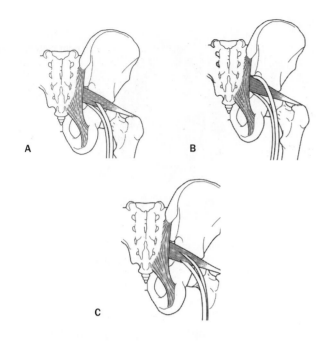

Figure 7.21 Variations of the sciatic nerve divisions as they pass the piriformis muscle: peroneal division through the muscle, tibial division below (A); peroneal division above, tibial below (B); both divisions passing through piriformis muscle (C). (Used with permission from Lowe, W. Orthopedic Massage: Theory & Technique. Edinburgh: Mosby;2003).

to include *superior gluteal nerve entrapment*, although the symptoms differ slightly. Pressure can be exerted on the superior gluteal nerve between the piriformis muscle and the **greater sciatic notch** (Figures 7.19 & 7.20). The superior gluteal nerve is primarily a motor nerve that supplies the **gluteus medius, minimus**, and **tensor fasciae latae**. Compression of the nerve can produce gluteal pain or a functional weakness in the abductors of the hip, but radiating pain down the posterior leg is unlikely as the nerve is confined to the gluteal region. If neurological symptoms are confined to the posterior thigh and do not extend below the knee, compression of the *posterior femoral cutaneous nerve* could be the reason. The posterior femoral cutaneous nerve lies adjacent to the **sciatic nerve** and can also be compressed by the **piriformis muscle**.[20]

There is an anatomical variation in the **tibial** and **peroneal divisions of the sciatic nerve** that occurs in about 15% of the population. Usually these nerves run together within the outer sheath of the sciatic nerve and pass inferior to the piriformis muscle. In some cases, these nerves split as they pass the piriformis and the peroneal division runs through the piriformis muscle while the tibial division runs inferior to it (Figure 7.21a). In other cases the peroneal portion runs superior to the piriformis muscle, while the tibial division runs inferior to it (Figure 7.21b). In less than 1% of the population both divisions of the sciatic nerve pass directly through the piriformis muscle (Figure 7.21c).[21] While it seems likely that passage of either division of the sciatic nerve through the piriformis

would exacerbate symptoms, this is not always the case. In fact, many people with these anatomic variations are asymptomatic.[17]

Nerve compression in piriformis syndrome can result from external pressure, such as sitting on a wallet. In rare cases piriformis syndrome results from a direct blow to the buttock area.[22] As a result of trauma, adhesions can develop between the **piriformis muscle**, the **sciatic nerve**, and the roof of the **greater sciatic notch**.

Myofascial trigger points in the piriformis or other gluteal muscles can create *hypertonicity* and lead directly to nerve compression. Trigger points in the **gluteus minimus** are known to reproduce symptoms identical to *sciatica* and could be confused with nerve entrapment by the piriformis muscle.[21] *Sacroiliac joint dysfunction* can also perpetuate trigger points in the piriformis muscle and increase the likelihood of nerve compression.[16] A sudden load, such as falling on the sacroiliac region or piriformis muscle could be the initial source of trigger point problems. Ongoing hypertonicity then leads to nerve compression.

History

A client with piriformis syndrome complains of pain in the low back, gluteal region, or the posterior lower extremity. The pain is described as sharp, shooting, or electrical in nature. Pain from nerve compression is felt in either the entire region innervated by that nerve or only a part of it. For example, it is possible for pain from a proximal nerve compression to be felt in the lower leg and foot, but not in the thigh. If pain is limited to the gluteal region only, it may be due to pressure on one of the gluteal nerves and not the sciatic or posterior femoral cutaneous nerves.

The client may report an exaggeration of pain when sitting for long periods. Ask about sitting habits, as increased pressure on the affected nerves results from sitting on a wallet or other objects placed in back pockets. Simultaneous symptoms of low back or sacroiliac pain are typical as well.

Observation

Visual signs are rarely evident with piriformis syndrome. If nerve compression has affected the inferior gluteal nerve, it is possible that some size difference in the gluteal region due to muscle atrophy might be perceived when the affected side is compared with the unaffected side.

Palpation

Pressure applied to the gluteal region generally reproduces characteristic neurological pain. The piriformis muscle and the gluteus maximus are frequently hypertonic. Note the specific anatomic location that reproduces symptoms to determine if additional pressure on the piriformis muscle and sciatic nerve aggravate symptoms. Sciatica-like symptoms also occur with referrals from gluteus minimus trigger points.

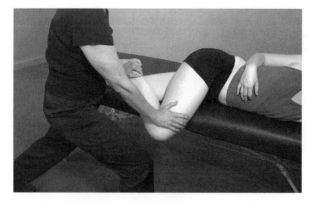

Figure 7.22 Piriformis (or FAIR) test

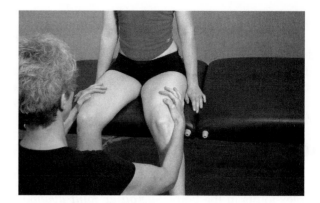

Figure 7.23 Pace abduction test

Range-of-Motion and Resistance Tests

AROM: If the piriformis muscle is tight, there may be discomfort or limitation to medial rotation when the hip is in extension due to stretching of the piriformis. Pain is sometimes felt at the end of hip flexion when the sciatic nerve is stretched, especially if the knee is extended.
PROM: The same principles apply as for active motion.
MRT: Pain is sometimes felt with resisted abduction, if performed in a seated position (see Pace abduction test below). Weakness in abduction from a neutral position may be evident if the superior gluteal nerve is compressed. Pain may also be evident from resisted lateral rotation with the starting position of neutral extension and full medial rotation.

Special Tests
Piriformis Test

The client lies on the side opposite the one being tested and close to the edge of the table so the upper leg can be dropped past the edge of the table. The practitioner brings the client's hip on the test side into at least 60⁰ of flexion and then into full adduction with the knee flexed (Figure 7.22). This test is sometimes called the FAIR test—an acronym for the hip positions of flexion, adduction, and internal rotation. If there is radiating pain in the gluteal region or down the posterior leg, piriformis syndrome is probable. Increased tension can be applied to the sciatic nerve by extending the knee, thereby making the test more sensitive.

Explanation: When the hip is flexed past 60⁰, the piriformis muscle changes its action. The muscle's primary action at this point is abduction of the hip. The piriformis muscle is stretched with the hip in a flexed and adducted position. Stretching the muscle pulls it taut against the nerve and increases nerve compression symptoms.

Pace Abduction Test

The client is seated on the edge of the treatment table with the hips partially abducted. The practitioner places each hand on the lateral sides of the client's knees. The client is instructed to hold this position as the practitioner

attempts to press the client's knees together (Figure 7.23). If there is radiating pain in the gluteal region or down the posterior leg, there is a good likelihood of piriformis syndrome.

Explanation: In this test the piriformis muscle is being contracted instead of stretched. If the piriformis is pressing on a nerve, contracting the muscle against resistance can reproduce the primary symptoms. In a seated position the hip is flexed to 90⁰. When the hip is past 60⁰ of flexion, abducting the hip against resistance engages the piriformis.

Differential Evaluation

Lumbar radiculopathy, lumbar facet joint dysfunction, sacroiliac joint dysfunction, spondylolysis, spondylolisthesis, trochanteric bursitis, myofascial trigger point referral, other peripheral neuropathy.

Box 7.4 Clinical Notes

Clarifying sciatic nerve pain

Pain in the posterior leg is routinely ascribed to lumbar nerve root pathology and often called sciatica. However, entrapment of the sciatic nerve by the piriformis muscle could produce the same symptoms. Thorough evaluation of neurological signs and symptoms through testing procedures helps discriminate between the two.

Evaluation is enhanced by increasing the sensitivity of the side-lying (FAIR) piriformis test. This test is most commonly performed with the knee in a flexed position. If the knee is brought into extension, there is increased tensile stress on the sciatic nerve. Additional tensile stress on the sciatic nerve while the piriformis muscle is simultaneously being stretched may elicit symptoms when the normal position does not.

Suggestions for Treatment

The best treatment method is soft-tissue manipulation and stretching aimed at reducing hypertonicity in the piriformis muscle. Myofascial trigger points should also be treated. Caution should be used in applying deep pressure in the area as it can exacerbate the symptoms by increasing pressure on the nerve.

SACROILIAC JOINT DYSFUNCTION

The **sacroiliac (SI) joint** is one of the most biomechanically complex joints in the body. *Sacroiliac joint dysfunction* develops for several reasons including *joint misalignment, ligament sprain,* and *irritation at the contact surfaces*. The condition produces pain primarily in the low back and upper sacral region. Due to the complexity of structures in the SI region, accurately identifying the root of pain in SI joint dysfunction is challenging.

Characteristics

There are two SI joints, one between the **sacrum** and **ilium** on each side. The SI joints are an important biomechanical transition region as these joints are the location at which weight is transmitted from the axial skeleton into the pelvis. Appropriate load transfer from the upper skeletal structures to the lower requires a great deal of stability in the joint. The SI joints are tightly bound with a dense webbing of ligaments on both the anterior and posterior sides. The primary stabilizing ligaments are the **anterior sacroiliac, posterior sacroiliac, sacrotuberous**, and **sacrospinous ligaments** (Figure 7.24).

Additional stability in the joint is provided by the irregular contact surface between the **sacrum** and **ilium** on each side (Figure 7.25). The roughened contact surface lets the bones of the articulation fit together like puzzle pieces. While the irregular contact surface is effective for increasing stability, it becomes a painful problem if the sacrum is displaced in relation to the ilium and the contoured surfaces are no longer congruent.

Because of the need for stability, there is very little motion possible at the SI joint. There is a slight degree of motion in the sagittal plane. The forward tipping of the superior surface of the sacrum is called **nutation** and the backward tipping is called **counternutation**; the range for both is only 7–8 degrees. This motion is essential for proper mechanics during walking, bending over, and other motions because each innominate must rotate independently. Motion at a joint is usually controlled by muscles that span directly between the two bones of the joint. At the SI joint no muscles span directly from the sacrum to the ilium. Instead joint motion is controlled by a collection of muscles, ligaments, and fascia in the lumbosacral region.

The superior attachment of the **hamstrings** is through a conjoined tendon to the **ischial tuberosity**. There is continuity in the connective tissue of the hamstring tendons and the **sacrotuberous ligament**.[25] Tension in the

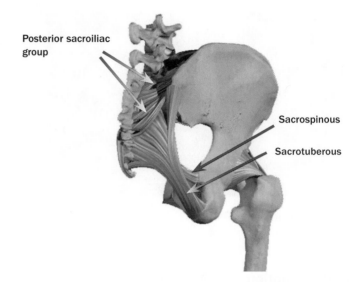

Posterior sacroiliac group

Sacrospinous

Sacrotuberous

Figure 7.24 Primary stabilizing ligaments of the sacroiliac joint. Anterior sacroiliac ligaments are on the anterior surface of the sacrum and not visible in this image. (3-D anatomy image courtesy of Primal Pictures Ltd. www.primalpictures.com.)

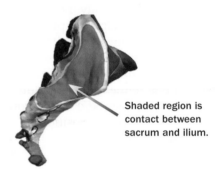

Shaded region is contact between sacrum and ilium.

Figure 7.25 Irregular contact surfaces of the ilium and sacrum. (3-D anatomy image courtesy of Primal Pictures Ltd. www.primalpictures.com.)

hamstring muscles is transmitted to the sacrotuberous ligament and eventually to the **sacrum,** where the tension can alter SI joint position or function. There is also a connection between the posterior **sacroiliac ligaments** and the lower fascia of the **erector spinae muscles**. Tension in the erector spinae can affect sacral position as well.

The **sacrotuberous ligament** has fascial connectivity with the **gluteus maximus muscle**, which also contributes to stability of the SI joint. Stress forces on these connections do not have to be large to have an effect. Due to the rich innervation of the SI region, even minor loads of tensile stress can create irritation of the pain receptors and produce back or SI joint pain.[2, 23, 24]

Several factors can be responsible for producing SI joint pain. The sacrum and ilium are designed to fit together in a specific manner. Misalignment of the contact surfaces between the sacrum and ilium can produce SI joint pain. The dense web of ligaments spanning the joint is also vulnerable to sprain, especially from acute injuries. Stress to the muscles, tendons, and fascial connections in the region also produces SI joint pain.

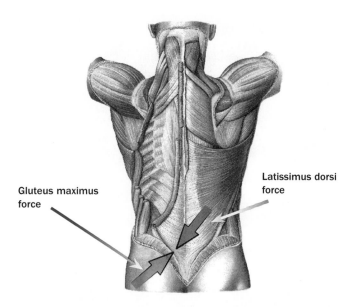

Gluteus maximus force

Latissimus dorsi force

Figure 7.26 Force closure at the sacroiliac joint. (Mediclip image copyright, 1998 Williams & Wilkins. All rights reserved.)

Gravity is another factor that adds stress to the SI joint. Gravity's pull on the upper body produces a shear force on the SI joint because the contact surface between the **ilium** and **sacrum** is almost vertical and the joint supports the weight of the upper body. In order to improve stability and resist the vertical shear force there is a coupled action between the **gluteus maximus** on one side and the **latissimus dorsi** on the other. These muscles work to hold the sacrum and the ilia tightly together creating what is called a **force closure** (Figure 7.26).[26] The pulling force of the two muscles squeezes the SI joint together to enhance stability. The piriformis is another muscle that contributes to force closure of the SI joint. The pull of the piriformis on its two attachment sites, the sacrum and femur, is such that it contributes lateral compressive force to the SI joint.

Other factors that contribute to SI joint dysfunction include unequal forces on the joint, such as *leg length discrepancies, pelvic tilting, scoliosis, muscle tightness, immobility of the SI joint,* improper shoes, running on uneven surfaces, awkward sitting postures, or other *biomechanical distortions.*[27] In some cases, there may be different dysfunctions on either side. In most cases, SI dysfunction develops gradually. However, acute injuries such as *sprains* to the supporting ligaments may occur. For example, falling on stairs and hitting one innominate but not the other could produce forces sufficient to cause ligament tearing.

History

A client with SI joint dysfunction reports pain in the lower lumbar or upper sacral and/or gluteal region. Sometimes the pain will refer down the posterior lower extremity. Pain is generally diffuse and aching, but could be described as sharp or shooting. SI joint pain is some-

times similar to that of *sciatic nerve compression.* A single event may initiate the pain, such as a fall or an automobile accident, but more often pain arises gradually. Ask about any biomechanical factors that can be correlated with the onset of symptoms. Biomechanical stress, such as leg-length inequality, vigorous activities on an uneven surface, or prolonged sitting in awkward positions should be thoroughly investigated in the history.

Observation

In many cases there are no clear visual indicators of sacroiliac joint dysfunction. Visible pelvic alignment problems, such as lateral tilting or rotation of one or both innominates, could be a contributing factor. However, the presence of one or more postural distortions in the pelvis is not necessarily indicative of SI joint dysfunction.

Palpation

Tenderness is sometimes felt in the soft tissues of the lower lumbar, gluteal, or upper sacral region. When palpated, active myofascial trigger points in the lumbar or gluteal regions can reproduce the client's pain. Despite pain or tenderness that might be felt in the area, lack of pain with palpation does not necessarily indicate absence of SI joint dysfunction. If pain is not reproduced with palpation, it could be because the pain-producing tissues are too deep. Dysfunction in the anterior sacroiliac ligaments or the contact surface between the sacrum and ilium are examples regions not easily accessible to palpation.

Range-of-Motion and Resistance Tests

AROM: Pain is present with several active motions of the hip or lumbar region including trunk flexion or extension, as well as hip flexion, abduction, or extension. In some cases pain also results from adduction or rotational movements of the hip, but not often.

PROM: The same principles apply as for AROM.

MRT: Due to the location of attachments of the lower lumbar erector spinae group in the SI region, pain may be felt with resisted extension of the lumbar spine. Due to fascial continuities in the region, pain could also be felt with resisted flexion, extension, lateral rotation, or abduction of the hip.

Special Tests

Special tests designed to evaluate SI joint dysfunction focus on one of three factors: positional distortions of associated bones based on static palpation; identification of motion disturbances based on palpation during movement; or pain provocation tests intended to reproduce the client's primary pain.[28] Tests that require palpating bony landmarks during motion or static position of the hip, pelvis, or lumbar spine are not always accurate.[3, 29-31] Pain provocation tests tend to be have the highest accuracy and are discussed in this section.[28, 29, 32, 33] The best approach for evaluating SI joint dysfunction is to compare and contrast the results of several tests.[3]

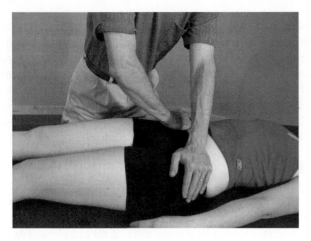

Figure 7.27 Gapping test.

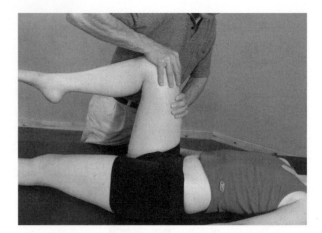

Figure 7.28 Thigh thrust test.

Gapping (Distraction) Test

The client is supine on the table. The practitioner places the flat aspect of the palm over each ASIS. To prevent discomfort, do not place the base of the hand against the ASIS. Crossing the arms to put the hands on the same side ASIS (right hand on right ASIS, left hand on left ASIS) provides a better angle of force during the test (Figure 7.27). A moderate amount of pressure is applied to each ASIS in a posterior and lateral direction (pressing down and out). If SI joint dysfunction is present, this movement can reproduce the client's primary pain.

Explanation: In this procedure the innominates are pressed in a downward (posterior) and outward (lateral) direction. As pressure is applied, there is tensile stress on the anterior sacroiliac ligaments and compression on the posterior aspects of the SI joint. It will not be immediately clear if pain is from ligament stress or joint compression.

Thigh Thrust Test

The client is supine on the table. The hip is brought actively or passively into 90⁰ of flexion. The practitioner applies a posterior shear force to the SI joint by pressing down toward the table along the long axis of the femur (Figure 7.28). The force is applied gradually until a moderate degree of pressure is reached. If symptoms are reproduced, SI joint dysfunction is likely.

Explanation: This test uses the femur to apply force to the ligaments and surface of the SI joint. The downward pressure on the femur produces anterior to posterior shear force on the SI joint. If there is irritation of the joint surface on the test side, the client's pain is reproduced.

Compression Test

The client is side-lying on the table. The practitioner places both hands on the lateral sides of the client's pelvis over the upper iliac crest. A moderate amount of pressure is gradually applied directly down toward the treatment table (Figure 7.29). The pressure is sustained for a few moments to identify if the client's pain is reproduced, which would indicate SI joint dysfunction.

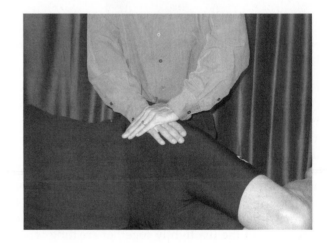

Figure 7.29 Compression test.

Explanation: When there is articular dysfunction at the SI joint, pressing the joint contact surfaces closer together reproduces the client's pain.

Gaenslen's Test

The client lies on the side opposite that being tested and brings the thigh closest to the table into full flexion near the chest. The practitioner uses one hand to stabilize the pelvis and the other hand to bring the upper leg into full hyperextension (Figure 7.30). Pain reproduced in this position is an indicator of SI joint irritation. Pain is most likely to be reproduced on the upper side where the hip is in hyperextension. The test should be repeated on the other side to compare the symptoms.

Explanation: In the test position one hip is in full flexion while the other is in (hyper)extension. This position produces significant stress on the SI joints, as the motions between the sacrum and ilia on each side are opposite. A normal SI joint should not have any pain with this procedure, but if there is ligament damage or joint misalignment, pain is felt.

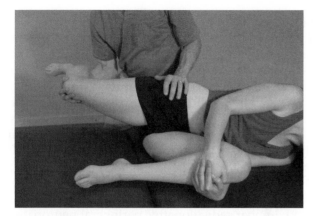

Figure 7.30 Gaenslen's test.

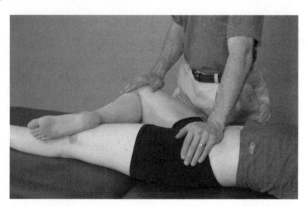

Figure 7.31 FABER (Patrick's) test.

FABER (Patrick's) Test

The client is supine on the table. This test gets its name from the acronym of the positions of the hip. The hip on the affected side is put in a position of flexion, abduction, and external rotation with the knee flexed and the foot resting on the opposite distal thigh. The practitioner places one hand on the medial side of the client's knee (on the test side) and the other hand on the opposite side ASIS (Figure 7.31). A slight amount of pressure is applied to the knee on the test side so the thigh is pushed away from the opposite side ASIS. Pain in the SI region indicates SI joint pathology.

Explanation: The FABER position applies tensile stress across the anterior sacroiliac ligaments and compressive force to the posterior SI joint, similar to the gapping test. The leg on the test side is used as a fulcrum and generally puts greater tensile stress on the ligaments of the SI joint on the ipsilateral side than on those of the contralateral side. However, the opposite side ligaments can be stretched as well and reproduce pain if a problem exists. If the adductors are tight, pain or discomfort may be felt in the adductors before there is adequate stress on the SI joints, reducing the accuracy of the test. This test is also used to identify *hip joint capsule pathology*. Because flexion and abduction are limited in the capsular pattern of the hip, the test can produce pain in the hip joint if there is capsular pathology.

Differential Evaluation

Hip joint pathology, lumbar radiculopathy, iliotibial band friction syndrome, trochanteric bursitis, lumbar facet joint dysfunction, peripheral sciatic nerve entrapment, superior or inferior gluteal nerve entrapment, arthritic changes in the SI joint.

Suggestions for Treatment

Treatment of SI joint dysfunction varies depending on the nature of the disorder. Posterior ligament sprains can be treated with deep friction massage that encourages tissue remodeling and repair. Ligament sprains to the anterior sacroiliac ligaments are difficult to treat with massage because the ligaments cannot be safely palpated. Joint alignment problems are often treated with manipulation or mobilization techniques that are performed by a physical therapist, osteopath, chiropractor, or other manipulative therapist. Soft-tissue treatment to other muscles spanning the joint is a valuable adjunct therapy. Consider the connections of the soft tissues that cross the SI joint when designing appropriate treatment strategies. For example, treatment of hypertonic hamstrings could be helpful for a hypomobile SI joint as fascial connections from the hamstrings through the sacrotuberous ligament restrict sacral movement.

TROCHANTERIC BURSITIS

Trochanteris bursitis is usually an overuse problem caused by repetitive friction. The condition occurs more frequently in older people and those performing repetitive flexion and extension activities of the hip.

Characteristics

There are two bursae that lie directly over the **greater trochanter of the femur** and reduce friction of the overlying **gluteal muscles** (Figure 7.32). One bursa sits between the distal fibers of the **gluteus medius** and the **iliotibial band**, and the other between the **gluteus maximus** and **iliotibial band**. **Trochanteric bursitis involves painful inflammation of one or both bursae.** The bursa under the gluteus maximus is more regularly irritated due to its location close to the tendinous insertion of the gluteus medius muscle. The iliotibial band can produce compression and irritation of the bursae during various hip movements because it courses directly over the bursae.

Trochanteric bursitis could result from a direct blow to the lateral hip, but usually results from activities of repetitive hip flexion in which the iliotibial band moves back and forth across the trochanter, such as in running or climbing stairs.[35] In rare cases, the condition can result from a systemic disorder such as *rheumatoid arthritis*.[36] Biomechanical alterations such as a *broad pelvis* or *leg-length discrepancy* may also create iliotibial band tightness sufficient to compress and irritate the bursae. In some cases the condition appears in the absence of any specific trauma or repetitive irritation.[34] *Enthesitis* (irrita-

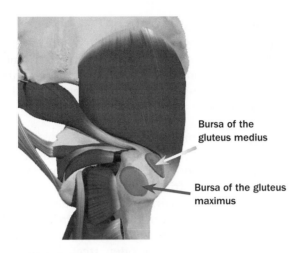

Figure 7.32 Posterior view of the right hip showing bursae affected in trochanteric bursitis. (3-D anatomy image courtesy of Primal Pictures Ltd. www.primalpictures.com.)

tion of the tendon attachment) of the gluteus medius is sometimes mistaken for trochanteric bursitis.[35]

History
If the bursitis is chronic the client reports a gradual onset of lateral hip pain typically associated with activities involving repetitive flexion and extension of the hip. The condition can be painful at night if the person lies on the affected hip during sleep. If the condition is acute, ask about incidents involving direct compression of the lateral hip that initiated the symptoms. Pain is frequently exaggerated when the hip is maintained in a flexed position for long periods, such as sitting in a car or a movie theater.

Observation
Visual signs are unlikely if the trochanteric bursitis is chronic. Postural distortions sometimes contribute to the development of chronic bursitis. For example, a broad pelvis with a large Q angle could produce exaggerated tensile stress on the iliotibial band and pull the band taut over the greater trochanter compressing the bursa. If the condition is acute, signs of bruising from the impact trauma are sometimes visible.

Palpation
Palpation is a primary method for identifying trochanteric bursitis. When the region around the greater trochanter of the femur is palpated, the client feels pain that is out of proportion to the amount of pressure applied. Depending on the degree of inflammation, the region may feel puffy or swollen as well.

Range-of-Motion and Resistance Testing
AROM: Pain can occur with hip flexion or extension as the iliotibial band rubs over the irritated bursa. Pain could be felt in abduction or adduction, but not typically.

PROM: Pain patterns are the same as for active motion. In some cases there is less pain with PROM than AROM because the muscles overlying the bursa do not generate enough tension to create compression of the bursa.

MRT: There can be pain with resisted abduction or extension due to tension on the iliotibial band that compresses the bursa. Weakness is possible due to reflex muscular inhibition.

Differential Evaluation
Femoral or hip fractures, avascular necrosis, iliotibial band friction, lumbar radiculopathy, peripheral neuropathy of lateral femoral cutaneous nerve, gluteus medius tendinopathy, osteoarthritis of the hip, iliopectineal bursitis.

Suggestions for Treatment
Treatment of chronic bursitis requires activity modification. Direct soft-tissue manipulation of the bursa will not treat the condition and could hinder the rate of healing. Tension should be relieved in the tensor fasciae latae muscle as well as the gluteal muscles in order to reduce compression of the bursa. Acute cases are treated with rest from offending activities and anti-inflammatory strategies, such as ice or medications. In cases that do not respond to conservative treatment, corticosteroid injections are used.

GENERAL NEUROMUSCULAR DISORDERS

In many cases, soft-tissue dysfunctions are not given a specific name. Adequate assessment is required to determine the tissues most likely involved and to take into account pathologies that may or may not have specific titles. Chapter 4 provides a discussion of the pathological processes of hypertonicity, myofascial trigger points, muscle strains, nerve compression and tension, tendinosis, tenosynovitis, ligament sprains, and osteoarthritis in any region of the body. Chapter 4 also includes the history, observation, palpation, relevant tests, and treatment suggestions sections for these conditions. The principles are the same for these conditions wherever they occur in the body.

Included in this section are specific tables and graphics for the hip and pelvis, including dermatomes, cutaneous innervation, trigger point referral patterns, and findings for MRTs. Tenosynovitis is not an issue in the hip and pelvis as there are no tendons surrounded by a synovial sheath in this area. Tendinosis is also rare in this region due to the structure and function of the muscles and tendons.

Nerve compression or tension pathologies produce symptoms in the hip and pelvis from either a lumbar radiculopathy (spinal nerve root compression) or a peripheral neuropathy (peripheral lower extremity nerve injury). Some of the locations in the hip and pelvis where peripheral neuropathies occur are discussed above as

Box: 7.5 Locations of Possible Nerve Entrapment

Sciatic nerve
  Between the greater sciatic notch and piriformis muscle
  Between the sacrospinous ligament & piriformis muscle
  Within the piriformis muscle

Superior gluteal nerve
  Between the greater sciatic notch and piriformis muscle

Inferior gluteal nerve
  Between the sacrospinous ligament & piriformis muscle

Posterior femoral cutaneous nerve
  Between the greater sciatic notch and piriformis muscle

Femoral nerve
  Underneath the inguinal ligament

Lateral femoral cutaneous nerve
  Underneath the inguinal ligament

Pudendal nerve
  Near the perineum

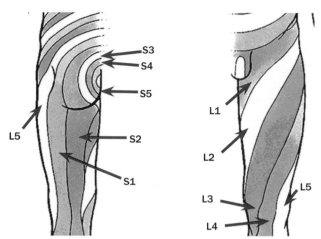

Figure 7.33 Dermatomes of the hip and pelvis (Mediclip image copyright, 1998 Williams & Wilkins. All rights reserved).

discrete nerve compression pathologies. Other regions of common nerve compression are listed in Box 7.5.

Sensory symptoms from a lumbar radiculopathy may be felt in the hip and pelvis and are experienced within the dermatome associated with that nerve root (Figure 7.33). Sensory symptoms of peripheral neuropathy are felt in the region of cutaneous innervation for the nerve affected (Figure 7.34). Radiculopathies or peripheral neuropathies can cause motor dysfunction and produce weakness in the muscles innervated by the affected nerve (Box 7.6).

Muscular hypertonicity develops in the hip and pelvis as a result of repetitive motion or postural stress. Myofascial trigger points can develop in the affected muscle(s) due to chronic muscular tension or trauma and refer pain or characteristic neurological sensations to various areas of the hip and pelvis. Common myofascial trigger point referral patterns for the major muscles in this region are shown in Figures 7.35 and 7.36.

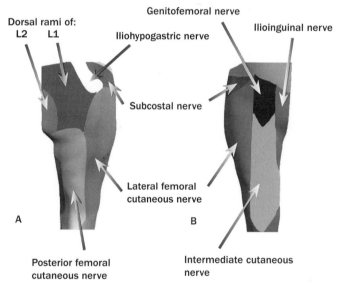

Figure 7.34 Cutaneous innervation of the posterior (A) and anterior (B) pelvic regions. (3-D anatomy image courtesy of Primal Pictures Ltd. www.primalpictures.com.)

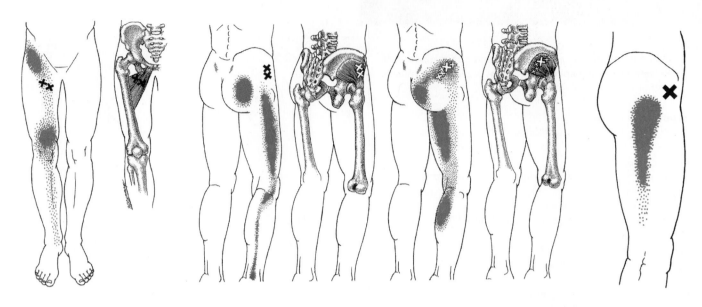

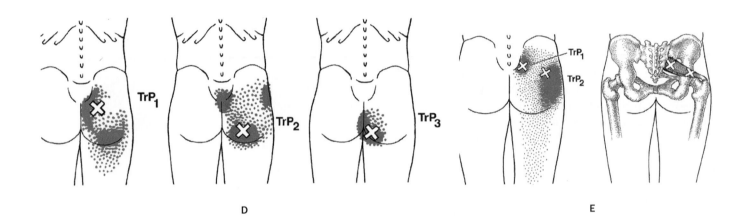

Figure 7.35 Myofascial trigger point referral patterns: Adductor brevis & longus (A), Gluteus minimus (B), Tensor fasciae latae (C), Gluteus maximus (D), Piriformis (E), Gluteus medius (F), Adductor magnus (G). (Images courtesy of Mediclip, copyright 1998 Williams & Wilkins. All rights reserved.)

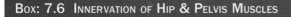

Box: 7.6 Innervation of Hip & Pelvis Muscles

Femoral Nerve	Superior Gluteal Nerve	Obturator Nerve	Muscles innervated directly from lumbar or sacral plexus
Iliopsoas	Gluteus minimus	Adductor longus	Quadratus femoris
Pectineus	Gluteus medius	Adductor brevis	Gemellus superior
	Tensor fasciae latae	Gracilis	Gemellus inferior
		Adductor magnus	Obturator internus
	Inferior Gluteal Nerve	superior, middle fibers	Obturator externus
	Gluteus maximus	Obturator externus	Piriformis

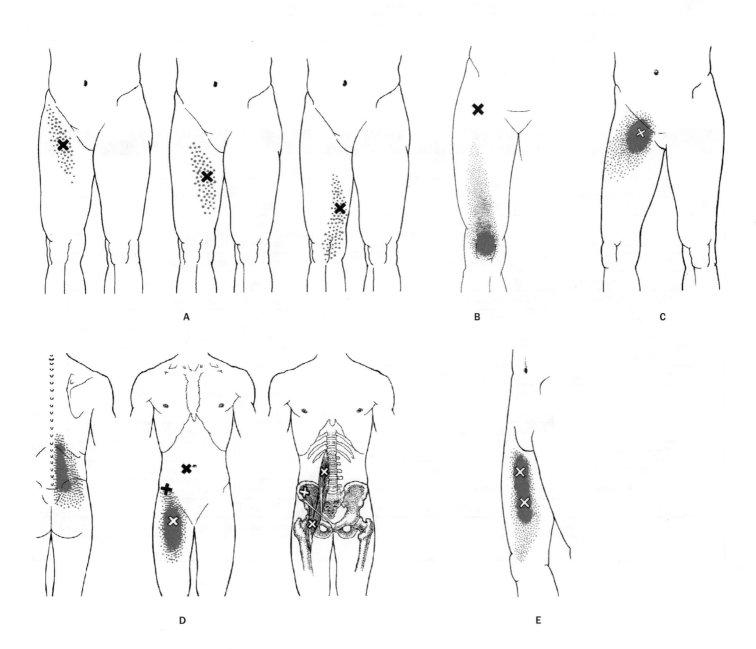

Figure 7.36 Myofascial trigger point referral patterns: Sartorius (A), Rectus femoris (B), Pectineus (C), Iliopsoas (D), Gracilis (E). (Images courtesy of Mediclip, copyright 1998 Williams & Wilkins. All rights reserved).

TABLE 1 JOINTS, ASSOCIATED MOTIONS, PLANES OF MOTION IN ANATOMICAL POSITION, AXIS OF ROTATION, AND AVERAGE ROM

Joint	Motion	Plane of Motion	Axis of Rotation	Avg. ROM (degrees)
Hip	Flexion	Sagittal	Medial-lateral	120
	Extension	Sagittal	Medial-lateral	30
	Abduction	Frontal	Anterior-posterior	45
	Adduction	Frontal	Anterior-posterior	30
	Medial rotation	Transverse	Superior-inferior	45
	Lateral rotation	Transverse	Superior-inferior	45

TABLE 2 WEAKNESS WITH MANUAL RESISTIVE TEST AND POSSIBLE NERVE INVOLVEMENT

Muscle	RESISTED ACTION	POSSIBLE NERVE INVOLVEMENT IF ACTION WEAK
Adductor Brevis	Hip adduction	obturator (L2-L3)
Adductor Longus	Hip adduction	obturator (L2 or L3-L4)
Adductor Magnus	Hip adduction	obturator (L2-L4)
Gemellus Inferior	Hip lateral rotation	nerve to quadratus femoris (L5-S1)
Gemellus Superior	Hip lateral rotation	nerve to obturator internus (L5-S1)
Gluteus Maximus	Hip extension	inferior gluteal (L5-S2)
Gluteus Medius	Hip abduction	superior gluteal (L4-S1)
Gluteus Minimus	Hip abduction	superior gluteal (L4-S1)
Gracilis	Hip adduction	obturator (L2-L3)
Obturator Externus	Hip lateral rotation	obturator (L3-L4)
Obturator Internus	Hip lateral rotation	nerve to obturator internus (L5-S1)
Pectineus	Hip adduction	femoral (L2 - L3)
Piriformis	Hip lateral rotation	nerve to piriformis (S1-S2)
Iliopsoas	Hip flexion	femoral (L2 - L4)
Quadratus femoris	Hip lateral rotation	nerve to quadratus femoris (L5-S1)
Rectus Femoris	Hip flexion	femoral (L2 - L4)
Sartorius	Hip flexion, abduction, & external rotation	femoral (L2 - L3)
Tensor Fasciae Latae	Hip abduction	superior gluteal (L4-S1)

Reference Table for Condition Assessment

This table lists a number of pathological conditions along the left-hand column. The top of the table lists common evaluation procedures. A ◆ in the box associated with a pathological condition and an evaluation procedure indi-cates the procedure is commonly used to identify that pathology. A ● in the box associated with the condition and a range-of-motion or resistance test, indicates pain is likely with that test for that pathology. Conditions are listed alphabetically.

TABLE 3 REFERENCE TABLE FOR CONDITION ASSESSMENT

	AROM	PROM	MRT	Compression test	FABER test	Gaenslen's test	Gapping test	Pace abduction test	Piriformis (FAIR) test	Thigh thrust test
Muscle Strains	●	●	●							
Muscular Hypertonicity	●	●								
Nerve Compression & Tension	●	●								
Piriformis Syndrome	●	●	●					◆	◆	
Sacroiliac Joint Dysfunction	●	●		◆	◆	◆	◆			◆
Trochanteric Bursitis	●	●								

References

1. Adams M, Bogduk N, Burton K, Dolan P. *The Biomechanics of Back Pain*. Edinburgh: Churchill Livingstone; 2002.
2. DonTigny RL. Anterior dysfunction of the sacroiliac joint as a major factor in the etiology of idiopathic low back pain syndrome. *Phys Ther.* 1990;70(4):250-265; discussion 262-255.
3. Cibulka MT, Koldehoff R. Clinical usefulness of a cluster of sacroiliac joint tests in patients with and without low back pain. *J Orthop Sports Phys Ther.* 1999;29(2):83-89; discussion 90-82.
4. Broadhurst NA, Bond MJ. Pain provocation tests for the assessment of sacroiliac joint dysfunction. *J Spinal Disord.* Aug 1998;11(4):341-345.
5. Laslett M, Williams M. The reliability of selected pain provocation tests for sacroiliac joint pathology. *Spine.* 1994;19(11):1243-1249.
6. Kokmeyer DJ, Van der Wurff P, Aufdemkampe G, Fickenscher TC. The reliability of multitest regimens with sacroiliac pain provocation tests. *J Manipulative Physiol Ther.* Jan 2002;25(1):42-48.
7. Lee D. *The Pelvic Girdle*. 3rd ed. Edinburgh: Churchill Livingstone; 2004.
8. Chaitow L, Delany J. *Clinical Application of Neuromuscular Techniques*. Vol 2. Edinburgh: Churchill Livingstone; 2002.
9. Neumann DA. *Kinesiology of the Musculoskeletal System*. St. Louis: Mosby; 2002.
10. Burkett LN. Causative factors in hamstring strains. *Med Sci Sports.* 1970;2(1):39-42.
11. Cibulka MT. Understanding sacroiliac joint movement as a guide to the management of a patient with unilateral low back pain. *Man Ther.* 2002;7(4):215-221.
12. DonTigny RL. Function and pathomechanics of the sacroiliac joint. A review. *Phys Ther.* Jan 1985;65(1):35-44.
13. Sprigle S, Flinn N, Wootten M, McCorry S. Development and testing of a pelvic goniometer designed to measure pelvic tilt and hip flexion. *Clin Biomech (Bristol, Avon).* Jun 2003;18(5):462-465.
14. Greenman P. *Principles of Manual Medicine*. 2nd ed. Baltimore: Williams & Wilkins; 1996.
15. White SC, Gilchrist LA, Wilk BE. Asymmetric limb loading with true or simulated leg-length differences. *Clin Orthop Relat Res.* Apr 2004(421):287-292.
16. Magee D. *Orthopedic Physical Assessment*. 3rd ed. Philadelphia: W.B. Saunders; 1997.
17. Dawson D, Hallett M, Wilbourn A. *Entrapment Neuropathies*. 3rd ed. Philadelphia: Lippincott-Raven; 1999.
18. Barton PM. Piriformis syndrome: a rational approach to management. *Pain.* 1991;47(3):345-352.
19. Silver JK, Leadbetter WB. Piriformis syndrome: assessment of current practice and literature review.

Orthopedics. 1998;21(10):1133-1135.

20. Moore K, Dalley A. *Clinically Oriented Anatomy.* 4th ed. Philadelphia: Lippincott Williams & Wilkins; 1999.

21. Travell J, Simons, D. *Myofascial Pain and Dysfunction: The Trigger Point Manual.* Vol 2. Baltimore: Williams & Wilkins; 1992.

22. Benson ER, Schutzer SF. Posttraumatic piriformis syndrome: Diagnosis and results of operative treatment. *J Bone Joint Surg Amer Vol.* 1999;81A(7):941-949.

23. Brolinson PG, Kozar AJ, Cibor G. Sacroiliac joint dysfunction in athletes. *Curr Sports Med Rep.* Feb 2003;2(1):47-56.

24. Bernard TN, Jr., Kirkaldy-Willis WH. Recognizing specific characteristics of nonspecific low back pain. *Clin Orthop Relat Res.* Apr 1987(217):266-280.

25. Vleeming A, Mooney V, Dorman T, Snijders C, Stoeckart R. *Movement, Stability, & Low Back Pain.* New York: Churchill Livingstone; 1999.

26. Snijders C, Vleeming A, Stoeckart R, Mens J, Kleinrensink G. Biomechanics of the Interface Between Spine and Pelvis in Different Postures. In: Vleeming A, Mooney V, Dorman T, Snijders C, Stoeckart R, eds. *Movement, Stability, & Low Back Pain.* New York: Churchill Livingstone; 1999.

27. Basmajian J, Nyberg R. *Rational Manual Therapies.* Baltimore: Williams& Wilkins; 1993.

28. Freburger JK, Riddle DL. Using published evidence to guide the examination of the sacroiliac joint region. *Phys Ther.* May 2001;81(5):1135-1143.

29. Potter NA, Rothstein JM. Intertester reliability for selected clinical tests of the sacroiliac joint. *Phys Ther.* 1985;65(11):1671-1675.

30. Dreyfuss P, Michaelsen M, Pauza K, McLarty J, Bogduk N. The value of medical history and physical examination in diagnosing sacroiliac joint pain. *Spine.* Nov 15 1996;21(22):2594-2602.

31. Tullberg T, Blomberg S, Branth B, Johnsson R. Manipulation does not alter the position of the sacroiliac joint. A roentgen stereophotogrammetric analysis. *Spine.* 1998;23(10):1124-1128; discussion 1129.

32. Laslett M. Pain Provocation Sacroiliac Joint Tests: Reliability and Prevalence. In: Vleeming A, Mooney V, Snijders C, Dorman T, Stoeckart R, eds. *Movement, Stability, and Low Back Pain.* New York: Churchill Livingstone; 1999.

33. Slipman CW, Sterenfeld EB, Chou LH, Herzog R, Vresilovic E. The predictive value of provocative sacroiliac joint stress maneuvers in the diagnosis of sacroiliac joint syndrome. *Arch Phys Med Rehabil.* Mar 1998;79(3):288-292.

34. Shbeeb MI, Matteson EL. Trochanteric bursitis (greater trochanter pain syndrome). *Mayo Clin Proc.* 1996;71(6):565-569.

35. Browning KH. Hip and pelvis injuries in runners. *Physician Sportsmed.* 2001;29(1).

36. Raman D, Haslock I. Trochanteric bursitis--a frequent cause of 'hip' pain in rheumatoid arthritis. *Ann Rheum Dis.* Dec 1982;41(6):602-603.

8 Lumbar & Thoracic Spine

Low back pain (LBP) is a pervasive orthopedic problem and in the United States it is estimated to affect more than 70% of the population at some point in life.[1] The causes of LPB are often poorly understood and treatment for the condition can be inadequate. For many years LBP was thought to result primarily from structural disorders, such as *herniated discs*.[1] While disc pathology does exist in some cases, many LBP complaints do not involve disc herniation. Many low back pain problems do not have easily identifiable structural or organic sources; these disorders are referred to as *non-specific low back pain*. LBP frequently involves functional impairment of the richly innervated soft tissues that govern movement in the spine.

The spine is a complex biomechanical structure designed to function like a flexible rod. Each vertebral segment has four articulations: a **superior** and **inferior articular facet** on the left and right sides. Each articulation is a normal synovial joint encapsulating a large number of pain receptors. With many richly innervated joints in the spine, pain-producing joint disorders are commonplace. There are also numerous muscles, tendons, and ligaments responsible for creating and limiting movement in the spine. Many of the muscles in this region are small, some only spanning one vertebral segment. Despite their small size these muscles are essential in proper spinal function and when impaired contribute to various pathological conditions.

A large percentage of LBP complaints can be resolved with conservative treatments such as massage because muscles are a primary source of pain. Due to the seriousness of some conditions in this region, such as *bone spurs* and *spinal tumors*, the practitioner must distinguish between general soft-tissue LBP complaints and disorders that need referral to other health care providers. Several conditions are not identifiable with physical examination and it is advisable to consult with other health care professionals for evaluation and treatment requirements.

Movements and Motion Testing

SINGLE-PLANE MOVEMENTS

Range-of-motion evaluation in the lumbar and thoracic spine includes four primary movements: flexion, extension, lateral flexion, and rotation. Lateral flexion and rotation occur to each side. Because it is the axial skeleton that moves, movements are termed left or right instead of medial and lateral (e.g. left or right rotation, not medial or lateral rotation). In rotational movements the point of reference is the anterior side of the vertebral body. Rotational movements can be confusing because the anterior part of the vertebra rotates right while the spinous process rotates left.

Due to the number of articulations, spinal movement does not occur around a single axis as it does in most other joints. Instead there are a few degrees of motion at each functional unit. A functional unit includes two adjacent vertebrae and the intervertebral disc between them. Range-of-motion evaluations generally test cumulative motion of the lumbar and thoracic spine instead of motion at a single articulation. For example, range-of-motion values are given for thoracolumbar flexion and not for flexion at the L4-L5 articulation. In this text, movement occurring past full extension or anatomical position is considered hyperextension. The associated motions, planes, axes of rotation, and range of motion values for the lumbar and thoracic spine are listed in Table 3 at the end of the chapter.

Thoracolumbar spine

Flexion and **extension** occur in the **sagittal plane** (Figure 8.1). In anatomical position, flexion takes place as the trunk is brought toward the anterior surface of the thighs. Extension is the return to anatomical position from any flexed position with any motion past anatomical position considered hyperextension. Average range of motion is 75^0–85^0 for flexion; 25^0–35^0 for extension.

Lateral Flexion, or side bending, occurs in the **frontal plane** as the trunk moves toward the lateral aspect of the thigh (Figure 8.2). Average range of motion in lateral flexion is 35^0–45^0.

Rotation is movement in the **transverse plane** around the central axis of the spine (Figure 8.2). The spine rotates as the trunk is twisted to either side. Average range of motion in rotation to each side is 35^0–45^0.

Capsular Patterns

In most cases the joint capsules in the spine do not restrict motion the same way they do in extremity joints. When present, the capsular pattern is inconsistent and usually only apparent with severe arthritic changes.[2]

RANGE-OF-MOTION & RESISTIVE TESTS

Results from single-plane movement analysis form the basis for further evaluation procedures. Movement testing should be performed in a certain order, allowing for an efficient evaluation and the least amount of accumulated discomfort or pain to develop. It is also general practice to leave movements known or expected to be painful to the end of the evaluation. When possible, the pain-free side is evaluated first.

Active range-of-motion (AROM) movements are performed first to establish the client's movement abilities and pain symptoms. Passive range of motion (PROM) is performed next and manual resistive tests (MRT) follow. PROM evaluations are challenging in the lumbar and thoracic spine because the practitioner has to hold the entire weight of the client's torso. Some modifications in position may be necessary when attempting to perform passive movements. AROM results may make PROM assessment procedures unnecessary. If no pain occurs with active movement, pain is unlikely with passive movement. The practitioner should be familiar with the full step-by-step instructions and guidelines for how to interpret ROM and resistive test results as explained in Chapter 3.

Active Range of Motion

Active trunk flexion and extension are evaluated with the client in a standing position. When performing AROM evaluations, take into consideration the position of the torso to ensure the target tissues are engaged. For example, when the client actively flexes the torso from a standing position by bending forward at the waist, the

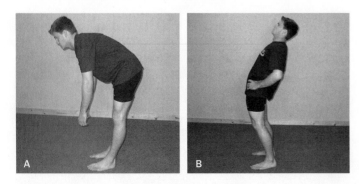

Figure 8.1 Thoracolumbar flexion (A) and extension (B).

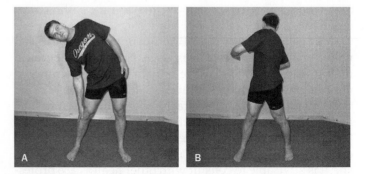

Figure 8.2 Thoracolumbar lateral flexion (A) and rotation (B).

Box 8.1 MUSCLE ACTIONS OF THE THORACOLUMBAR SPINE

Spine		
Flexion		**Extension**
Iliopsoas		Iliocostalis (thoracis and lumborum)
Obliquus externus abdominis		Longissimus thoracis
Obliquus internus abdominis		Spinalis thoracis
Rectus abdominis		Semispinalis thoracis
		Multifidi
Lateral flexion		Quadratus lumborum
Quadratus lumborum		Rotatores (thoracis and lumborum)
Intertransversarii (thoracis and lumborum)		Interspinales (thoracis and lumborum)
Obliquus externus abdominis		Intertransversarii (thoracis and lumborum)
Obliquus internus abdominis		
Iliopsoas		**Rotation (contralateral)**
		Obliquus externus abdominis
Rotation (ipsilateral)		Multifidi
Obliquus internus abdominis		Rotatores (thoracis and lumborum)

---

spinal extensors are engaged eccentrically. Engaging the trunk flexors requires a change in body position or in the way the resistance of gravity affects the movement.

Pain with active movement indicates problems in either the contractile or inert tissues associated with that movement. Factors prematurely limiting active movement in this region include *ligamentous or capsular damage, muscle tightness, pain from nerve compression or tension, disc pathology, fibrous cysts*, previous surgeries, or *joint disorders* such as *arthritis*.

Compare AROM test results with those from PROM and manual resistive tests to identify possible reasons for movement restriction. The muscles used to perform actions of the lumbar and thoracic spine are listed in Box 8.1. Note that other muscles can contribute to the motion and subsequent dysfunction.

Passive Range of Motion

Passive motion is performed after active. Pain during passive movement predominantly implicates inert tissues. However, muscles and tendons that contract in the opposite direction are stretched at the end range of passive movement. Evaluating passive motion in the lumbar and thoracic spine is difficult because the practitioner must often hold the entire weight of the client's torso while attempting to produce these movements. For this reason it may be difficult to get adequate information with certain positions.

PROM testing also evaluates end feel. Box 8.2 lists the primary joint locations and their normal end feel. Review Chapter 3 for a discussion of normal and pathological end feel descriptions. Factors that could prematurely limit passive movement are the same as for active movement.

Manual Resistive Tests

A manual resistive test (MRT) produces pain when there is a mechanical disruption of tissue. Pain with an MRT indicates that one or more of the muscles and/or tendons performing that action are involved. Testing all of a muscle's actions is not necessary, as a muscle's secondary actions recruit other muscles and make the test results less accurate. Palpation elicits more information if the test alone does not produce pain or discomfort. Refer to Box 8.1 for the list of primary muscles involved with each action. Table 1 at the end of the chapter lists actions commonly used for testing muscles in the lumbar and thoracic spine.

In some cases weakness is evident with MRTs. Factors that produce weakness include *lack of use, fatigue, reflex muscular inhibition,* and possibly a neurological pathology (*radiculopathy, peripheral neuropathy,* or a systemic neurological disorder). The nerves or nerve roots that may be involved are listed in Table 1 at the end of the chapter.

Box 8.2 JOINT REGION, ASSOCIATED MOTION, & END FEEL

Thoracolumbar Spine

Flexion	Tissue stretch
Extension	Tissue stretch (firm)
Lateral flexion	Tissue stretch
Rotation	Tissue stretch

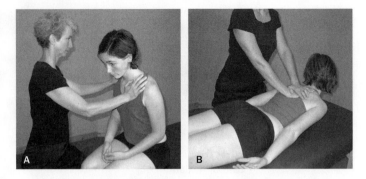

Figure 8.3 Resisted thoracolumbar flexion (A) and extension (B).

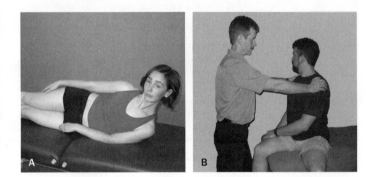

Figure 8.4 Resisted thoracolumbar lateral flexion (A) and rotation (B).

Thoracolumbar Spine
RESISTED FLEXION AND EXTENSION
To test flexion, the client is seated on the end of the treatment table. The practitioner's hands are placed on the client's upper chest. The client leans forward as the practitioner resists the movement (Figure 8.3). To test extension, the client is prone on the treatment table and attempts to lift the torso without using the arms (Figure 8.3). The weight of the torso provides enough resistance for this test, but if greater resistance is desired the practitioner can place one or both hands on the client's upper back to offer resistance.

RESISTED LATERAL FLEXION
The client is side-lying on the treatment table with the hips and knees extended. The client attempts to raise the trunk as far as possible (Figure 8.4). If the side-lying position is too difficult for the client to perform, the test can be performed with the client standing and the feet slightly more than shoulder width apart. The practitioner places one or both hands on the lateral aspect of the client's shoulder, covering the deltoid muscle. The client attempts to side-bend toward the practitioner. The standing version of the MRT is easier for the client, but not as effective in isolating the action of the quadratus lumborum and other lateral flexors of the spine.

RESISTED ROTATION
The client is in a seated position on the treatment table. The practitioner faces the client with a hand on each of the client's shoulders (Figure 8.4). The client is instructed to turn the torso to the side as the practitioner holds the

torso in the starting (neutral) position. The ipsilateral and contralateral rotators are involved in the movement. For example, left rotation uses left side ipsilateral rotators and right side contralateral rotators.

Structural and Postural Deviations
The following section covers common structural or postural deviations unique to the lumbar and thoracic spine. Under each condition there is a brief description of its characteristics followed by likely HOPRS findings. If applicable, orthopedic tests are included in the special tests section. If there is no special orthopedic test listed for that condition, evaluation should focus on other portions of the assessment process, such as range-of-motion testing.

KYPHOSIS

Kyphosis **is an abnormally increased convexity in the curvature of the thoracic spine**, also called *hunchback*.[3] Mild kyphosis routinely occurs with advanced age and can also develop from chronically poor posture or degenerative changes such as *osteoporosis*. The condition can adversely affect other physiological processes such as digestive function and breathing.[4]

Characteristics
There is a natural slight **kyphotic curvature** in the thoracic region located between the **lordotic curves** of the **cervical** and **lumbar spine**. The primary function of these

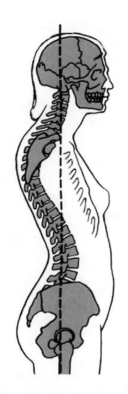

Figure 8.5 Lateral view of the torso showing upper thoracic kyphosis. (Mediclip image copyright, 1998 Williams & Wilkins. All rights reserved.)

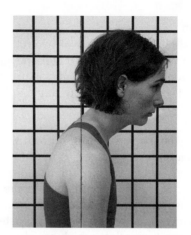

Figure 8.6 Kyphosis is evident with a postural grid chart for reference.

curves is shock absorption. Kyphosis occurs when the curvature is exaggerated and a subsequent postural distortion develops (Figure 8.5).

When the kyphotic curvature is increased, the head naturally tilts toward the floor. At the same time the body's righting reflex attempts to keep the eyes horizontal by contracting the cervical extensor muscles. The attempted postural compensation produces exaggerated compressive loads on the anterior aspect of the thoracic vertebrae and the posterior aspect of the cervical vertebrae. In some cases, the increased loads are enough to create *vertebral stress fractures*.[5]

An individual with kyphosis is likely to have an exaggerated cervical lordosis and forward head posture. Biomechanical patterns of muscular dysfunction, such as the *upper crossed syndrome* discussed in Chapter 9, are common in the client with kyphosis. In addition there is increased tensile load on ligaments and muscle tissues in the posterior thoracic region.

Some degree of kyphosis results naturally with age and is magnified by poor posture. Psychosocial factors can also play a role in the development of the disorder. For example, adolescents who feel too tall compared to their counterparts may hunch over in an effort to appear shorter. The postural patterns that are initiated at this age can be carried through adulthood, establishing a neuromuscular pattern of kyphosis.

Pathological kyphosis that causes clinical problems

usually results from *trauma, tumors, infection, tuberculosis, chronic postural stress, developmental disorders, rheumatoid arthritis,* or other *systemic conditions.*[6] Bone weakness pathologies, such as *osteoporosis* or *Scheuermann's disease*, are common causes of kyphosis. Osteoporosis involves a loss of bone density and is most prevalent in the elderly. Scheuermann's disease is a hereditary condition involving vertebral end-plate weakening and predominantly affects juveniles.[7]

Kyphosis can aggravate other disorders including *rib head subluxation, spinal stenosis, disc pathology,* or *facet joint irritation*. Other postural compensations can appear simultaneously with kyphosis. *Hypertonicity* in the anterior chest muscles, such as the **pectoralis major**, pulls the arm into medial rotation and a corresponding scapular protraction also develops. The altered scapular position limits function in the shoulder girdle, reducing range of motion and contributing to structural problems, such as *shoulder impingement syndrome*.[8]

Kyphosis does not necessarily produce pain or discomfort, but prolonged postural stress or more severe cases can produce a number of symptoms. *Myofascial trigger points* are typical in the upper thoracic or posterior cervical muscles and produce characteristic referral patterns. Pain in the upper thoracic region is typical and due to fatigue and overexertion in the upper thoracic spinal muscles. Pain could also result from any of the associated conditions mentioned above.

History

Ask the client about systemic bone disorders including Scheuermann's disease, osteoporosis, former vertebral fractures, or rheumatoid arthritis. Find out if the client is involved in long periods of static sitting postures or other postural patterns that exaggerate the kyphosis. Also inquire about the length of time that the kyphotic posture has been evident. Pain and fatigue may be described after long periods of sitting due to compressive and tensile loads on the vertebral structures.

Observation

Visual analysis is the best way to evaluate kyphosis. A visual reference such as a plumb line and grid chart are helpful (Figure 8.6). Forward head posture accompanies kyphosis and is evident in the lateral view as well.

Palpation

Depending on the severity of the kyphosis, the prominence of the thoracic spinous processes may be exaggerated. When palpated, the muscles of the upper back are likely to feel tight, due to their being pulled taut (stretched) and not because they are hypertonic and thus shortened. Palpable tightness is also possible in the posterior cervical and anterior chest muscles, which are chronically shortened. When palpated, myofascial trigger points produce characteristic referral patterns.

Range-of-Motion and Resistance Testing

AROM: Thoracic extension is generally more limited than flexion because the muscles and fascia of the anterior torso are chronically shortened, although there is little flexion or extension in the thoracic region even in a normal spine. There is sometimes loss in rotation due to the adverse effect on spinal mechanics.

PROM: The principles are the same as for AROM.

MRT: There is no pain with MRTs, but there may be weakness in muscles of the upper back.

Suggestions for Treatment

If the excessive kyphosis is from a bony disease such as osteoporosis, treatment should be coordinated with input from the client's physician. Be particularly careful about applying pressure to the posterior thoracic region if the client has osteoporosis as it is possible to produce damage to the delicate bone structure. In severe forms of kyphosis, a brace is sometimes necessary to keep the spinal structures in alignment. If the kyphosis is caused by chronic postural strain, then postural retraining is the cornerstone of treatment. Soft-tissue treatments should focus on lengthening the shortened muscles of the anterior upper torso. Massage of the upper back muscles reduces discomfort and myofascial trigger points as well.

SCOLIOSIS

Scoliosis is a **lateral/rotary curvature in the spine and is relatively common, especially in children.**[6] Most children grow out of scoliosis without need for further intervention. If the condition persists into adulthood, it can become seriously debilitating. The condition can be caused by various diseases or muscular distortion.

Characteristics

There are two types of scoliosis: **structural** and **functional**. **Structural scoliosis is caused by a fixed bony deformity, which can be inherited or acquired.** The deformity could result from structural irregularities in the spine or a

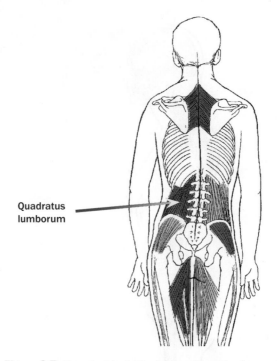

Figure 8.7 Hypertonicity in the left quadratus lumborum that creates a functional scoliosis. (Mediclip image copyright, 1998 Williams & Wilkins. All rights reserved.)

number of *systemic disorders* or *neuromuscular pathologies* such as an upper or lower *motor neuron lesion*.[9] Structural scoliosis is hard to correct and has detrimental long-term effects on spinal mechanics.

Functional scoliosis develops from excessive muscle tension and not from deformity in the bones of the spine. For example, *hypertonicity* in the **quadratus lumborum** and **iliocostalis lumborum** produce a lateral pelvic tilt to the opposite side, creating functional scoliosis in the lumbar region (Figure 8.7).

A thorough understanding of scoliosis requires a comprehensive understanding of the interaction of anatomy and biomechanics of the **lumbar** and **thoracic spine**. Spinal movements are governed by the orientation of the **facet (zygapophysial) joints**. In the thoracic region, the facet joints allow rotation and small amounts of lateral flexion, forward flexion, and extension. In the lumbar region, motion is predominantly sagittal plane flexion and extension with limited amounts of rotation and lateral flexion. Scoliosis involves both lateral flexion and rotation in the lumbar and thoracic spine.

Because the spine is like a flexible rod, it must partially rotate when it is side-bent (laterally flexed). In a normal upright position when the lumbar spine is laterally flexed to one side, the vertebrae simultaneously rotate to the opposite side (Figure 8.8). The coordinated and simultaneous movements are called **coupled motions**.

In the lumbar spine, lateral flexion is coupled with rotation to the opposite side. In the cervical spine, the movement is reversed so that lateral flexion is coupled with rotation to the same side. In the thoracic spine cou-

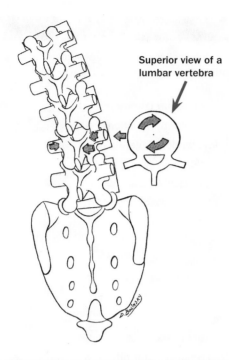

Superior view of a lumbar vertebra

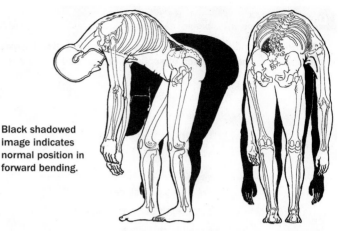

Black shadowed image indicates normal position in forward bending.

Figure 8.9 Left side rib hump from the rotational distortion of a thoraco-lumbar levoscoliosis. (Mediclip image copyright, 1998 Williams & Wilkins. All rights reserved.)

Figure 8.8 Coupling pattern in the lumbar spine during left lateral flexion. Lumbar vertebrae are laterally flexed left and rotated right. (Mediclip image copyright, 1998 Williams & Wilkins. All rights reserved.)

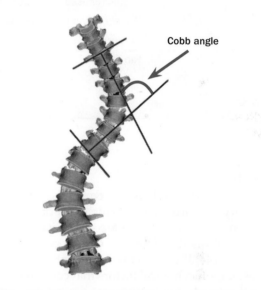

Cobb angle

Figure 8.10 Cobb method for measuring scoliotic curve. The Cobb angle is created at the intersection of two lines. One line is perpendicular to the superior surface of the uppermost vertebra that is a prominent part of the curve. The other is perpendicular to the inferior surface of the lowest vertebra that is a prominent part of the curve. (3-D anatomy image courtesy of Primal Pictures Ltd. www.primalpictures.com.)

pled motion is not as consistent. It appears that coupled motions can vary with certain pathological conditions. Generally, the lower thoracic region follows the coupling pattern of the lumbar vertebrae while the upper thoracic region follows the pattern of the cervical vertebrae.[6] The intricacies of coupling patterns in the spine demonstrate that scoliosis must be considered not only as a lateral curvature of the spine, but as a rotary dysfunction as well.

In severe cases of scoliosis, especially structural forms, the characteristic **rib hump** is sometimes visible (Figure 8.9). The hump is pronounced in the thoracic region due to the ribs and vertebrae's transverse processes being pushed posteriorly from the rotary distortion. A similar hump may exist on the convex side of the lateral curve in the lumbar region. The hump is most evident when the individual bends forward from a standing position.

If there is a single scoliotic curve it is called a *C curve*. In other cases there will be two curves that are convex in opposite directions and the distortion is called an *S curve*. The scoliotic curve is named for the convex side of the curve. If, for example, the right quadratus lumborum is in spasm and the pelvis tilts to the left, a functional scoliosis in the lumbar region results that is convex on the left and concave on the right. When the convex side of the curve is to the left, the condition is called a *levoscoliosis*; if the convex side of the curve is to the right the condition is called a *dextroscoliosis*.

Scoliosis could be confined to either the lumbar or thoracic region, or curves could appear in both sections of the spine. The severity of the curve is frequently evaluated by the **Cobb method** after taking a spinal x-ray (Figure 8.10).[6] The greater the angle, the more serious is the scoli-

osis. Cobb angles of greater than 50^0 are considered much more serious and could require surgical treatment. When Cobb angles are greater than 60^0 in the thoracic region, scoliosis is likely to adversely affect lung function and cause significant rib pain.[10]

Many cases of scoliosis begin as mild structural disorders, but can progress to serious complaints because of the functional adaptation of muscles to the distorted postures. There is a focus on the role of **paraspinal muscles** and the **quadratus lumborum** in creating or perpetuating the lateral bending, but the small intrinsic spinal muscles should not be overlooked as critical components of scoliosis. Muscles such as the **multifidi, rotatores**, and **transversospinalis** govern spinal rotary movement and may play an important role in developing the condition.

Box 8.3 Conditions Caused By or Related to Scolioisis

Numerous conditions and disorders are known to be associated with or to cause scoliosis. 85-90% of scoliosis cases are idiopathic.[6] Known causes of scoliosis are divided into the following categories[6, 10, 47]

Alteration of Structure
- Rickets
- Tumors
- Infection
- Disfigured vertebrae
- Fractures or dislocations
- Leg-length discrepancies
- Small hemi-pelvis
- Marfan syndrome

Iatrogenic (caused by other treatments)
- Vertebral end-plate destruction from radiation
- Surgery
- Rib removal

Neuromuscular Disorders
- Muscular dysfunction
- Myofascial trigger points
- Cerebral palsy
- Friedreich's ataxia
- Muscular dystrophy
- Torticollis
- Polio
- Syringomyelia
- Visual disturbances

Congenital
- Infantile scoliosis
- Sprengel's deformity
- Genetic disorders

History

Identify structural or systemic diseases in the client's history that are related to the onset of scoliosis. The conditions listed in Box 8.3 are of particular interest. Ask if the scoliosis developed in childhood or if its onset was later in life. If the scoliosis is recent, ask about back injuries or biomechanical factors that could have led to spasm in the quadratus lumborum, iliocostalis, paraspinals, or intrinsic spinal muscles.

The client with scoliosis may complain of pain or restricted range of motion in the lumbar or thoracic region. In some cases there are no specific symptoms as the individual has learned to compensate for the biomechanical dysfunction. In severe cases of structural scoliosis, the client will complain of chronic, general back pain.

Observation

If the scoliosis is severe, the lateral curvature is visible when viewing the individual from the posterior direction. A postural grid chart is helpful as a point of reference. Look for the presence of a rib hump or posterior protrusion of the paraspinal muscles when the individual bends forward from the waist. The protrusion will usually be on the convex side of the curve.

Palpation

Scoliosis is sometimes evident by running the fingers along each of the spinous processes to determine if there is a lateral deviation representing a scoliotic curve. A single spinous process that appears out of alignment is not enough to designate a lateral spinal curvature. There must be a succession of adjacent vertebrae in a curved distortion to indicate the condition.

There may be palpable tightness in the muscles on the concave side of the curve due to hypertonicity. Muscles on the convex side are also apt to feel tight, due to being stretched taut. The rotational dysfunctions mentioned above that produce visible humps on the convex side of the scoliotic curve are palpable as well. The tissue in these humps feels dense as it is pressed posteriorly by bones underneath the hump. Ribs may also feel farther apart on the convex side of the curve and closer together on the concave side.

Range-of-Motion and Resistance Testing

AROM: Some movements of the spine are limited due to the lateral curvature. Pain may or may not limit movement. In a functional scoliosis, range of motion in lateral flexion toward the convex side is more limited by shortened and hypertonic muscles on the concave side than by bony restrictions within the spinal structures. In a structural scoliosis, motion may be limited in several directions from alterations in skeletal mechanics.

PROM: The same principles apply as for AROM.

MRT: Pain is rare with MRTs unless the scoliosis has created severe postural distortions. Muscular weakness from chronic postural strain may be evident.

Suggestions for Treatment

Structural scoliosis can often be prevented by detection early in life and use of corrective braces or surgery. A physician might also recommend spinal fusion and corrective devices such as Harrington rods that are surgically placed along each side of the spine and attached to the vertebral bodies. The rods help correct the lateral/rotary curvature and prevent the curvature from affecting other structures, such as spinal nerve roots or internal organs.

Treatment of a functional scoliosis requires identification of biomechanical factors that led to the distortion. For example, if the functional scoliosis results from a lateral pelvic tilt caused by muscular hypertonicity, attention should focus on reducing tightness or myofascial trigger points in the muscles on the concave side of the curve.

In certain cases a functional disorder results from a structural leg-length discrepancy (Chapter 7). The skeletal imbalance must be addressed first and then muscular compensations can be treated with massage. While massage treatments for scoliosis have not been adequately researched, there is reason to believe that treating hypertonic muscles on the concave side of the curvature is beneficial. Massage is valuable for reducing general hypertonicity and overall pain reduction.

EXCESSIVE LUMBAR LORDOSIS

An *excessive lumbar lordosis* (or hyperlordosis) **is an exaggerated curvature in the lumbar spine and is also called** *swayback*. The condition can have detrimental effects on the kinetic chain both above and below the lumbar region. In most cases, the condition is a muscular distortion created by chronic muscle tightness, fatigue, and poor posture.

Characteristics

There is a natural **lordotic curve** in the lumbar region that is necessary for shock absorption. The lordotic curve is exaggerated during extension and is reduced during flexion. The primary muscles that produce spinal extension are the **erector spinae group, quadratus lumborum,** and several small intrinsic spinal muscles including the **multifidi, rotatores, interspinales,** and **intertransversarii.** *Low back pain* and *myofascial trigger points* can develop from hypertonicity in these muscles and exaggerate the lordosis.

In a normal lumbar lordosis the vertebral body is the primary weight-bearing structure. With an *excessive lumbar lordosis,* more of the body's weight is transferred to the posterior portion of the vertebrae (Figure 8.11). Increased weight is then borne by posterior vertebral arch structures such as the **lamina, pedicle, pars interarticularis, posterior portion of the intervertebral disc,** and **facet joints.** These structures are not designed for the weight increase and pathologies such as *facet joint dysfunction, disc herniation, spondylolysis,* or *spondylolisthesis* can result. Lumbar extension also narrows the

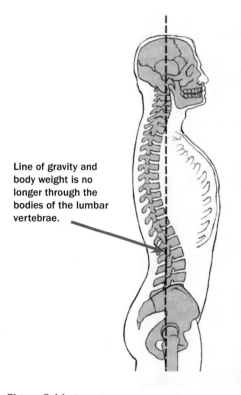

Line of gravity and body weight is no longer through the bodies of the lumbar vertebrae.

Figure 8.11 Posterior vertebral arch structures bear a greater percentage of weight in hyperlordosis. (Mediclip image copyright, 1998 Williams & Wilkins. All rights reserved.)

intervertebral foramen and can lead to *spinal nerve root compression.*

Excessive lordosis can develop from wearing high-heeled shoes. Lifting the heels throws the body weight forward and anteriorly rotates the pelvis. The natural reflex to maintain an upright posture activates the lumbar extensor muscles and brings the upper torso back to an erect position. Because the pelvis remains anteriorly rotated, the net effect is an excessive lumbar lordosis.

Dysfunctional patterns of muscular activation and poor posture routinely perpetuate an excessive lordosis. An example is the *lower crossed syndrome,* originally described by Vladimir Janda.[11] Many of the body's muscles fall into one of two categories, **postural** or **phasic muscles,** which differ in their fiber type and activation patterns.[12] When overused and fatigued, postural muscles tend to become hypertonic, while phasic muscles tend to become weak and inhibited. The phasic muscles are antagonists to postural muscles. Because postural muscles tend toward hypertonicity, they create a functional weakness in the phasic muscles through the process of **reciprocal inhibition.**[13]

Postural muscles in the lumbar spine include the **erector spinae, quadratus lumborum,** and **iliopsoas.** Phasic muscles in this region include the **abdominals, gluteus maximus** and **medius.** A graphical comparison of their position and functional relationships with each other shows how they interact and where the term *crossed syndrome* originates from (Figure 8.12). The postural muscles

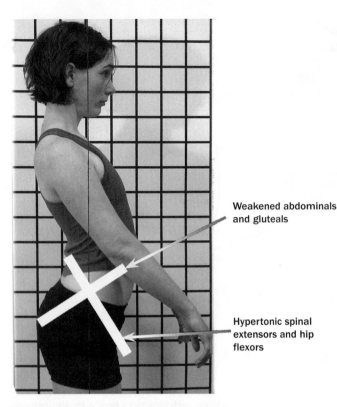

Figure 8.12 The lower crossed syndrome.

Weakened abdominals and gluteals

Hypertonic spinal extensors and hip flexors

are known to house active *myofascial trigger points* and refer characteristic symptoms when palpated. Continual tightness in the postural muscles maintain an *anterior pelvic tilt* and exaggerated lumbar lordosis.

In some cases excessive lumbar lordosis results from a congenital bone deformity or disease, such as *osteoporosis*. The postural distortion could also result from a significant weight gain in the abdominal region, such as pregnancy. In pregnancy the postural change is exacerbated by the increased elasticity of ligaments, resulting from elevated hormone levels.

History

Excessive lordosis does not always produce pain or characteristic symptoms. The client may complain of pain directly along the spine, which could be due to arthritic changes in the facet joints, increased compressive load on the posterior vertebral structures, or muscular hypertonicity. Ask about chronic postural factors, such as sitting positions at work or wearing of high-heeled shoes.

Observation

Excessive lumbar lordosis is best viewed from the side. A plumb line and postural reference grid are helpful (Figure 8.12). Excessive lordosis can also be viewed when the individual lies supine on a surface without soft cushioning. Typically there is just enough space to fit the fingers between the lumbar region and surface. With exaggerated lumbar lordosis, there is more space and a flat hand can fit between the client's back and the surface.

Palpation

Muscular hypertonicity is generally present and palpable in the iliopsoas, quadratus lumborum, and lumbar erector spinae muscles. Myofascial trigger points may be evident with palpation as well. The spinous processes may seem recessed in an anterior direction.

Range-of-Motion and Resistance Testing

AROM: The spine is in extension in an excessive lumbar lordosis. Further extension is sometimes limited by pain or discomfort. There is often muscular pain and limitation in forward flexion due to hypertonicity of the spinal extensor muscles.

PROM: The same principles apply as for AROM.

MRT: Pain is unlikely with MRTs, except for pain from myofascial trigger points. There could be functional weakness in the phasic muscles.

Suggestions for Treatment

Excessive lordosis can usually be treated with soft-tissue therapy. Massage techniques and stretching procedures are an effective method for reducing hypertonicity in the affected muscles. Postural re-education is an essential part of the treatment regimen as well.

DECREASED LUMBAR LORDOSIS

A *decreased lumbar lordosis* results when **the natural lordotic curve in the lumbar spine is reduced or absent.** The condition usually results from prolonged periods of poor sitting posture and may or may not produce pain or discomfort.

Characteristics

The spine is designed to have a natural **lordotic curve**, which is essential for proper shock absorption (see *excessive lumbar lordosis*). The bodies of the intervertebral discs are shaped in such a way that the lordotic curve is normally maintained. When the curvature in the lumbar spine is reduced, the vertebrae lose their shock-absorbing abilities because they become more vertically positioned (Figure 8.13). Once vertically stacked, the vertebrae increase pressure on the **intervertebral discs**, which can lead to *pain, disc degeneration,* or *herniation of the nucleus pulposus.*

Biomechanical studies have shown a difference in compressive loads on the intervertebral discs when the person is in different positions, such as standing, lying down, bending forward, and sitting in a slouched position. The greatest degree of disc compression is in a slumped sitting posture where there is a reduction in the lordotic curve.[14] The key characteristic of poor sitting that exaggerates the compressive load on the intervertebral discs is the loss of lumbar lordosis. Consequently, disc compression is increased in clients who have lost the proper lumbar curve not only in sitting, but also in their normal postural alignment. Disc compression is magnified even further if

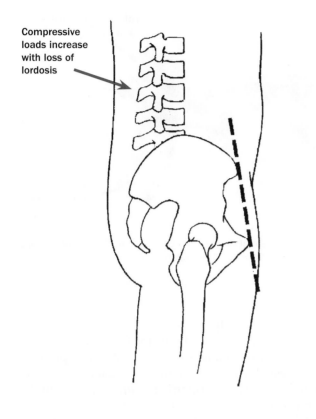

Compressive loads increase with loss of lordosis

Figure 8.13 Vertically stacking of the vertebrae in a loss of lumbar lordosis increases compression loads on them. (Mediclip image copyright, 1998 Williams & Wilkins. All rights reserved.)

the individual with a decreased lordosis engages in lifting activities.[15]

Recent studies in spinal biomechanics provide evidence of small nerve endings in the disc that are sensitive to compressive loads.[16] Back pain can result from compressive loads on the disc that activate these nerve endings in the disc. A loss of lumbar lordosis could then produce back pain due to disc pressure, but without the characteristic herniation that is so frequently considered the source of back pain.

Long periods of increased compressive load on the intervertebral disc can eventually lead to *disc degeneration* or *herniation of the nucleus pulposus* (see Herniated Nucleus Pulposus later in this chapter). Most disc herniations occur not from sudden loads, but from long periods of compression, as occur in this postural distortion. Loss of lumbar lordosis should be considered an important factor when investigating the cause of a lumbar disc herniation.

Decreased lumbar lordosis primarily results from prolonged periods of poor sitting or work postures.[6] *Posterior pelvic rotation* and the corresponding *hypertonicity* in the abdominal or hamstring muscles can also lead to a

loss of lumbar lordosis. Muscular reactions are either a cause or a result of the postural distortion and include fatigue, hypertonicity, and over-lengthening. The stresses on the lumbar muscles frequently cause them to develop active *myofascial trigger points*.

The postural distortion can also be brought on by previous surgical procedures, such as spinal fusion. Spinal fusion surgeries are often performed as an effort to reduce facet joint compression or maximize space in the intervertebral foramen. In order to accomplish these objectives, the spinal segments are fused in a position that decreases the lumbar lordosis.

History
The client might report pain, but it is common for there to be no pain or discomfort. If present, pain is generally felt close to the spine or as diffuse soft-tissue pain in the lumbar musculature. Ask the client about postural or mechanical factors at work, home, or in recreational activities that might contribute to the distortion. Ask about surgical procedures that might have compromised spinal mechanics and decreased the natural lumbar lordosis.

Observation
A decrease in the lumbar lordosis is visually evident. The low back has a flat appearance and there is *posterior pelvic rotation* (Chapter 7). The buttocks generally have a tucked under appearance and there can be a corresponding degree of *upper thoracic kyphosis*.

Palpation
The spinous processes are sometimes more palpable in the lumbar region than in a normal lordotic curvature due to the loss of lordosis. The lumbar muscles may feel tight and house active myofascial trigger points.

Range-of-Motion and Resistance Testing
AROM: Limitations are expected in forward trunk flexion due to tight hamstrings. There could also be limitation in extension due to increased disc compression.
PROM: The same principles apply as for AROM.
MRT: MRTs do not produce pain with a decreased lumbar lordosis. Functional muscle weakness could result from the postural distress. Myofascial trigger points could produce pain during various MRTs, but not always.

Suggestions for Treatment
A decreased lumbar lordosis is harder to treat than an exaggerated lumbar lordosis. Habitual postural patterns must be addressed through postural re-training if this condition is to improve. Muscular fatigue and/or hypertonicity can be effectively addressed with soft-tissue therapy. Attention should also focus on the hamstring muscles, which are routinely hypertonic in this condition. Training in proper occupational body mechanics is an important part of reducing or eliminating back pain associated with a decreased lumbar lordosis.

Common Injury Conditions

LUMBAR FACET SYNDROME

Lumbar facet syndrome is **low back pain that originates from articular dysfunction of the facet (or zygapophysial) joints**. The condition is difficult to verify and is often overlooked as a possible source of low back or lower extremity pain.

Characteristics

Despite advances in technology there is still no accurate method of positively identifying lumbar facet syndrome, even with high-tech diagnostic studies. Difficulty in identification has led some to question whether or not the condition even exists.[17] Other sources cite facet joint dysfunction as a possibility in any low back pain complaint and claim facet irritation could be involved in as many as 15% of cases.[15]

The *facet joints* are the only location where adjacent vertebrae articulate with each other. Each vertebra has four facet joints: one superior and one inferior facet on each side (Figure 8.14). Each facet joint has a joint capsule. The joint's purpose is to guide appropriate movement in the spine. The majority of movement in the lumbar spine is flexion or extension, with minor amounts of rotation and lateral flexion.

In normal movement, joint compression occurs **bilaterally during hyperextension** and to the **ipsilateral side when laterally flexing**. The joints are slightly compressed during rotational movements and opened during forward flexion or lateral flexion to the opposite side. The primary weight-bearing structures in the lumbar spine are the **vertebral bodies** and the **intervertebral discs**. The **posterior vertebral structures**, which include the facet joints, also bear a certain percentage of weight.

Facet syndrome could result from an acute injury, although it is more common as a chronic condition. The facet joints and their **synovial capsules** are richly innervated, so even minor levels of irritation could produce pain. A probable source of the disorder is *biomechanical stress* in the posterior vertebral structures. When activities exaggerate spinal motions, compressive loads can be produced on the facet joints sufficient to cause pain.

The facet joints support greater amounts of weight in certain postural distortions. *Anterior pelvic tilt* and *exaggerated lumbar lordosis* frequently occur concurrently with facet syndrome.[6] For example, the more exaggerated is the lumbar lordosis, the greater is the degree of weight-bearing by the lumbar facet joints (Figure 8.12) and the more likely the person is to have facet joint irritation.

Hypertonicity and increased *myofascial trigger point* activity in the **hip flexors** and **spinal extensors** are typical in facet joint syndrome.[15] *Sacroiliac joint dysfunction* can also appear with the syndrome.[18] The increased compressive loads may contribute to *intervertebral disc degeneration*. When the disc loses height, there are greater

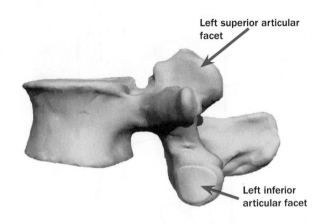

Figure 8.14 Left lateral view of a lumbar vertebra. (3-D anatomy image courtesy of Primal Pictures Ltd. www.primalpictures.com.)

compressive loads on the facet joints. Similar to synovial joints in other regions of the body, the facet joints are susceptible to arthritic changes from repeated compressive loads or excessive friction. Irritation of the facet joints can lead to *hypertrophy* (enlarging) and *inflammation* of the joint, which can then produce *stenosis* (narrowing) of the intervertebral foramen and increase pressure on nearby nerve roots.

Facet syndrome can refer pain to other regions of the body, such as the **low back, buttock, groin, posterior thigh**, and **foot**.[17, 19, 20] Pain referral complicates identification of the condition. Due to similar location and patterns, pain referred from facet joint dysfunction could easily be confused with *nerve root compression* or *myofascial trigger point pain* referrals from low back or gluteal muscles.

History

A client may complain of deep aching pain close to the spine or referred distally. Pain is aggravated when the joints are further compressed. Ask about the frequency and onset of pain. Ask the client about previous injuries that might have involved hyperextension or rotation of the spine. With acute injury, the client reports an immediate onset of pain at the time of injury. Acute injuries can linger and become chronic.

Long periods of immobility, especially with the spine in a degree of extension, can aggravate symptoms. Morning pain is common and results from lack of spinal movement during the night. This may improve as the person moves around. Sleeping in a prone position or sitting for long periods could also aggravate symptoms.

Observation

Lumbar facet syndrome is not identifiable with observation. A visibly exaggerated lumbar lordosis might be a contributing factor.

Palpation

The facet joints are not easily palpated due to adipose tissue and the paraspinal muscles, but palpation deep in the lamina groove near the joints sometimes reveals exaggerated tenderness. Hypertonicity and myofascial trigger points in the lumbar extensors, such as the erector spinae and quadratus lumborum, are common.

Range-of-Motion and Resistance Testing

AROM: Pain results during motions that further compress the facet joints, including hyperextension, ipsilateral side bending (lateral flexion), or rotational movements. Flexion opens the facet joints and decreases pain. Contralateral side bending also reduces pain.

PROM: The same principles apply as in AROM.

MRT: There are usually no specific findings with MRTs. Myofascial trigger points in the paraspinal muscles could become symptomatic during resisted extension.

Differential Evaluation

Muscular low back pain, spondylolisthesis, herniated nucleus pulposus, spinal tumor, spondylolysis, myofascial trigger point pain, degenerative disc disease, radiculopathy, spinal ligament sprain, piriformis syndrome, sacroiliac joint dysfunction.

Suggestions for Treatment

The primary focus of treatment for lumbar facet syndrome is to reduce compressive forces on the facet joint. Activity modification and postural re-training are an essential part of the rehabilitation process. Massage can be applied to the paraspinal muscles to address joint irritation or myofascial trigger points. Massage is also helpful for structural and postural problems. Spinal manipulation and injection of corticosteroids are used by other health professionals to treat this problem.

SPONDYLOLYSIS & SPONDYLOLISTHESIS

Spondylolysis and *spondylolisthesis* are closely related and are therefore addressed together. The names for these conditions are derived from Greek; *spondylos* meaning vertebrae, *lysis* to break down or dissolve, and *olisthesis* a slippage or sliding down an incline.

Characteristics

Spondylolysis **is a vertebral stress fracture that results from excessive loads.** Spondylolysis stress fractures develop most often in a region of the vertebra called the **pars interarticularis,** which is located between the **superior** and **inferior articular facets** on the posterior arch of each vertebra (Figure 8.15). Spondylolysis is generally a precursor to spondylolisthesis. Left untreated, the stress fracture may fully separate causing one vertebra to slip forward in relation to another. The **forward slippage of a vertebra is** *spondylolisthesis* **and typically occurs at the L5-S1 junction** (Figure 8.16). If the stress fracture of the

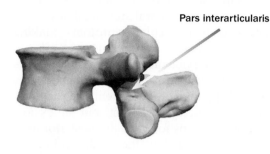

Figure 8.15 **Pars interarticularis of the lumbar vertebra. (3-D anatomy image courtesy of Primal Pictures Ltd. www.primalpictures.com.)**

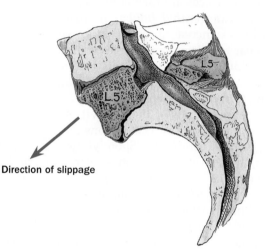

Figure 8.16 **Lateral cross-sectional view of the lumbar region showing forward slippage of L5 on S1 in spondylolisthesis (Mediclip image copyright, 1998 Williams & Wilkins. All rights reserved.)**

spondylolysis is bilateral and progressively worsens, the **vertebral arch** separates from the **anterior vertebral body** and a forward slippage of the anterior body results.

Spinal mechanics and weight distribution in the spine play an important role in the development of this condition. The forward slippage is exacerbated by the downward pull of gravity and made worse by the anterior and inferior sloping L5-S1 junction. Gravity and upright posture are important in creating the forward slippage and spondylolisthesis has never been observed in quadrupeds or in bedridden individuals.[21]

Spondylolysis and the subsequent *listhesis* are sometimes attributed to weakness or defects in the pars interarticularis, which might have existed since birth. Stress loading on the pars is the primary cause of these conditions, regardless of any existing weakness. Pain results from fatigue in the bones or when the lysis or listhesis become advanced enough to affect richly innervated structures such as **nerve roots** or **dura mater**.[23] However, there is a poor correlation between pars defects and symptoms in these conditions. Many individuals appear to have vertebral arch breakdown or forward slippage and no particular symptoms, making connection between pars defects and pain unclear.[22]

In a small percentage of spondylolisthesis cases, there is no apparent stress fracture at the pars, but there is still forward slippage of the vertebra. In these cases the entire vertebral structure is intact, but slides forward. When the vertebra slips forward the posterior arch can pull on nerve roots and irritate the **cauda equina,** causing serious neurological symptoms.[23, 24]

Repetitive flexion and extension of the spine produce cumulative stress on the posterior vertebral structures. The compressive forces are further magnified if the individual has an *exaggerated lumbar lordosis*. When the lumbar lordosis is increased, the posterior vertebral arch structures bear a greater percentage of the upper body weight. In addition, the posture tilts the lower lumbar vertebrae even farther in an anterior and inferior direction, making forward slippage more likely.

Due to the mechanics of their activities, individuals engaged in certain sports or occupations are particularly susceptible to both conditions. Spondylolysis and spondylolisthesis are prevalent in gymnastics, rowing, diving, swimming (especially the butterfly), tennis, wrestling, weight lifting, and football. Running or jumping on a hard, unyielding surface can also cause problems. An increased incidence appears in loggers and soldiers carrying heavy backpacks.[21, 22] Both conditions are prevalent in adolescents due to the extremes of physical exertion in athletics and bones that are not fully formed.[23] Females are affected more often than males, possibly due to strength differences in bone structure. Young females involved in vigorous athletics are at the highest risk. Young female gymnasts have an incidence of spondylolisthesis four times that of their age-matched counterparts not in gymnastics.[25]

Some occurrence patterns are related to ethnicity, although the reason is not determined. Vertebral arch defects that lead to spondylolisthesis have appeared in as much as 50% of the Eskimo population. Back pain is not reported anywhere near 50% within that group so the correlations between the neural arch defects, pain, and spondylolysis or spondylolisthesis are unclear.

Hamstring tightness is present in many individuals with spondylolisthesis. There is a strong proprioceptive function of the hamstrings as the body attempts to adjust to the forward slippage of the lower lumbar vertebra. The hamstrings tighten in an effort to posteriorly rotate the pelvis. The posterior pelvic rotation decreases the potential for forward slippage of the lower lumbar vertebra and helps stabilize the lumbar region.[21]

Conditions that can occur alongside spondylolysis or spondylolisthesis that may also need evaluation include: *stretching of supporting ligaments* due to forward slippage, *local muscle spasm, neural tension or compression, disc irritation, facet joint irritation,* or *myofascial trigger point pain* from hypertonic muscles.[26] Accurate identification of spondylolysis or spondylolisthesis requires an x-ray. The fracture is usually evident in the x-ray and forward slippage of the vertebra can be seen as well as measured.

History

Both conditions can produce dull aching pain in the lower lumbar or upper sacral region. Pain also extends into the buttocks or down the lower extremity in some cases. Pain typically increases with activity and decreases with rest. A supine position is more comfortable than prone due to stress on the vertebral arch. Spondylolisthesis is sometimes asymptomatic.

The client frequently reports repetitive flexion or extension activities prior to the onset of symptoms. In other cases there may be mechanical stress on the spine, particularly if the client has an exaggerated lumbar lordosis. For example, the client might report wearing a very heavy backpack or running on hard concrete surfaces. Consider the client's report of recent activities that produce aggravating stress on the posterior vertebral arch.

Observation

There are no direct visual cues for spondylolysis or spondylolisthesis. An excessive lumbar lordosis could contribute to the condition. Hamstring tightness might produce a visible gait alteration; for example a shortened stride length, limited hip flexion, or an appearance of waddling.

Palpation

There is tenderness in the soft tissues in the lower lumbar and upper sacral region, but it is often a secondary factor and not caused by the stress fracture or vertebral slippage. Attempting to palpate tissues in this region produces anterior pressure to the vertebral structures. The pressure can push the vertebra further into the position of slippage, causing pain. In addition to tenderness, hypertonicity in the lumbar erector spinae, quadratus lumborum, gluteals, and hamstring muscles is typical.

Box 8.4 Clinical Notes

A physician identifies spondylolisthesis through a posterior-lateral x-ray image called a scottie dog.

When viewed from this angle the transverse and spinous processes resemble the head and body of a Scottish terrier. When the dog image looks as if the head is separated from the body, it is considered evidence of forward slippage of the vertebral body (spondylolisthesis).

Range-of-Motion and Resistance Testing

AROM: In spondylolisthesis, pain increases with lumbar hyperextension because extension pushes the vertebral structures further in an anterior direction. Flexion decreases pain because flexion pushes the vertebra back toward the normal position. The same pattern is present in spondylolysis, but is related to the amount of compression on the posterior vertebral structures and not slippage of the vertebral bodies. In either condition, pain can be aggravated during lateral flexion or rotation, although there is not a clearly established pain pattern. Hip flexion with the knee in extension can be limited due to hamstring tightness.

PROM: The findings are the same as those in AROM.

MRT: Some weakness in resisted spinal extension might be evident due to reflex muscular inhibition. Myofascial trigger point activity could become apparent during the resisted muscle contractions, particularly in the paraspinal muscles.

Special test

One Leg Lumbar Extension

The client balances on one leg, while attempting to bend backward, extending the spine (Figure 8.17). The test is repeated on the opposite side. If pain is felt, there is a strong likelihood of a stress fracture in the pars interarticularis. If the stress fracture is only on one side, standing on the ipsilateral leg produces greater pain.

Explanation: As spinal extension increases, so does the amount of weight borne by the posterior arch of the vertebrae. Standing on one foot increases the degree of compressive load on the ipsilateral side. If there is a bony disruption such as spondylolysis or spondylolisthesis, pain is apt to be reproduced in this position. The standing extension also increases anterior translational force on the vertebrae if spondylolisthesis is present.

Differential Evaluation

Muscular low back pain, herniated nucleus pulposus, facet joint syndrome, spinal tumor, myofascial trigger point pain, degenerative disc disease, radiculopathy, spinal ligament sprain, lumbar muscle spasm, sacroiliac joint dysfunction, cauda equina syndrome.

Suggestions for Treatment

Massage is helpful in reducing overall muscular hypertonicity. Caution should be used when applying pressure to the lumbar region in an anterior direction as pressure on the low back can aggravate the problem. In traditional medical approaches, spondylolysis and spondylolisthesis are treated with rest from the offending activity and rehabilitative exercise. Therapeutic exercise is aimed at correcting the biomechanical dysfunction that led to the stress fracture and/or vertebral slippage. In more severe cases of slippage, a surgical procedure might be necessary to stabilize the vertebral structures while the bones heal.

HERNIATED NUCLEUS PULPOSUS

The *herniated nucleus pulposus (HNP)* is routinely referred to as a *herniated disc*. The lay term for the condition is *slipped disc*, which is a misnomer because the disc does not slip. Herniated discs in the lumbar spine can produce back pain as well as pain down one or both lower extremities.

Characteristics

For many years a large number of low back pain problems were thought to originate from herniated discs. The focus on disc herniation led to a dramatic increase in back surgery. Many of these surgeries are now considered questionable due to limited effectiveness.[1] Research shows that presence of a herniated disc does not necessar-

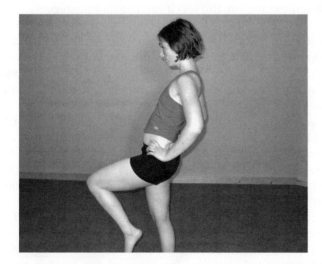

Figure 8.17 One-leg lumbar extension.

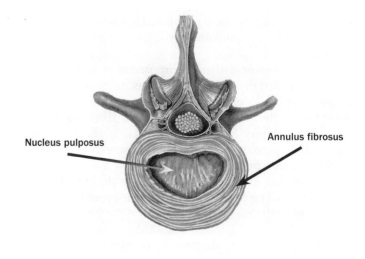

Figure 8.18 Components of an intervertebral disc. (Mediclip image copyright, 1998 Williams & Wilkins. All rights reserved.)

Nucleus pulposus

Annulus fibrosus

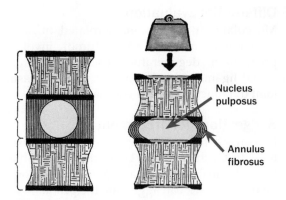

Figure 8.19 Compressive loads push the nucleus pulposus against the walls of the annulus fibrosis. (Mediclip image copyright, 1998 Williams & Wilkins. All rights reserved.)

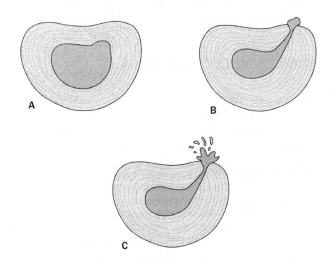

Figure 8.20 Different degrees of disc herniation: protrusion (A), prolapse/extrusion (B) and sequestration (C). (Used with permission from Lowe W. Orthopedic Massage: Theory and Technique. Edinburgh: Mosby; 2003.)

ily indicate a pathological problem. Disc herniations have been found in a significant percentage of asymptomatic individuals.[27, 28]

The *intervertebral disc* is composed of an inner gel-like substance called the **nucleus pulposus**, and is surrounded by overlapping layers of collagen that make up the outer boundary of the disc called the **annulus fibrosus** (Figure 8.18). The primary function of the disc is shock absorption in the spine. In cases of HNP, biomechanical loads on the nucleus pulposus force it against the outer walls of the annulus fibrosus and eventually deform the disc (Figure 8.19). The term *herniation* means *pushing through* and refers to the nucleus pushing into the boundaries of the annulus.

There are varying degrees of herniation, which are assessed by how far the nucleus pushes into the annulus. In a *protrusion*, the disc bulges but does not tear or rupture annulus fibers. A *prolapse* is a partial, but not

complete, rupture of the annulus. An *extrusion* occurs when the pulposus breaks through the outer walls of the annulus and protrudes into the spinal canal. The most severe injury, a *sequestration*, involves complete rupture of the annulus, with elements of the annulus and the nucleus protruding outside the disc (Figure 8.20).[9] Assessing the degree of herniation requires a diagnostic evaluation, such as an MRI; physical examination is not sufficient, although certain symptoms are identified during the process.

Due to the proximity of sensitive neurological structures, such as **spinal nerve roots** and the **spinal cord**, any degree of disc protrusion may press on these structures and cause pain. Other factors could also play a role in back and leg pain from disc protrusions. The nerve fibers in the intervertebral disc are also sensitive to pressure and pain can come from compressive loads, without the disc actually pressing on a nerve root.[6, 16] Back pain can result from disc pressure on the sinuvertebral nerve, which is immediately adjacent to the anterior motor nerve root. Pressure on the sinuvertebral nerve would produce back pain, but there would be no pain or neurological symptoms down the lower extremity.[29]

The structure of nerve roots affects the symptoms felt from the HNP. The **epineurium** is a connective tissue membrane around the nerve that provides additional protection. Spinal nerve fibers can have either a poorly developed epineurium or could be devoid of an epineurium altogether.[30] The lack of a solid epineurium makes the spinal nerves more susceptible to low levels of compression.

In HNP, the nucleus pulposus usually protrudes in a posterior-lateral direction. Straight posterior protrusions are rare, because the **posterior longitudinal ligament** directly behind the disc prevents a protrusion in this direction (Figure 8.21). However, there is evidence that the posterior longitudinal ligament can be narrower in the lumbar region, providing less resistance to a straight posterior protrusion.[31] The narrower the ligament is in the lumbar region, the less it can prevent posterior-lateral protrusions.

If there is a straight posterior protrusion, the disc presses on the **cauda equina** producing a serious pathology called *cauda equina syndrome*. Cauda equina syndrome is marked by pain that is predominantly confined to the buttocks and posterior leg along with widespread numbness all the way to the feet. These symptoms are ordinarily felt bilaterally. Bowel, bladder, or sexual dysfunction are general symptoms.[32] If these symptoms are present, the client needs to be referred immediately to a physician for proper evaluation. A delay in identifying this condition can produce irreversible neurological damage.[33]

Disc herniations are rare in the thoracic region. The greatest number are in the lumbar spine at the L4–L5 and L5–S1 junctions.[34] Positions that involve exaggerated and prolonged compressive loads of the lumbar spine characteristically produce the herniation. Compressive

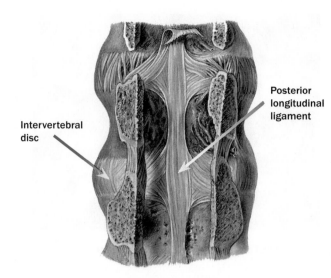

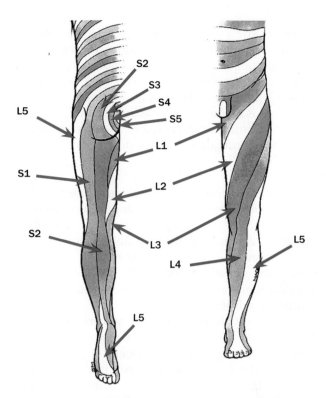

Figure 8.21 Posterior view of the spine with the spinous and transverse processes removed. The posterior longitudinal ligament prevents most straight posterior protrusions of intervertebral discs. (Mediclip image copyright, 1998 Williams & Wilkins. All rights reserved.)

Figure 8.22 Dermatomes related to the lumbar and sacral nerve roots. (Mediclip image copyright, 1998 Williams & Wilkins. All rights reserved.)

loads on the lumbar spine are least while lying down and greatest during poor sitting postures, such as a slouched position.[14] Heavy lifting is assumed to be a primary cause of HNP, but in many situations lifting is not the source of the problem. A study evaluating 115 pairs of identical twins found that familial or genetic patterns of disc weakness were a better indicator for disc herniation than was heavy lifting.[35] This study reinforces the suggestion that compressive loads are rarely the sole reason for disc herniations.

Researchers found interesting results when attempting to identify the level of compressive load on the spine required to create a disc herniation. When the spine is loaded with high compressive forces, either suddenly or slowly, the **vertebral end-plates** normally *fracture* before the disc herniates.[6, 32, 36] These results do not support the theory of a sudden herniation to a normal disc from a single traumatic event. A sudden load is more likely to fracture the vertebral end plates than produce a disc herniation. In the majority of acute HNP cases, a degree of disc degeneration probably already existed. Consequently, it is customary to have several episodes of low back pain prior to an event that produces severe or debilitating symptoms.[37]

When pressure is applied to a nerve root, sensation generally decreases in the area supplied by that nerve root. Severe numbness in the lower extremity is usually the result of a *peripheral nerve lesion* or *neuropathy*, not disc herniation.[29] Pressure on nerve roots also affects muscles innervated by the affected nerve and can produce *muscle atrophy* or *weakness*. Muscle weakness occurs more frequently with disc protrusions affecting the lower lumbar nerve roots, rather than the upper. Weakness is usually less apparent than sensory symptoms. In addition, *myofascial trigger points* sometimes develop in

muscles innervated by the damaged nerve root. Active trigger points can lead to an overlay of symptoms on top of the pain from nerve root compression.[38]

If the disc protrusion is in the upper lumbar region, the **femoral nerve** is primarily affected and symptoms are felt in the anterior thigh dermatomes. If the protrusion is in the lower lumbar region, the **sciatic nerve** is affected and symptoms are felt primarily in the dermatomes of the posterior thigh and leg (Figure 8.22). Disc protrusions are more common in the lower lumbar region. The client may have a tendency to lean toward or away from the side affected with a lower lumbar protrusion. This postural adaptation is referred to as a *sciatic scoliosis*.[32] In severe cases the client demonstrates an unwillingness to put weight on the affected leg when standing, preferring instead to hold the leg in slight flexion which decreases tension on the nerve roots.

Other pathological conditions in the spine can result from disc herniations and produce symptoms similar to HNP. The space between adjacent vertebrae decreases as the disc herniates and loses its size. Loss of **intervertebral disc volume** is called *degenerative disc disease*. A related problem is *spinal stenosis*, in which the **intervertebral foramen** becomes narrower (stenosis means narrowing). With a narrower opening for the nerve root, there is greater likelihood for nerve compression within the foramen. No specific degree of stenosis has been identified as more likely to cause symptoms.[39]

The primary symptoms from HNP include pain, paresthesia, or weakness in the low back or lower extremities. Pain or paresthesia can skip regions throughout a dermatome or area of cutaneous innervation.[32] For example, pain or paresthesia from a lumbar disc herniation could be felt in the lower leg and foot, but not in the upper leg. Disc herniation pain is made worse by activities that increases intraspinal and intradiscal pressure, such as sneezing, coughing, and bearing down during defecation.[32]

History

The client with an HNP may complain of deep aching back pain. If a herniated disc is pressing on a nerve root, symptoms might include sharp, shooting pain described as electrical or stabbing in nature. Pain can occur in the back, but frequently extends down the lower extremity. Pain is ordinarily unilateral because the disc protrudes to one side. Pain is bilateral in more serious cases, such as in cauda equina syndrome.

Clients routinely describe pain being worse after prolonged sitting. Pain dissipates as the individual moves around, as long as the client does not engage in heavy lifting and refrains from compromised postures. There are certain positions or movements that aggravate the pain and others that relieve pain. Bed rest generally decreases pain as the compressive loads on the spine are reduced.

Observation

There are no definitive visual signs for a herniated nucleus pulposus, although postural distortions could indicate disc involvement. Watch for postural adaptations such as sciatic scoliosis or reluctance to put weight on an affected leg. Atrophy of lower extremity muscles innervated by the affected nerve root(s) might be visible.

Palpation

Tenderness or hypertonicity in muscles of the lumbar or sacral regions is prevalent when there is disc herniation. However, this tenderness is not the same pain that the client feels with the nerve compression. Exaggerated sensitivity of the muscles in the lower lumbar and sacral regions is typical. Pressure on the lower back muscles can reveal myofascial trigger point referrals that result from nerve irritation.[38] Caution is advised as pressure applied to the lumbar region, particularly when the client is in a prone position, could initiate movement of the lumbar vertebrae and amplify pressure on the affected nerve root.

Range-of-Motion and Resistance Testing

AROM: Pain or other neurological symptoms can be aggravated with active motion in any direction of lumbar movement. Nerve roots can be stretched taut against protruding structures during lateral flexion to the opposite side or compressed by narrowing of the intervertebral foramen during lateral flexion to the same side. Symptoms could also be elicited from either flexion or extension.

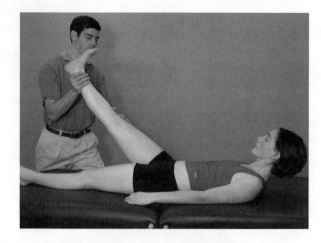

Figure 8.23 Final position in the straight leg raise test.

PROM: Principles are the same as for AROM.
MRT: There are no significant findings with MRTs. Muscles innervated by fibers from the affected nerve root(s) sometimes appear weak during MRTs.

Special Tests

Due to the potential seriousness of these conditions, referral to a physician for an accurate diagnosis is advised. The following special orthopedic tests are used to identify disc herniations primarily in the lumbar region. Obstructions near the nerve roots such as bone spurs, tumors, or spinal stenosis can produce similar symptoms with these tests. While information from physical examination is crucial in evaluating the tissues involved, other high-tech diagnostic methods may be necessary to identify the source of the client's symptoms.

Straight Leg Raise Test

This test gradually increases tensile stress on the sciatic nerve roots and is specific to obstructions in the lower lumbar region. There are several steps in this test. The client is asked about changes in sensation or increases in symptoms after each step is performed. Increases in neurological symptoms indicate the likelihood of nerve root compression in the lumbar region.

The client is supine on the treatment table. The practitioner raises the leg of the affected side (the side where symptoms are felt) as if attempting to stretch the hamstring muscles. The practitioner continues to raise the leg on this side until the client reports a reproduction of symptoms (Figure 8.23). The sciatic nerve is fully stretched at about 70^{0} of hip flexion, so symptoms are usually present by this point. The leg is slightly lowered to determine if symptoms decrease. This slight movement helps differentiate the symptoms from hamstring tightness when the next step is performed. At this position, the client dorsiflexes the foot and the head and neck are then flexed.

A variation of the straight leg raise test is the **well leg test.** In this procedure the same process is used as in the straight leg raise test, except the test is performed on the unaffected side (assuming the client is only feeling symptoms on one side). If performance of the straight leg raise on the unaffected side produces symptoms on the affected side, it is further validation of lumbar radiculopathy.

Explanation: The straight leg raise test places tensile stress on the lumbar nerve roots from both superior and inferior directions. If a structure is protruding against a nerve root, increasing tensile stress on the nerve root pulls the nerve taut against the protruding structure and increases symptoms. Due to the way the nerve roots are stressed in this procedure, the test is most effective in evaluating disc pathology at the L5 and S1 nerve roots.[32] When the sciatic nerve is pulled taut at 70^0 of hip flexion, any further stretching of the entire neural axis stretches the connective tissue elements of the nerve.

In the well leg test, tension applied to the lumbar nerve roots on one side is transmitted to the opposite side. When performing the test, distinguish between neurological symptoms and those produced by hamstring stretching (symptoms of hamstring stretching are not a positive result).

Slump Test

The slump test provides information about sciatic nerve pathology, as well as nerve compression or tension throughout the upper extremities and neck. Several steps are performed either actively or passively, with each step placing additional tensile stress on the nervous system. After each step, the practitioner asks about changes in sensation or increases in symptoms.

The client is seated on the treatment table with hands clasped behind the back. From this position the client slumps forward with the upper thoracic region. Next, the head and neck are fully flexed. The leg on the affected side is then extended at the knee. Once the leg is fully extended, the foot is dorsiflexed (Figure 8.24). These motions are performed actively or passively. Some pain or discomfort from neural tension is expected to be felt at the end of this series of movements, even in a normal individual. If pain or discomfort is felt prior to the end of the movement series, or if the symptoms are severe, there is a good chance of neural pathology.

If a person is unable to perform this test in a seated position, a variation known as the **side-lying slump test** can be performed (Figure 8.25). The side-lying position is helpful in the evaluation of lower lumbar nerve root problems. In the normal slump test position, symptoms can be aggravated from increased compressive loads on the disc while sitting in a poor posture. The side-lying slump position decreases disc compression so neural dynamics can be examined independent of disc compression.

Explanation: As with the straight leg raise test, the slump test puts progressive tension on specific segments of the peripheral nervous system. The brachial plexus is stretched with the client's hands behind the back. Further tension on the upper region of the peripheral nervous system is produced by the upper thoracic slump followed by head and neck flexion. The lower neural structures (sciatic nerve in particular) are stretched with the knee extension and ankle dorsiflexion. The slump test is biased toward the sciatic nerve and does not put tensile stress on the femoral nerve, which is derived from the upper lumbar nerve roots.

Because tension is generated in the cervical nerve roots as well as the lower lumbar, this test is used to identify neural compression or tension pathologies in the upper or lower extremities. The location of the neural pathology is determined by where the symptoms are felt. For example, if symptoms are felt in the upper extremity during this test, then attention should focus on the cervical nerve roots. If symptoms increase in the sciatic nerve distribution in the lower extremity, then a lower lumbar nerve root problem would be expected.

Prone Knee Bend Test

The client is prone on the treatment table. The practitioner places the client's knee in a fully flexed position, as if stretching the quadriceps (Figure 8.26). The client is

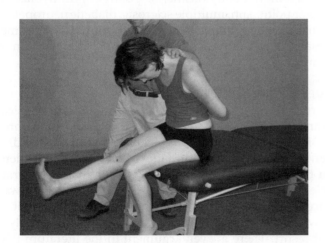

Figure 8.24 Final position in the slump test.

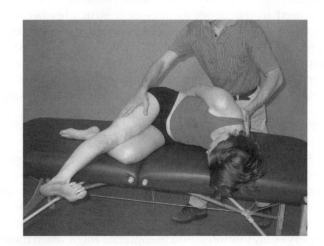

Figure 8.25 Side-lying slump test.

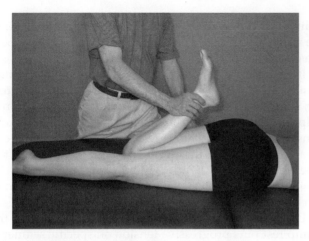

Figure 8.26 **Prone knee bend test.**

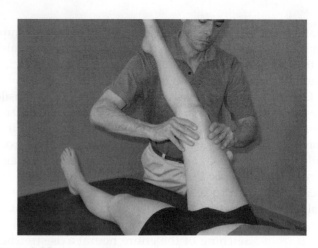

Figure 8.28 **Bowstring test.**

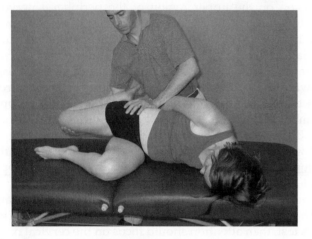

Figure 8.27 **Side-lying prone knee bend test variation.**

asked about changes in symptoms, especially increases in neurological symptoms (pain, paresthesia, or numbness) in the anterior thigh. Distinguish neurological symptoms felt in the anterior thigh from sensations of quadriceps stretching.

The prone knee bend test is not as sensitive as the straight leg raise or slump tests. Tension cannot be increased in the upper neurological structures because the client is prone on the table. A variation of the prone knee bend test combines it with the side-lying slump position, and thereby increases tension on the affected neural structures and makes the test more accurate. In the side-lying slump position, add hip extension and knee flexion while the upper torso, head, and neck are flexed (Figure 8.27). This position creates the greatest degree of tension on the femoral nerve and its nerve roots.

Explanation: Nerve root compression in the upper lumbar nerve roots is identified with this test. The femoral nerve originates from nerve roots in the upper lumbar region. If a protrusion affecting the upper lumbar nerve roots exists, neurological symptoms are felt in the femoral nerve distribution down the anterior thigh when these nerve roots are stretched.

Bowstring Test

The client is supine on the treatment table. The practitioner raises the leg of the affected side as if performing the straight leg raise test. The leg is raised until the client reports a reproduction of symptoms. Once symptoms are reproduced the practitioner slightly flexes the client's knee (about 20^0) to reduce symptoms. The thigh is not lowered and is kept in the same degree of hip flexion. The practitioner presses the thumb or fingers into the client's popliteal region to reproduce symptoms (Figure 8.28). If symptoms are reproduced, there is a good likelihood of sciatic nerve involvement from neural tension or a protruding structure in the lumbar region.

Explanation: Once symptoms are reproduced after raising the leg, the knee is flexed to decrease tension on the neural structures. Pressure applied in the popliteal region pulls on the sciatic nerve without causing further lengthening of the hamstring muscles. Stressing the sciatic nerve distinguishes sciatic nerve pain from hamstring tightness.

Differential Evaluation

Spinal tumor, spondylolisthesis, spondylolysis, myofascial trigger point pain, multiple sclerosis, diabetic neuropathy, spinal infection, vertebral fracture, piriformis syndrome, tarsal tunnel syndrome, other regions of neural tension or compression, facet syndrome.

Suggestions for Treatment

Herniation severity cannot be determined by physical examination alone. Consult with other health care professionals for recommendations on how to treat the disc herniation, as the proper treatment method is dependent on the degree of herniation. Numerous treatment strategies have been advocated for HNP. While surgery was once considered almost essential for this problem, it is now considered less necessary and in some cases only a last resort. There is even argument in the literature that the majority of disc herniations heal spontaneously without surgery or other invasive procedures.[40] Rehabilitative exercises are now used with a high degree of success.

While massage is not absolutely contraindicated for disc herniations, treatment methods should be used cautiously to prevent aggravation of symptoms. Symptoms can be aggravated by minor vertebral movements that occur from pressure applied to the low back region. Although the transverse processes protect the nerve roots from further direct compression, movement can cause pain. Massage can be helpful to decrease muscle tension in the area and subsequently reduce compressive loads on the disc. Any massage treatment should be done with great caution and should not aggravate symptoms.

SPINAL LIGAMENT SPRAIN

The **lumbar spine** stabilizes the torso and handles significant force loads during bending and rotation. The structure of the spine makes it vulnerable to injury from motion in multiple directions. **Ligaments** play a fundamental role in maintaining stability and preventing excessive motion in the spine. *Sprains* result when excess tensile stress causes the ligaments to overstretch or tear.

Characteristics
Ligaments are dense connective tissue structures composed of **elastin** and **collagen**. Elastin gives them some degree of pliability, while collagen gives them strong tensile strength. Ligaments are designed to withstand tensile loads along the direction that their fibers run.[6] Because there are so many different forces to which the

spine is subjected, there is a complex webbing of ligaments throughout the spine designed to resist excessive movement in multiple directions (Figure 8.29, 8.21). In addition, these ligaments have an important protective role in preventing excessive stress to the **spinal cord**, especially in sudden traumatic movements.

Spinal ligaments have different anatomical characteristics depending on their location and primary function. For example, the **ligamentum flavum** is located on the inside of the vertebral canal and is designed to hold the **laminae** of adjacent vertebrae together. It elongates during flexion and shortens during extension. It is composed of a high degree of elastin, making it capable of stretching and retracting without buckling and pressing on the dura mater. Its high degree of elastin also prevents it from being sprained as often as other spinal ligaments because it is so flexible.

Other ligaments have important functional roles in limiting movement but vary in their structure or function. For example, the **intertransverse ligaments** are considered too small to function as true ligaments in the lumbar spine. The dorsal portion of the **supraspinous ligaments** are primarily composed of tendinous fibers from the **erector spinae** muscles so they are really more tendinous than ligamentous.[16]

An important supporting ligament in the lumbar region is the **iliolumbar ligament**. This ligament anchors the **L5 vertebra** to the **pelvic girdle** and helps prevent forward sliding and rotational distortions of the lower lumbar vertebrae. Due to its position and mechanical vulnerability the iliolumbar ligament is susceptible to *sprain* from sudden forces to the lower lumbar or sacral regions.[16]

An overwhelming sudden tensile load is the cause of a ligament sprain. However, prolonged stress on the ligaments can weaken them and make them more susceptible to injury from smaller loads. Box 8.5 lists the primary ligaments in the lumbar and thoracic spine along with the motions they are designed to resist. When evaluating an injury to the spine, determine if the force of the injury could have caused tensile stress on a particular spinal lig-

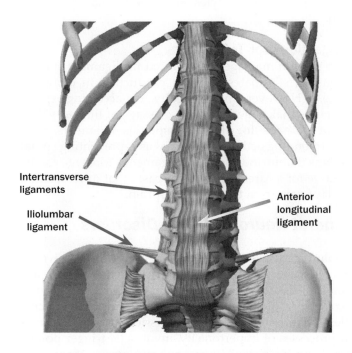

Intertransverse ligaments
Iliolumbar ligament
Anterior longitudinal ligament

Figure 8.29 Anterior view of the lumbar spine showing several of the primary stabilizing ligaments. (3-D anatomy image courtesy of Primal Pictures Ltd. www.primalpictures.com.)

BOX 8.5 STABILIZING THORACOLUMBAR LIGAMENTS	
Ligament	**Motion Resisted**
Anterior longitudinal	Extension
Posterior longitudinal	Flexion
Ligamentum flavum	Flexion
Intertransverse	Lateral flexion
Interspinous	Flexion
Iliolumbar	Rotation/forward translation
Supraspinous	Flexion
Lateral costotransverse	Rib movement

ament. For example, a sudden and forceful lateral flexion of the torso to the left could cause a sprain to the right intertransverse or iliolumbar ligaments.

Spinal ligament sprains are more prevalent in people with systemic disorders such as *Ehlers-Danlos* or *Marfan syndromes*, because these conditions involve connective tissue weakness.[9] The connective tissue weakness makes the individual more susceptible to tearing of the ligament fibers. Women in the later stages of pregnancy experience a greater number of spinal ligament sprains due to increased ligamentous laxity resulting from elevated levels of the hormone relaxin.

Identifying specific ligament sprains through physical examination is difficult due to the depth of the spinal ligaments and the abundance of soft tissues around the spine. A high-tech diagnostic procedure such as MRI is usually required although familiarity with characteristics of ligament sprains helps in the identification process.

Chapter 2 includes a comprehensive discussion of the physiology of ligament sprains as they pertain to all regions of the body. Chapter 4 contains details about assessing sprains including the history, observation, palpation, as well as range-of-motion, and resistance testing of ligaments in any region of the body. The discussion in the section below is limited to specifics about spinal ligaments, but the reader is encouraged to consult these other sections for a more thorough understanding of the pathology and assessment of ligament sprains.

History

The client describes an acute injury or accident prior to the onset of symptoms. Identify as clearly as possible the forces and motions associated with the injury to determine which tissues had the excess tensile load placed upon them. The client reports pain close to the spine that is aggravated by movements that pull on the damaged fibers. The client may also report tightness of muscles in the area near the ligament sprain. Ask the client about systemic disorders that may involve ligamentous laxity.

Box 8.6 Clinical Notes

Injuries to the soft tissues in the lumbar region are one of the most common reasons for people to visit their physician. In many cases the patient is given a diagnosis of lumbar sprain/strain, indicating damage to the musculotendinous unit and/or spinal ligaments. However, the diagnosis does not usually specifiy the exact muscles or ligaments affected.

From a massage therapy perspective it is important to know which muscles and/or ligaments are involved so treatment can be targed to the affected tissue. In massage assessment and treatment tissue-specific palpatory techniques are used, making it sometimes easier to locate the tissues involved and to adjust treatment for those tissues.

Observation

There are no significant visual cues to the presence of a spinal ligament sprain. There may be inflammation, but it is rarely visible. Gait alterations or movement distortions might develop as a result of pain avoidance.

Palpation

Most spinal ligaments are difficult to palpate and some, such as the anterior or posterior longitudinal ligaments, are not palpable at all. A few ligaments are superficial, such as the supraspinous and interspinous ligaments, and palpation would reproduce the client's pain if an injury was present. Palpable tightness in muscles near the sprain is common.

Range-of-Motion and Resistance Testing

AROM: AROM increases pain when the motion stretches the affected ligament (Box 8.5). For example, active lateral flexion to the left produces pain near the end of the movement with a sprain of the right intertransverse ligaments. Motion that shortens the ligament decreases pain.
PROM: The same principles apply as for AROM.
MRT: There are fascial and tendinous connections between the supraspinous ligaments and the parallel fibers of the erector spinae muscles. Pain could be expected when the erector spinae contract during resisted spinal extension movements if the supraspinous ligaments are injured.

Differential Evaluation

Spinal tumor, spondylolisthesis, spondylolysis, muscle strain, myofascial trigger point pain, vertebral fracture, acute nerve injury, facet syndrome, arthritis, lumbar radiculopathy, osteophytes, stenosis, herniated nucleus pulposus.

Suggestions for Treatment

Deep friction massage is advocated for ligament sprains because it stimulates collagen production in damaged tissue.[41] However the difficulty of accessing spinal ligaments makes deep friction massage of limited value, except perhaps for the supraspinous ligaments. Rest from offending activities is crucial as is preventing spinal motions that further stress the ligaments. Massage can be effective for addressing muscle spasm that develops as a result of pain from the ligament sprain.

General Neuromuscular Disorders

In many cases, soft-tissue dysfunctions are not given a specific name. Adequate assessment is required to determine the tissues most likely involved and to take into account pathologies that may or may not have specific titles. Chapter 4 provides a discussion of the pathological processes of hypertonicity, myofascial trigger points, muscle strains, nerve compression and tension, tendinosis, tenosynovitis, ligament sprains, and osteoarthritis in any region of the body. Chapter 4 also includes the history, observation, palpation, relevant tests, and treatment suggestions sections for these conditions. The principles are the same for these conditions wherever they occur in the body.

Included in this section are specific tables and graphics for the lumbar spine, including dermatomes, cutaneous innervation, trigger point referral patterns, and findings for MRTs. Tenosynovitis is not an issue in the lumbar region as there are no tendons surrounded by a synovial sheath in this area. Tendinosis is also rare in this region due to the structure and function of the muscles and tendons. Nerve compression and tension pathologies affect nerve roots and not peripheral nerves in the lumbar and thoracic spine.

Muscular hypertonicity and myofascial trigger points are two of the most common causes of back pain. Back pain ranks second only to upper respiratory illness as a reason for office visits to physicians.[42] Muscular sources of back pain can be overlooked in favor of joint disorders or other structural problems that are more easily identifiable with diagnostic testing procedures.[43, 44] A comprehensive approach to back pain must consider the frequent occurrence of pain that originates from muscular dysfunction.[1, 45] Considering the muscular contribution to pain in the low back is essential and should not be underemphasized.

Muscular hypertonicity and myofascial trigger points develop in the lumbar or thoracic regions especially as a result of postural stress. Myofascial trigger points refer pain or characteristic neurological symptoms to various regions of the torso or extremities. Myofascial trigger point referral patterns for the major muscles in this region are shown in Figures 8.30, 8.31.

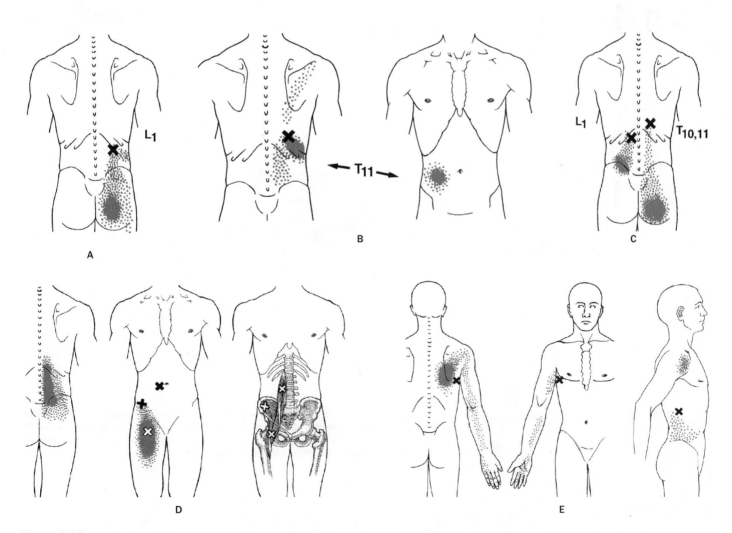

Figure 8.30 Myofascial trigger point referral patterns: Iliocostalis lumborum (A), Iliocostalis thoracis (B), Longissimus thoracis (C), Iliopsoas (D), Latissimus dorsi (E) (Images courtesy of Mediclip, copyright 1998 Williams & Wilkins. All rights reserved).

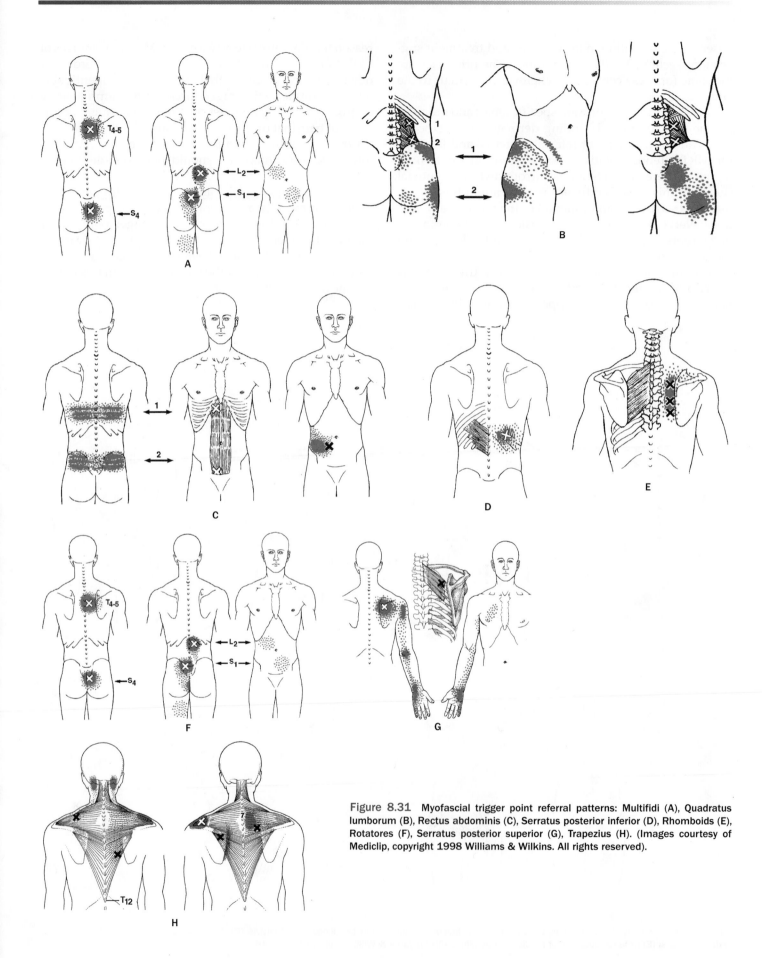

Figure 8.31 Myofascial trigger point referral patterns: Multifidi (A), Quadratus lumborum (B), Rectus abdominis (C), Serratus posterior inferior (D), Rhomboids (E), Rotatores (F), Serratus posterior superior (G), Trapezius (H). (Images courtesy of Mediclip, copyright 1998 Williams & Wilkins. All rights reserved).

TABLE 1 WEAKNESS WITH MANUAL RESISTIVE TEST AND POSSIBLE NERVE INVOLVEMENT

Muscle	Resisted Action	Possible Nerve Involvement if Action Weak
Iliocostalis lumborum	Trunk extension	Lumbar spinal nerves (variable)
Iliocostalis thoracis	Trunk extension	T1-T12 (variable)
Iliopsoas	Hip flexion	L1-L4
Interspinalis lumborum	Trunk extension	Lumbar spinal nerves (variable)
Interspinalis thoracis	Trunk extension	T1-T3, T11-T12 (variable)
Intertransversarii lumborum	Lateral trunk flexion	Thoracic spinal nerves (very variable)
Intertransversarii thoracis	Lateral trunk flexion	Thoracic spinal nerves (very variable)
Longissimus thoracis	Trunk extension	T1-L1
Multifidi	Trunk extension	T1-T12 spinal nerves; whole spine
Obliquus externus abdominis	Contralateral trunk rotation	T7-T12
Obliquus internus abdominis	Ipsilateral trunk rotation	T7-L1
Quadratus lumborum	Lateral trunk flexion	T12-L3
Rectus abdominis	Trunk flexion	T7-T12
Rotatores lumborum	Contralateral trunk rotation	Lumbar spinal nerves (variable)
Rotatores thoracis	Contralateral trunk rotation	T1-T12 (variable)
Semispinalis thoracis	Trunk extension	T1-T12
Spinalis thoracis	Trunk extension	T1-T12 (variable)

Reference Table for Condition Assessment

This table lists a number of pathological conditions along the left-hand column. The top of the table lists common evaluation procedures. A ◆ in the box associated with a pathological condition and an evaluation procedure indicates that the procedure is commonly used to identify that pathology. A ● in the box associated with the condition and a range-of-motion or resistance test, indicates that pain is likely with that test for that pathology. Conditions are listed alphabetically.

TABLE 2 REFERENCE TABLE FOR CONDITION ASSESSMENT

	AROM	PROM	MRT	One leg lumbar extension	Straight leg raise test	Prone knee bend test	Slump test	Bowstring test
Facet Joint Dysfunction	●	●						
Spondylolysis & Spondylolisthesis	●	●		◆				
Herniated Nucleus Pulposus	●	●			◆	◆	◆	◆
Spinal Ligament Sprain	●	●						
Muscular Hypertonicity	●	●			◆			
Muscle Strains	●	●	●				◆	

TABLE 3	JOINTS, ASSOCIATED MOTIONS, PLANES OF MOTION IN ANATOMICAL POSITION, AXIS OF ROTATION, AND AVERAGE ROM

Back	Motion	Plane of Motion	Axis of Rotation	Avg. ROM (degrees)
	Flexion	Sagittal	Medial-lateral	75-80
	Extension	Sagittal	Medial-lateral	20-30
	Lateral flexion	Frontal	Anterior-posterior	35
	Rotation	Transverse	Superior-inferior	45

References

1. Waddell G. *The Back Pain Revolution*. Edinburgh: Churchill Livingstone; 1998.

2. Berryman Reese N, Bandy WD. *Joint Range of Motion and Muscle Length Testing*. Philadelphia: W.B. Saunders Co.; 2002.

3. *Dorland's Illustrated Medical Dictionary*. 30th ed. Philadelphia: W.B. Saunders; 2003.

4. Di Bari M, Chiarlone M, Matteuzzi D, et al. Thoracic kyphosis and ventilatory dysfunction in unselected older persons: an epidemiological study in Dicomano, Italy. *J Am Geriatr Soc*. Jun 2004;52(6):909-915.

5. Neumann DA. *Kinesiology of the Musculoskeletal System*. St. Louis: Mosby; 2002.

6. White A, Panjabi M. *Clinical Biomechanics of the Spine*. 2nd ed. Philadelphia: Lippincott Williams & Wilkins; 1990.

7. Nowak J. Scheuermann Disease. *eMedicine*. September 1, 2004. Available at: www.emedicine.com. Accessed May 26, 2005.

8. Bullock MP, Foster NE, Wright CC. Shoulder impingement: the effect of sitting posture on shoulder pain and range of motion. *Man Ther*. Feb 2005;10(1):28-37.

9. Magee D. *Orthopedic Physical Assessment*. 3rd ed. Philadelphia: W.B. Saunders; 1997.

10. Rattray F, Ludwig L. *Clinical Massage Therapy: Understanding, Assessing and Treating over 70 Conditions*. Toronto: Talus Incorporated; 2000.

11. Janda V. Muscles as a pathogenic factor in back pain. Paper presented at: IFOMT, 1980; New Zealand.

12. Janda V. Postural and Phasic Muscles in the Pathogenesis of Low Back Pain. Paper presented at: XIth Congress ISRD, 1968; Dublin.

13. Chaitow L, DeLany J. *Clinical Application of Neuromuscular Techniques*. Vol 1. Edinburgh: Churchill Livingstone; 2000.

14. Nachemson A. The load on lumbar disks in different positions of the body. *Clin Orthop Relat Res*. Mar-Apr 1966;45:107-122.

15. Liebenson Ce. *Rehabilitation of the Spine*. Baltimore: Williams & Wilkins; 1996.

16. Adams M, Bogduk N, Burton K, Dolan P. *The Biomechanics of Back Pain*. Edinburgh: Churchill Livingstone; 2002.

17. Jackson RP. The facet syndrome. Myth or reality? *Clin Orthop*. 1992(279):110-121.

18. Schwarzer A, April C, Bogduk N. The sacroiliac joint in chronic low back pain. *Spine*. 1995;20:20.

19. Dreyer SJ, Dreyfuss PH. Low back pain and the zygapophysial (facet) joints. *Arch Phys Med Rehabil*. 1996;77(3):290-300.

20. Mooney V, Robertson J. The facet syndrome. *Clin Orthop*. 1976(115):149-156.

21. Amundson G, Edwards C, Garfin S. Spondylolisthesis. In: Herkowitz H, Garfin S, Balderston R, Eismont F, Bell G, Wiesel S, eds. *Rothman-Simeone: The Spine*. Vol 1. 4th ed. Philadelphia: W.B. Saunders; 1999:835-885.

22. Moller H, Sundin A, Hedlund R. Symptoms, signs, and functional disability in adult spondylolisthesis. *Spine*. 2000;25(6):683-689; discussion 690.

23. McCulloch J, Transfeldt E. *Macnab's Backache*. 3rd ed. Baltimore: Williams & Wilkins; 1997.

24. Esses S. *Textbook of Spinal Disorders*. Philadelphia: J.B. Lippincott Company; 1995.

25. Wiltse LL, Jackson DW. Treatment of spondylolisthesis and spondylolysis in children. *Clin Orthop Relat Res*. Jun 1976(117):92-100.

26. Grobler L, Wiltse L. Classification, and Nonoperative and Operative Treatment of Spondylolisthesis. In: Frymoyer JW, ed. *The Adult Spine*. Vol 2. Philadelphia: Lippincott-Raven; 1997:1865-1921.

27. Jensen MC, Brant-Zawadzki MN, Obuchowski

N, Modic MT, Malkasian D, Ross JS. Magnetic resonance imaging of the lumbar spine in people without back pain. *N Engl J Med.* 1994;331(2):69-73.

28. Boden SD, Davis DO, Dina TS, Patronas NJ, Wiesel SW. Abnormal magnetic-resonance scans of the lumbar spine in asymptomatic subjects. A prospective investigation. *J Bone Joint Surg Am.* 1990;72(3):403-408.

29. Durrant DH, True JM. *Myelopathy, Radiculopathy, and Peripheral Entrapment Syndromes.* Boca Raton: CRC Press; 2002.

30. Rydevik B, Brown MD, Lundborg G. Pathoanatomy and pathophysiology of nerve root compression. *Spine.* 1984;9(7).

31. Cailliet R. *Low Back Pain Syndrome.* Philadelphia: F.A. Davis; 1988.

32. Wisneski R, Garfin S, Rothman R, Lutz G. Lumbar disc disease. In: Herkowitz H, Garfin S, Balderston R, Eismont F, Bell G, Wiesel S, eds. *Rothman-Simeone: The Spine.* Vol 1. Philadelphia: W.B. Saunders Company; 1999:613-679.

33. Markham DE. Cauda equina syndrome: diagnosis, delay and litigation risk. *Current Orthopedics.* 2004;18:58-62.

34. Spangfort EV. The lumbar disc herniation. A computer-aided analysis of 2,504 operations. *Acta Orthop Scand Suppl.* 1972;142:1-95.

35. Battie MC, Videman T, Gibbons LE, Fisher LD, Manninen H, Gill K. 1995 Volvo Award in clinical sciences. Determinants of lumbar disc degeneration. A study relating lifetime exposures and magnetic resonance imaging findings in identical twins. *Spine.* Dec 15 1995;20(24):2601-2612.

36. Jayson MI, Herbert CM, Barks JS. Intervertebral discs: nuclear morphology and bursting pressures. *Ann Rheum Dis.* Jul 1973;32(4):308-315.

37. Weber H. Lumbar disc herniation. A controlled, prospective study with ten years of observation. *Spine.* Mar 1983;8(2):131-140.

38. Baldry PE. *Myofascial Pain and Fibromyalgia Syndromes.* Edinburgh: Churchill Livingstone; 2001.

39. Fardon D. Differential Diagnosis of Low Back Disorders. In: Frymoyer J, Ducker T, Hadler N, Kostuik J, J. W, eds. *The Adult Spine.* Vol 2. 2nd ed. Philadelphia: Lippincott-Raven; 1997:1745-1768.

40. Benoist M. The natural history of lumbar disc herniation and radiculopathy. *Joint Bone Spine.* 2002;69(2):155-160.

41. Gehlsen GM, Ganion LR, Helfst R. Fibroblast responses to variation in soft tissue mobilization pressure. *Med Sci Sport Exercise.* 1999;31(4):531-535.

42. Deyo RA, Rainville J, Kent DL. What can the history and physical examination tell us about low back pain? *Jama.* 1992;268(6):760-765.

43. Craton N, Matheson GO. Training and clinical competency in musculoskeletal medicine. Identifying the problem. *Sports Med.* 1993;15(5):328-337.

44. Freedman KB, Bernstein J. The adequacy of medical school education in musculoskeletal medicine. *J Bone Joint Surg Am.* 1998;80(10):1421-1427.

45. Simons D, Travell J, Simons L. *Myofascial Pain and Dysfunction: The Trigger Point Manual.* Vol 1. 2nd ed. Baltimore: Williams & Wilkins; 1999.

46. Garrett WE. Muscle strain injuries. *Am J Sports Med.* 1996;24(6 Suppl):S2-8.

47. Mehlman C. Idiopathic Scoliosis. *eMedicine.* 6-30-2004. Available at: www.emedicine.com. Accessed February 12, 2006.

9 Cervical Spine

The cervical spine is a complex biomechanical region containing many bones, joints, muscles, ligaments, and tendons that provide structural protection for the spinal cord, arteries and nerves. Given the mobility and biomechanics of the area, pain in the cervical region is common. Poor posture, faulty ergonomics, muscle exhaustion, and stress can all cause pathological conditions of the neck, as can a number of injuries including *impact trauma, whiplash,* and overuse.

Neck muscles not only produce motion of the head and neck, but also maintain the head in an upright position. Muscle conditions involving chronic *hypertonicity* and *myofascial trigger points* are common. Muscle conditions are difficult to detect with high-tech diagnostic procedures and a detailed physical examination remains one of the most effective methods for accurately evaluating these pathologies.

Due to the proximity of the **brachial plexus** and other sensitive neurological tissues, nerve compression and tension syndromes are seen regularly in the neck. Pain and/or neurological symptoms can be felt in the neck or radiate down the upper extremity. Accurate assessment helps distinguish *peripheral nerve entrapments* in the upper extremity from those caused by cervical pathology. A detailed assessment should identify injuries, especially in the acute stage, needing evaluation by a physician.

Movements and Motion Testing

SINGLE-PLANE MOVEMENTS

There are four primary movements in the cervical spine: flexion, extension, lateral flexion, and rotation. Motion is divided into two regions: cranial and cervical. Motion at the neck is called **craniocervical** because it involves movement of the cranial and cervical regions. **Cranial** motion is movement of the head and occurs at the **atlanto-occipital joint** where the head moves on the atlas (C1). Motion at the **atlanto-axial joint** (between C1 and C2) is also considered cranial motion because C1 is anatomically tethered to the cranium. **Cervical** motion occurs at each vertebral segment between C2 and C7, the **intracervical region**. For ease of analysis cranial and cervical motions are considered together in the assessment process.

Lateral flexion and rotation are described as left or right, instead of medial or lateral, because the axial skeleton is what is being rotated or laterally flexed. In rotational movements, the point of reference is the anterior aspect of the vertebral body. Notice that when the anterior face of the vertebra rotates right, the spinous process rotates left. In this text, movement past full extension or anatomical position is considered hyperextension. The associated motions, planes, axes of rotation, and range-of-motion values for the cervical spine are listed in Table 1 at the end of the chapter.

Neck

Flexion and **extension** take place in the **sagittal plane** (Figure 9.1). Flexion occurs when the chin is brought toward the upper chest. Extension is the return to anatomical position from a flexed position. Average range of motion for craniocervical flexion is 45^0–50^0, with approximately 10^0 in cranial movement at the atlanto-occipital and atlanto-axial joints and the remaining movement (approximately 35^0) in the intracervical region (C2–C7).

Average range of motion for extension is 75^0–85^0. Motion is measured from anatomical position moving in a posterior direction and is called extension or hyperextension. Of that motion, an estimated 20^0 is cranial movement taking place at the atlanto-occipital and atlanto-axial joints and the remaining extension (55^0–65^0) is cervical motion in the intracervical region (C2–C7).

Lateral Flexion is in the **frontal plane** and occurs as the ear is brought toward the shoulder (Figure 9.2). Average range of motion in lateral flexion is 40^0–45^0. Nearly all lateral flexion takes place (35^0–40^0) in the intracervical region (C2–C7), with approximately 5^0 at the atlanto-occipital joint and a negligible amount at the atlanto-axial joint.

Rotation is around the **central axis** of the spine in the transverse plane and is movement of the head toward either side (Figure 9.2). Average range of motion in craniocervical rotation is about 90^0. There is cranial motion of approximately 45^0 at the atlanto-axial joint, with virtually no rotation at the atlanto-occipital joint. The remaining 45^0 is within the intracervical region (C2–C7).

Capsular Patterns

In most cases, joint capsules in the neck do not restrict motion the same way they do in extremity joints. When there is joint capsule involvement, the capsular pattern is inconsistent and rarely used as a clinical finding.[1]

RANGE-OF-MOTION & MANUAL RESISTIVE TESTS

Results from single-plane movement analysis form the basis for further evaluation procedures. Movement testing should be performed in a certain order, allowing for an

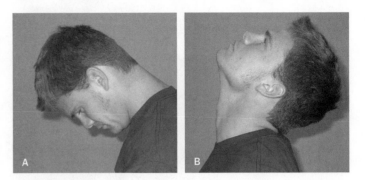

Figure 9.1 Neck flexion (A) and (hyper)extension (B).

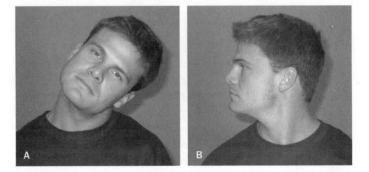

Figure 9.2 Lateral flexion (A) and rotation (B).

efficient evaluation and the least amount of accumulated discomfort or pain to develop. It is also general practice to leave movements known or expected to be painful to the end of the evaluation. When possible, the pain-free side is evaluated first.

Active range-of-motion (AROM) movements are performed first to establish the client's movement abilities and pain symptoms. Passive range of motion (PROM) is performed next and manual resistive tests (MRT) follow. AROM results may make PROM assessment procedures unnecessary. If no pain occurs with active movement, pain is unlikely with passive movement. The practitioner should be familiar with the full step-by-step instructions and guidelines for how to interpret ROM and resistive test results explained in Chapter 3.

Active Range of Motion

Active neck flexion and extension are usually evaluated with the client in a standing position. When performing AROM evaluations, take into consideration the position of the head and neck to ensure the target tissues are engaged. For example, from a standing position when the client actively flexes the neck by bringing the chin to the chest, the neck extensors are engaged eccentrically. Engaging the neck flexors concentrically requires a change in body position or in the way the resistance of gravity affects the movement. The neck flexors would be concentrically engaged if active flexion is performed from a supine position.

BOX 9.1 MUSCLE ACTIONS OF THE CERVICAL SPINE

Craniocervical

Flexion

Rectus capitis anterior
Rectus capitis lateralis
Longus capitis
Longus colli
Scalenes (all three)
Sternocleidomastoid (certain conditions)

Lateral flexion

Levator Scapulae
Trapezius (upper portion)
Scalenes (all three)
Sternocleidomastoid
Splenius capitis
Splenius cervicis
Longus Colli
Longus Capitis
Rectus capitis posterior major
Rectus capitis posterior minor
Obliquus capitis superior
Obliquus capitis inferior
Semispinalis capitis
Longissimus capitis
Multifidi

Ipsilateral Rotation

Levator scapulae
Splenius capitis
Splenius cervicis
Scalenes (all three)*
Rectus capitis posterior major
Obliquus capitis inferior
Longissimus capitis

Extension

Rectus capitis posterior major
Rectus capitis posterior minor
Obliquus capitis superior
Obliquus capitis inferior
Longissimus capitis
Splenius capitis
Semispinalis capitis
Spinalis capitis
Sternocleidomastoid (some conditions)
Trapezius (upper portion)
Longissimus cervic
Semispinalis cervicis
Iliocostalis cervicis
Splenius cervicis
Levator scapulae
Interspinales cervicis
Spinalis cervicis
Rotatores cervicis
Multifidi

Contralateral Rotation

Trapezius (upper portion)
Semispinalis capitis
Semispinalis cervicis
Rotatores cervicis
Longus colli
Sternocleidomastoid
Multifidi
Scalenes (all three)*

*The scalenes are listed in different sources as both ipsilateral and contralateral rotators due to their angle of pull. Their action is also dependent on other synergistic muscles.

Pain with active movement indicates problems in either the contractile or inert tissues associated with that movement. Factors prematurely limiting active movement in this region include *ligamentous* or *capsular damage, muscular hypertonicity,* pain from *nerve compression* or *tension, facet joint dysfunction, fibrous cysts* or *tumors* near the spine, or *joint disorders* such as *arthritis.*

Compare AROM test results with those from PROM and manual resistive tests to identify possible reasons for movement restriction. The primary muscles used to perform actions of the neck are listed in Box 9.1. Note that

other muscles can contribute to the motion and subsequent dysfunction.

Passive Range of Motion

Passive motion is performed after active. Pain during passive movement predominantly implicates inert tissues. However, muscles and tendons that contract in the opposite direction are stretched at the end range of passive movement. The primary goal of passive movement is to have minimal or no muscular activity. If performing these movements with the client in an upright position

Box 9.2 Joints, Associated Motion, & Normal End Feel		
Craniocervical	Flexion	Tissue stretch (soft)
	Extension	Tissue stretch (soft)
	Lateral Flexion	Tissue stretch (soft)
	Rotation	Tissue stretch (soft)

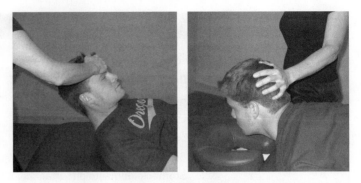

Figure 9.3 Resisted flexion (A) and extension (B).

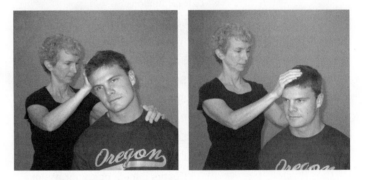

Figure 9.4 Resisted lateral flexion (A) and rotation (B).

does not adequately decrease muscular activity, use a supine position.

PROM testing also evaluates end feel. Box 9.2 lists the primary end feel for movements in the neck. The end feel is not specific to only one joint as several joints are moved. Review Chapter 3 for a discussion of normal and pathological end feel descriptions. Factors that could prematurely limit passive movement are the same as for active movement.

Manual Resistive Tests

A manual resistive test (MRT) produces pain when there is a mechanical disruption of tissue. Pain with an MRT indicates that one or more of the muscles and/or tendons performing that action are involved. Note that *tenosynovitis* is not a problem in the cervical region as there are no tendons surrounded by a synovial sheath. Due to the number of muscles in the cervical spine, most having multiple actions, it is difficult to simplify manual resistance testing to one muscle.

Testing all of a muscle's actions is not necessary, as a muscle's secondary actions recruit other muscles and make the test results less accurate. The following actions are the most common for assessing the cervical spine, however there are others. Some actions isolate muscles in the cervical region better than others; skill development in these procedures allows the practitioner to elicit more refined information.

In some cases weakness is evident with MRTs. Factors that produce weakness include *lack of use, fatigue, reflex muscular inhibition,* and possibly a neurological pathology (*radiculopathy, peripheral neuropathy,* or a *systemic neurological disorder*). Palpation elicits more information if the test alone does not create pain or discomfort. Refer to Box 9.1 for the list of primary muscles involved with each action. Table 2 at the end of the chapter lists actions commonly used for testing muscles in the cervical spine. The nerves or nerve roots that may be involved are also listed in this table.

Neck
Resisted Flexion
The client is supine on the treatment table. The client attempts to lift the head off the treatment table (Figure

9.3) with or without practitioner resistance. The weight of the client's head may be sufficient for the test. To increase muscular effort, the practitioner places a hand on the client's forehead to offer moderate resistance.

Resisted Extension
The client is prone on the treatment table. It is helpful to have the client in a face cradle to start this test so the neck muscles are fully relaxed. The practitioner places a hand on the back of the client's head to offer moderate resistance. The client lifts the head off the face cradle (Figure 9.3). If less muscular effort is desired, have the client lift the weight of the head without resistance.

Resisted Lateral Flexion
The client is seated on the treatment table with the head in neutral or slight lateral flexion. The practitioner places one hand on the client's shoulder and the other hand on the side of the client's head. The client holds this position while the practitioner attempts to push the client's head to the opposite side with moderate pressure (Figure 9.4).

Resisted Rotation
The client is seated on the treatment table with the head in a neutral position. The practitioner places one hand on the client's lateral forehead and the other hand on the occiput. The client holds this position while the practitioner attempts to rotate the client's head to the opposite side (Figure 9.4).

Structural and Postural Deviations

The following section covers common structural or postural deviations unique to the cervical spine. Under each condition there is a brief description of its characteristics followed by likely HOPRS findings. If applicable, orthopedic tests are included in the special tests section. If there is no special orthopedic test listed for that condition, evaluation should focus on other portions of the assessment process, such as range-of-motion testing.

MILITARY NECK

Military neck is the name given to a *loss of cervical lordosis* because the postural compensation looks like an exaggerated military attention posture. The postural distortion can alter biomechanics in the neck and contribute to certain pain complaints, but pain is not always present. Over time, loss of cervical lordosis could produce vertebral stress fractures due to increased compressive loads.

Characteristics

There is a natural lordotic curve in the cervical region that is essential for shock absorption and proper movement. The lordotic curvature is lost when **the lower cervical region is in extension and the upper cervical region is in flexion** (Figure 9.5). This is also the position of the head and neck when they are retracted.

Loss of the lordotic curve can lead to *facet joint irritation, muscular hypertonicity, myofascial trigger points*, and other dysfunctions. Military neck increases compressive loads on the **intervertebral discs**, which can then lead to *disc degeneration* or *herniation of the nucleus pulposus* (see herniated nucleus pulposus later in the chapter). Loss of cervical lordosis should be considered an important factor when investigating disc pathology in the neck.

Military neck can be hereditary or result from acquired poor postural habits. The upper cervical region is often in a greater degree of flexion due to hypertonicity in the cervical deep neck flexors, such as the **longus colli** and **longus capitis**. The postural distortion can also be brought on by previous surgical procedures, such as fusion of cervical vertebrae. Spinal fusion surgeries are performed to reduce facet joint compression or maximize space in the intervertebral foramen. In order to accomplish these objectives, the spinal segments are fused in a position that decreases the natural lordotic curve.

History

The client may complain of neck pain due to vertebral disc compression or facet joint irritation, but pain is not always present. Muscular pain or limited range of motion may also be reported.

Observation

Visual observation is the most effective means of identifying military neck. A postural grid chart is useful as a point

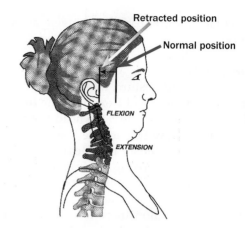

Figure 9.5 Military neck, loss of cervical lordosis. (Reproduced with permission from Neumann DA. Kinesiology of the Musculoskeletal System. St. Louis: Mosby; 2002.)

of reference. This condition is best viewed from the side and the posterior neck appears very straight. The chin also appears tucked under.

Palpation

The posterior and lateral cervical muscles generally feel tight. Though difficult to palpate, the deep flexors of the neck, especially the **longus colli**, could feel tight as well. Great caution should be used if attempting to palpate the deep neck flexors due to the proximity of the baroreceptors and the carotid sinus. In some cases the spinous processes of the cervical vertebrae may not feel evenly spaced due to the combination of flexion and extension through the cervical region.

Range-of-Motion and Resistance Testing

AROM: Limitation in active extension is possible due to positioning of the lower cervical vertebrae.
PROM: Limitations are the same as in active movement.
MRT: Pain or discomfort is not expected with MRTs. There may be muscular weakness.

Suggestions for Treatment

It is helpful to reduce tension in the neck, particularly the cervical deep neck flexors, although they are difficult to access with manual therapy. Stretching methods, such as muscle energy technique, are also effective. Soft-tissue treatment of the lower cervical extensor muscles may aid in the return to proper posture. Postural training and neuromuscular re-education are crucial elements of any rehabilitative strategy because the condition is usually a developed postural disorder.

FORWARD HEAD POSTURE

Because humans stand upright in a vertical gravity plane, we are susceptible to the distortion of a *forward head posture*. The condition primarily results from chronic dysfunctional postural patterns and usually involves muscular distortion in the thoracic as well as cervical regions.

Characteristics

In forward head posture, there is **extension in the upper cervical vertebrae and flexion in the lower cervical vertebrae** (Figure 9.6). When the head is positioned forward of the line of gravity, a tensile load is placed on the **posterior cervical extensor muscles**. These muscles function to keep the eyes looking straight ahead and prevent the head from falling forward. Even a slight degree of forward head posture increases stress on the posterior neck muscles. In addition there is an increased compressive load on the upper vertebral **posterior arch structures**. For every inch the head moves forward from its normal posture, the compressive load on the lower neck is increased by the additional weight of the head.[2]

In a forward head posture the posterior cervical muscles must work harder to keep the head upright. As a result *fatigue, tension,* and *myofascial trigger points* develop. Muscle tension and myofascial trigger point referrals can produce pain in the head, neck, upper back, or **temporomandibular joint**. Muscular irritation from forward head posture is at the root of numerous head and neck pain conditions. For example, myofascial trigger points that develop in the **sub-occipital muscles** from forward head posture frequently cause headache pain. The increased compressive loads can eventually lead to *vertebral stress fractures* or *cervical facet* **(zygapophysial)** *joint irritation.*

Chapter 8 discusses the lower crossed syndrome, a condition that involves the relationship between postural and phasic muscles in the lumbar region. A similar relationship exists in the cervical region and is referred to as the *upper crossed syndrome*.[3] The upper crossed syndrome often exists in conjunction with the *lower crossed syndrome*. Postural and phasic muscles differ in their fiber type and activation patterns. When overused and fatigued, postural muscles tend to become hypertonic, while phasic muscles tend to become weak and inhibited. The phasic muscles are antagonists to postural muscles. Because postural muscles tend toward hypertonicity, they create a functional weakness in the phasic muscles in a process called reciprocal inhibition. A graphical comparison of the muscles' positions and functional relationships with each other shows how they interact and where the term crossed syndrome originates from (Figure 9.7).

The postural muscles in the neck region prone to *hypertonicity* include the **upper trapezius, levator scapulae,** and **cervical extensors** on the posterior aspect, as well as the **pectoralis major** and **minor** in the front.[2] The postural muscles are known to house active myofascial trigger points and refer characteristic symptoms when palpated. Phasic muscles that are prone to weakness include the deep neck flexors such as the **longus colli** and **longus capitis**, as well as the **lower trapezius, rhomboids**, and **serratus anterior**.[2]

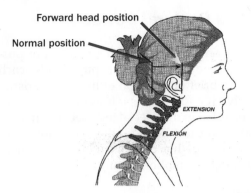

Figure 9.6 Forward head posture. (Reproduced with permission from Neumann DA. Kinesiology of the Musculoskeletal System. St. Louis: Mosby; 2002.)

Forward head posture results from poor postural habits, such as leaning forward toward a computer screen for long periods. Due to the postural compensations that naturally occur with age, forward head posture is seen more frequently in older clients.

History

The client might complain of aching pain in the posterior cervical or upper thoracic region due to increased stress on the muscles. In many cases the client has adapted to the postural distortion. Pain or discomfort might develop if the individual maintains a stressful posture for a prolonged period.

Observation

Forward head posture is most easily identified through visual observation from the lateral view. The head has an appearance of thrusting forward in relation to the torso. A postural grid chart aids in evaluating the degree of forward position. Normally the ear should be in line with the glenohumeral joint; with forward head posture the ear is forward of this position.

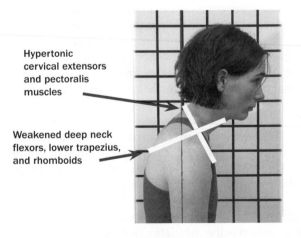

Hypertonic cervical extensors and pectoralis muscles

Weakened deep neck flexors, lower trapezius, and rhomboids

Figure 9.7 Upper crossed syndrome.

Palpation

Hypertonicity is common in the posterior cervical muscles, especially in the upper region. There is palpable tightness in the anterior and middle scalene muscles. Myofascial trigger points may refer pain to various areas of the head, neck, chest, or arm and are present in the posterior cervical and scalene muscles.

Range-of-Motion and Resistance Testing

AROM: There may be limitations to flexion and extension and pain due to hypertonicity, but not always. Hyperextension may be limited, due to chronic shortening in the anterior neck muscles.

PROM: The same principles apply as for active motion.

MRT: Pain is uncommon with MRTs, although some tests may produce myofascial trigger point pain. Muscle weakness is likely in the deep neck flexors from reciprocal inhibition. However, weakness during MRTs is not expected because of compensation by other neck flexors.

Suggestions for Treatment

The primary focus of treatment should be postural training and neuromuscular re-education. Repetitive dysfunctional patterns should be offset by repeated corrections that change the faulty biomechanics. Soft-tissue treatment is helpful for hypertonicity in the posterior cervical muscles, particularly the sub-occipital group. Chronic shortening in the lower cervical flexors, such as the longus colli, is improved with stretching. The longus colli is difficult to access safely and massage can apply adverse pressure to other structures, such as the baroreceptors in the carotid sinus.

Common Injury Conditions

THORACIC OUTLET SYNDROME

Thoracic outlet syndrome (TOS) is not a single condition; rather the term encompasses several variations of nerve or vascular compression near the base of the neck and upper rib cage. TOS is a complex condition and can be overlooked or misdiagnosed due to the difficulty in distinguishing between the variations.[4]

Characteristics

The **thoracic outlet** is the opening at the upper margin of the rib cage. It is called the thoracic outlet as it is the location where the **subclavian artery** exits the rib cage as it descends into the upper extremity. Ironically, this specific area does not factor into most cases of thoracic outlet syndrome as **the condition is primarily a** *nerve compression syndrome* and not a vascular disorder.

A bundle of upper extremity nerves called the brachial plexus passes near the thoracic outlet (Figure 9.8). The brachial plexus first passes between the anterior and middle scalene muscles, then underneath the clavicle and continues inferiorly underneath the pectoralis minor

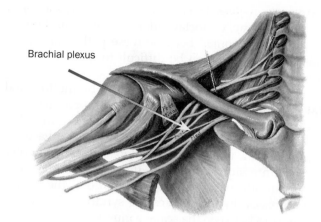

Figure 9.8 Brachial plexus passing near the thoracic outlet. (Mediclip image copyright, 1998 Williams & Wilkins. All rights reserved.)

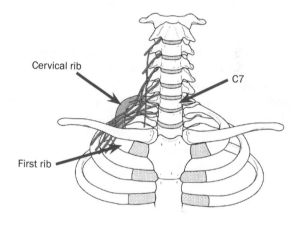

Figure 9.9 Anterior view of the upper thoracic region showing a cervical rib. (Reproduced with permission from Lowe W. Orthopedic Massage: Theory and Technique. Edinburgh: Mosby; 2003.

muscle before diverging along different paths down the upper extremity. The nerves of the brachial plexus can be compressed in several locations near the thoracic outlet. These various nerve compression pathologies have all come to be known as thoracic outlet syndromes.

There are four variations of thoracic outlet syndrome divided into two categories.[5] The first category contains one variation and is called *true neurologic thoracic outlet syndrome.* This condition occurs because of an anatomical anomaly called a **cervical rib**, which is a bony extension of the transverse process of the C7 vertebra (Figure 9.9). The cervical rib usually has a fibrous connection with the first rib . The existence of the cervical rib can place pressure on the brachial plexus, as it must cross over the cervical rib.

The second category, *non-specific thoracic outlet*

syndromes, involves three distinct conditions: anterior scalene syndrome, costoclavicular syndrome, and pectoralis minor syndrome.[6] Because these pathologies have similar symptoms, it can be difficult to distinguish one from the other.

Anterior scalene syndrome is caused by the **brachial plexus** and **subclavian artery** being entrapped between the **anterior** and **middle scalene muscles** (Figure 9.10). While it is possible to have either neurological or vascular compression, the majority of symptoms appear to involve nerve compression.[7] Although the subclavian vein is involved in other thoracic outlet conditions, the vein is not compressed in anterior scalene syndrome because it does not pass between the scalene muscles.

The second pathology of non-specific TOS, called *costoclavicular syndrome*, involves compression of the neurovascular structures between the **first rib** and the **clavicle** (Figure 9.10). Compression can affect the brachial plexus, subclavian artery, or subclavian vein. However, brachial plexus impingement remains the predominant concern and the symptoms are most frequently neurological.

In the third pathology, *pectoralis minor syndrome*, the neurovascular structures become compressed by the **pectoralis minor muscle**. The brachial plexus, subclavian artery, and vein pass underneath the pectoralis minor muscle. When the muscle is hypertonic, these structures can be compressed against the upper rib cage causing either neurological or vascular symptoms in the upper extremity. As with other variations of TOS, neurological

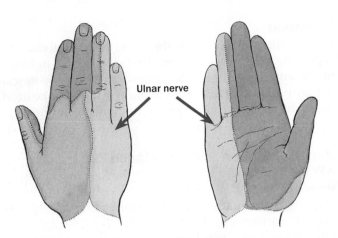

Figure 9.11 Ulnar nerve distribution in the hand. (Mediclip image copyright, 1998 Williams & Wilkins. All rights reserved.)

compression symptoms are more common than vascular.

Compression of the brachial plexus can affect any of the nerves that extend through the upper extremity. The medial cord of the brachial plexus is most vulnerable to impingement because of its anatomical position in the plexus. The majority of fibers in the medial cord come from the C8 and T1 nerve roots and eventually compose the **ulnar nerve**. As a result, TOS affects the ulnar nerve more than others and sensory symptoms are routinely felt in the ulnar nerve distribution in the hand (Figure 9.11).

While ulnar nerve involvement is typical, TOS can irritate any of the nerves derived from the brachial plexus. If fibers of the **median nerve** are involved, symptoms of brachial plexus compression are easily mistaken for *carpal tunnel syndrome*. Comprehensive assessment is necessary to identify the proper location of nerve compression and prevent a faulty interpretation of the condition. Inaccurate diagnosis that leads to treatment of carpal tunnel syndrome, rather than the TOS, is problematic and there are cases in which clients have been subjected to unnecessary surgery.

Thoracic outlet syndrome was originally described in the medical literature as a circulatory problem created by pressure on the arteries and veins in the upper shoulder region. For that reason, some tests focus on circulatory responses. Symptoms resulting from vascular compression can present alone or in conjunction with neurological symptoms. *Ischemia* of the nerves, for example, can aggravate neurological symptoms. Authors now agree that the majority of TOS symptoms, perhaps as much as 95%, arise from neurological impairment.[5, 7]

Any of the TOS variations may occur as an acute injury.[8] The condition is generally a chronic dysfunction induced by poor posture or faulty biomechanics. Postural distortion is more of a problem with non-specific TOS pathologies, versus true neurologic TOS. *Forward head posture* with an *exaggerated upper thoracic kyphosis* and internally rotated shoulders are seen regularly in those with TOS. Poor ergonomics in the workplace, such

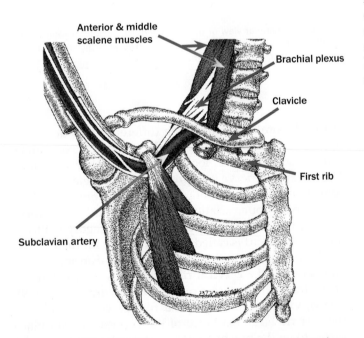

Figure 9.10 Brachial plexus compression can lead to anterior scalene or costoclavicular syndrome. (Mediclip image copyright, 1998 Williams & Wilkins. All rights reserved.)

as slumping over a keyboard, are also a frequent cause. Carrying heavy objects causes depression of the shoulder girdle and could contribute to either costoclavicular or pectoralis minor variations. Those who carry backpacks or equipment with shoulder straps are particularly susceptible to TOS because of shoulder girdle depression.

History

In some cases, the client reports an acute injury, but TOS is more likely to be a chronic postural problem. Primary neurological symptoms include pain, paresthesia, and burning or tingling sensations in the upper extremity. The client usually reports symptoms in the ulnar nerve distribution. The client might also report symptoms of coldness or a feeling of fullness or swelling in the upper extremity, which signifies vascular compression. Symptoms get worse the longer the condition is left untreated because nerve damage can result with even minor levels of prolonged compression.

Symptoms are aggravated by various activities, especially those that cause chronic postural stress of the upper thoracic or cervical regions. Sleeping positions may also aggravate symptoms. It is helpful to investigate whether the client is a side sleeper or sleeps with an arm draped over the head, as these positions can increase nerve compression. Inquire about other postural stresses, such as the wearing of a heavy knapsack, purse, or equipment strap that could cause shoulder girdle depression and compress the brachial plexus.

Observation

There are no directly observable signs that verify the presence of TOS. A cervical rib is rarely visible, though it would be visible on an x-ray. Vascular compromise might produce discoloration of the upper extremity. In severe cases, atrophy of muscles in the hand may be visible. Postural distortions may be present, but do not alone indicate TOS.

Palpation

A cervical rib, if present, is likely to be palpable near the lower margin of the scalene muscles. The existence of a cervical rib, however, must be verified through x-ray as palpation is not reliable. Cervical ribs may be bilateral or unilateral. The presence of a cervical rib does not signify nerve compression. In anterior scalene syndrome, it is common for the scalene muscles to feel hypertonic, particularly the anterior and middle scalenes. Because one of the functions of this muscle group is to lift the upper rib cage, hypertonic scalenes may also occur with costoclavicular syndrome. In pectoralis minor syndrome, either one or both pectoralis muscles (major and minor) are tight.

Palpation can reproduce symptoms in any of these conditions and the practitioner should be cautious with the level of pressure used. If symptoms are reproduced, discontinue pressure. Symptom reproduction with minimal

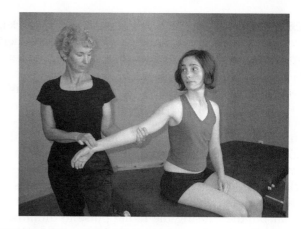

Figure 9.12 **Adson Maneuver.**

pressure is also a valuable finding, because it indicates the tissues are more sensitive than normal.

Range-of-Motion and Resistance Testing

AROM: Active motion may produce symptoms if the brachial plexus is stretched. This stretch is most likely when laterally flexing the neck to the opposite side. Although not frequent, there may be symptoms during neck extension or flexion due to tension developed in the upper dura mater that is transmitted to the nerve roots of the brachial plexus. If pectoralis minor syndrome is present, there may be an increase in symptoms during active or passive abduction of the shoulder (see Wright abduction test below).

PROM: The same principles apply as for AROM.

MRT: Pain is unlikely with MRTs. Muscle weakness is not as common with brachial plexus entrapment as it is with other ulnar nerve compression pathologies more distal along the length of the nerve, but symptoms are possible due to compression of fibers that supply the ulnar nerve. Consult Table 1 in Chapter 11 for upper extremity muscles supplied by the nerves of the brachial plexus.

Special Tests
Adson Maneuver

The Adson maneuver is considered a general test for TOS, but is more specific for anterior scalene syndrome. The client is seated or standing. The practitioner locates the client's radial pulse on the affected side and brings the client's arm into extension and lateral rotation. The client turns the head as far as possible to the affected side and tilts the chin up, which places the cervical region into extension and ipsilateral rotation (Figure 9.12). Once the head and neck are in this position, the client takes a deep breath and holds it. If the radial pulse diminishes in intensity (not rate), it is a positive test. Note whether neurological signs or symptoms increase. Sometimes it is recommended to turn the head to the opposite side, however this is a separate procedure called the Halstead maneuver.

Explanation: This test evaluates vascular blockage in the area of the thoracic outlet, which indicates nerve compression as well. The presence of neurological symptoms would confirm nerve compression. The position of the arm, head, and neck stretches the scalene muscles and the neurovascular bundle that travels distally in the upper extremity. Due to the action of the scalene muscles, the final position of the head could also include lateral flexion to the opposite side which would place more tensile stress on the scalenes. In the final stage of the test, the client's deep breath contracts the scalene muscles and lifts the rib cage, which can further compress the neurovascular bundle causing the radial pulse to diminish or disappear. Findings are not certain because the Adson's maneuver has a high number of false positives.

Allen Test

The Allen test is similar to the Adson maneuver in that it tests the presence of neurovascular compression by monitoring the radial pulse. The practitioner locates the radial pulse. The client is seated with the elbow flexed to 90^0 and the arm in 90^0 of abduction and externally rotated. The client rotates the head to the opposite side (Figure 9.13).

Explanation: A disappearance or diminishing of the radial pulse is indicative of TOS, specifically anterior scalene syndrome. The arm position puts significant tensile stress on the neurovascular structures of the brachial plexus. Contracting the anterior and middle scalene muscles can aggravate these structures and rotating the head to the opposite side may further pinch the neurovascular bundle between the muscles.

Military Brace Test

This test evaluates for costoclavicular syndrome. The client is seated or standing and pulls the scapulae together, so the arms are extended and the scapulae are fully retracted (Figure 9.14). The position is held for approximately 30-60 seconds. Do the test with varying degrees of shoulder abduction to produce different levels of pressure on the neurovascular structures.

Explanation: Reproduction of characteristic neurological symptoms in the distal upper extremity is considered a positive test for costoclavicular syndrome. Pulling the scapulae into a retracted position decreases the space between the clavicle and first rib causing increased brachial plexus compression. If the compression is significant, symptoms are felt almost immediately. If compression is not as severe it may take more time for symptoms to be felt.

Wright Abduction Test

This test evaluates for pectoralis minor syndrome. The client is seated with the arm on the affected side lifted as far into abduction as possible (Figure 9.15). The client holds the arm in this position for approximately one minute. If symptoms are exacerbated within 20 or 30 seconds it indicates a degree of compression of the brachial plexus, most

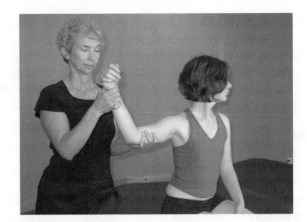

Figure 9.13 Allen test.

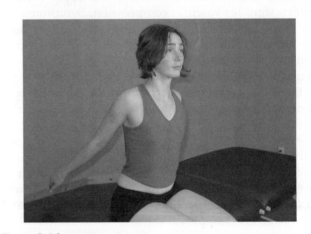

Figure 9.14 Military brace test.

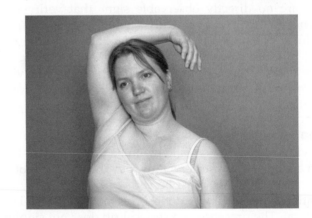

Figure 9.15 Wright abduction test.

likely underneath the pectoralis minor muscle. Several variations on the position of the elbow and wrist can be used to make the test more effective, depending on which nerve is most involved. For *ulnar nerve involvement*, the elbow is flexed and the wrist is fully extended. For *radial nerve involvement*, the elbow is extended and the wrist is flexed. With the median nerve, the elbow and wrist are fully extended.

Explanation: The brachial plexus travels in an inferior

direction from the thoracic outlet region, underneath the pectoralis minor muscle and distally through the upper extremity. When the arm is abducted, the neurovascular bundle changes direction almost 180⁰. The pectoralis minor muscle acts as a tether around which the neurovascular bundle must travel. If the muscle is hypertonic, the neurovascular bundle is further compressed against the upper rib cage, exacerbating symptoms.

Differential Evaluation

Carpal tunnel syndrome, rotator cuff injuries, myofascial trigger point pain, cervical disc herniation, cervical facet syndrome, other peripheral compression neuropathies, multiple sclerosis, diabetic neuropathy, coronary disorder, Raynaud's syndrome.

Suggestions for Treatment

Treatment should reduce compression on the neurovascular bundle whether that is from soft tissues or from bony encroachment. Reduce hypertonicity in the scalene and pectoralis minor muscles with static compression, stripping, active engagement, and stretching. Exercise caution so that additional pressure is not applied to the brachial plexus. Techniques that increase compression of the brachial plexus will exacerbate symptoms. Postural retraining is important because this condition is aggravated by postural distortions such as forward head posture and upper thoracic kyphosis.

CERVICAL FACET SYNDROME

Cervical facet syndrome is a dysfunction of the facet (zygapophysial) joints in the cervical region. The condition is difficult to identify and routinely occurs in situations involving rapid forces to the neck, as in whiplash injury. It also results from various postural distortions such as prolonged periods in a forward head posture.

Characteristics

Each vertebra has four **facet joints**: one superior and one inferior facet on each side (Figure 9.16). The joint's purpose is to guide appropriate movement in the spine. In the neck, the facet joints are angled so as to allow a significant amount of flexion, extension, lateral flexion, and rotation. Each facet joint is surrounded by a **joint capsule** that is composed of a richly innervated fibrous capsule and a synovial membrane. The facet joint capsules are more lax in the neck to allow for greater gliding during movement.[9] Greater laxity of the capsules makes the joints a little less stable and more susceptible to sprain injury.

Facet joint compression occurs **bilaterally during hyperextension** and to the **ipsilateral side when laterally flexing**. Rotational movements compress facet joints as well. During forward flexion or lateral flexion to the opposite side, the joints open up and there is tensile stress on the joint capsules. Increased force loads on the neck during high velocity movements, such as whiplash, cause facet joint damage from both compressive and tensile forces.[10, 11]

The primary weight-bearing structures in the cervical spine are the **vertebral bodies** and the **intervertebral discs**. The **posterior vertebral structures**, which include the facet joints, also bear a certain percentage of weight. Although the role of cervical facet joints in weight bearing is minor, they are further compressed in postural distortions such as *forward head posture* and *upper crossed syndrome.*[12]

There may be a relationship between facet joint irritation and *intervertebral disc pathology*, especially when the disc loses height.[13, 14] In some cases there may be a corresponding irritation of the facet joints and **uncovertebral joints** (joints of Luschka).[15] These joints are on the vertebral bodies of the cervical vertebrae where adjacent vertebrae articulate and appear to be most associated with guiding rotational movements (Figure 9.17).[9]

Facet syndromes in the cervical region have not been researched as thoroughly as in the lumbar region. The lack of clear signs and symptoms complicates the task of evaluating for this condition. Similar to the controversy around lumbar facet syndromes there are those who believe the condition is under-diagnosed and some who still question its existence.[16] Identifying the condition always involves excluding other causes as much as possible.

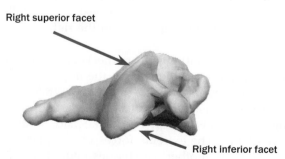

Figure 9.16 Lateral view of cervical vertebra with facet joints. (3-D anatomy image courtesy of Primal Pictures Ltd. www.primalpictures.com.)

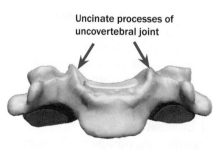

Figure 9.17 Anterior view of a cervical vertebra. (3-D anatomy image courtesy of Primal Pictures Ltd. www.primalpictures.com.)

Hypertonicity and increased *myofascial trigger point* activity is typical in facet joint syndrome. Facet joint irritation routinely produces headache pain, as well as neck pain and limitations in range of motion.[9] Dysfunctional cervical facet joints appear to refer pain in characteristic patterns much like myofascial trigger points.[9,17,18] Referred pain from the upper cervical facet joints extends into the head, while pain from lower facet joints can extend all the way to the inferior border of the scapula.

History

The client normally complains of neck pain that is aggravated by movement. The most painful movements are extension and lateral flexion to the same side. Pain is often described as a dull aching sensation, located in the posterior neck. Ask about the frequency and onset of pain. Pain can refer distally into the upper extremity or mid-back. Ask about neck injuries, such as whiplash, as they can precede facet joint syndrome. Morning pain is usual and results from lack of spinal movement during the night, which may improve as the person moves around. Sitting in certain positions could also aggravate symptoms.

Observation

There are no obvious visual signs of cervical facet syndrome. A forward head posture might be present and could indicate increased pressure on cervical facet joints.

Palpation

Tenderness often appears in muscles of the posterior cervical region. The facet joints are not easily palpated due to adipose tissue and the paraspinal muscles, but palpation deep in the lamina groove near the joints sometimes reveals exaggerated tenderness. Indirect pressure placed on the facet joints or their capsules may recreate the client's pain. Hypertonicity and myofascial trigger points in the cervical extensor muscles are typical.

Range-of-Motion and Resistance Testing

AROM: Pain is likely during motions that further compress the facet joints, such as hyperextension, lateral flexion to the same side, or rotational movements to either side. Flexion and lateral flexion to the side opposite the dysfunctional side is apt to decrease pain as the facet joints are opened.
PROM: The same principles apply as in AROM.
MRT: There are no specific patterns of pain or weakness with MRTs. Hypertonicity is expected in nearby paraspinal muscles and in some cases myofascial trigger points could become symptomatic during resisted contraction of these muscles.

Differential Evaluation

Cervical disc pathology, muscle strain, herniated nucleus pulposus, spinal ligament sprain, myofascial trigger point pain, spinal tumor, degenerative disc disease, radiculopathy, arthritis, spinal stenosis, spinal tumor.

Suggestions for Treatment

The primary focus of treatment is to reduce compressive forces on the facet joint. Activity modification and postural re-training are an essential part of the rehabilitation process. Massage can be applied to the paraspinal muscles to address joint irritation or myofascial trigger points. Massage is also helpful for structural and postural problems. Manipulation or joint mobilization may be used as well. Corticosteroids are sometimes used by other health professionals to treat this problem.

WHIPLASH

Whiplash is not a specific diagnostic term, but instead refers to a rapid acceleration or deceleration injury. The condition is also referred to as *whiplash-associated-disorder (WAD)*, which is considered more accurate due to the number of potential tissues involved and the variety of conditions that arise with the injury.[19] Due to the potential severity of whiplash disorders and their complexity, the client should be evaluated by a physician to rule out serious pathologies.

Characteristics

Any activity that results in **rapid acceleration or deceleration of the head and neck** could cause whiplash. Numerous tissues are at risk of injury with these forces and damage to the soft tissues is usually from either compressive or tensile stress resulting from the rapid acceleration or deceleration. Box 9.3 includes a list of neck movements and the tissues most likely injured from either compressive or tensile forces from the whiplash. Potential involvement of any of these tissues should be evaluated thoroughly with any client who has sustained a whiplash injury.

Automobile accidents are a primary cause of WAD, but recreational or occupational activities also produce the injury. During a rear impact, the most common type of whiplash injury, the head and neck are first rapidly forced into hyperextension and then recoil in flexion. In an impact from the front, the reverse happens and the head and neck are initially forced into flexion, and then recoil into extension. Side impacts cause force and recoil in lateral directions. For example, an impact from the left side creates a rapid left lateral flexion first, followed by recoil to the right. Impacts from the right side would be the reverse.

Accidents (automobile or other) occur with the head in any number of positions, with the impact forces coming from a number of possible directions. While it is customary to focus on acceleration and deceleration forces in the sagittal plane, whiplash injury take place in other or multiple planes. The extreme forces in one plane can cause instability in another. The tissues injured when hit from behind while the head is turned to the side are different than if the head is facing forward. Consider the mechanics of the injury carefully when evaluating a suspected

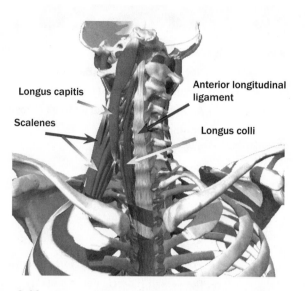

Figure 9.18 Anterior view of the cervical spine. (3-D anatomy image courtesy of Primal Pictures Ltd. www.primalpictures.com.)

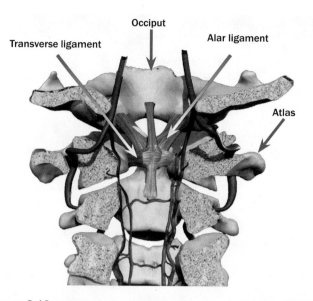

Figure 9.19 Anterior view of the deep suboccipital region with bodies of the vertebrae cut and removed. (3-D anatomy image courtesy of Primal Pictures Ltd. www.primalpictures.com.)

whiplash injury.

Various efforts have been made to classify WAD because of the potential number of tissues injured. One of the most significant classifications of WAD published to date comes from the Quebec Task Force on Whiplash-Associated Disorders.[19] The task force classifies WAD into four categories of severity. In category 1 there is complaint of neck pain or discomfort, but without musculoskeletal signs. With category 2 injuries, there is neck pain and musculoskeletal signs such as *loss of mobility, tenderness*, or *muscle spasm*. Category 3 disorders include the above, along with neurological signs such as *sensory deficit* or *diminished tendon reflexes*. Finally, in a category 4 there are the above symptoms plus *cervical fracture* or *dislocation*.

Muscle and *ligament damage* are a primary concern in whiplash injuries. Emphasis on damage to these tissues is evident with the frequency of *cervical strain/sprain* diagnoses for whiplash injury. Range of motion can also be lost due to *muscle spasm, joint binding*, or *instability*. Motion loss may not present immediately, but gradually progress to a final stage of impairment. In more severe injuries, *vascular compromise* and *nerve damage* may result, as well as *disc* or *vertebral damage*. *Contusions* to the brain are also possible.[12]

Extension in WAD causes stretching of the **deep neck flexors**. The **longus colli** and **scalenes** are two of the more frequently injured tissues in WAD. In addition, the **anterior longitudinal ligament, anterior aspect of the annulus fibrosus**, and the **anterior neck viscera** could be injured by over-stretching (Figure 9.18). On the posterior aspect, *stenosis* (narrowing) of the **intervertebral foramina** might compress the nerve roots. The **facet joints** or the posterior portion of the **intervertebral discs** may be damaged by compression. Rapid and extreme cervi-

cal flexion may be limited by the chin hitting the chest, depending on the flexibility of the tissues. The **cervical extensor muscles** may be strained in their attempt to control the flexion. See the beginning of the chapter for a complete list of cervical spine muscles.

Posterior vertebral structures are also at risk, such as the **ligamentum nuchae, posterior longitudinal ligament, facet joint capsules,** and the **interspinous ligaments**. Compressive forces may cause damage to the anterior portion of the intervertebral discs or **uncovertebral joints** (Figure 9.17). Extremes of lateral flexion cause tensile stress on tissues such as the **lateral flexor muscles**, the **brachial plexus, cervical nerve roots, facet joint capsules,** and **intertransverse ligaments** on the non-flexed side. On the laterally flexed side, compressive stress damage is possible to the **cervical facet joints**, nerve roots, **laminae**, intervertebral discs, or uncovertebral joints.

If the head and neck are in rotation at the time of acceleration or deceleration, greater degrees of injury could result. For example, in a lateral flexion whiplash injury with rotation there may be damage to the stabilizing support ligaments of the craniocervical region, such as the **alar** or the **transverse ligaments** (Figure 9.19). The alar ligaments are primarily responsible for limiting rotation of the cranium in relation to the axis. The transverse ligament is responsible for limiting forward translation of the atlas and cranium in relation to the axis.

Once instability develops from overstretching the support ligaments, vascular impairment can develop. Vascular compromise mainly develops from rotation or extension forces and can be dangerous due to lack of blood flow to the brain. Blood vessels such as the vertebral artery are particularly susceptible and may be damaged even with low levels of force.[20] Consequently practitioners should use particular caution during ROM evaluations.

Box 9.3 Tissues Injured During Rapid Acceleration & Deceleration

Flexion	Tensile Stress		Extension	Tensile Stress
	Cervical & cranial extensor muscles (Box 9.1)			Neck flexor muscles (Box 9.1)
	Ligamentum nuchae			Anterior longitudinal ligament
	Ligamentum flavum			Anterior aspect of the annulus fibrosus
	Facet joint capsules			Anterior neck viscera
	Posterior longitudinal ligament			Brachial plexus
	Interspinous ligaments			Cervical or thoracic nerve roots
				Cervical vascular structures
	Compression			
	Anterior aspect of the annulus fibrosus			**Compression**
	Uncovertebral joints			Cervical facet joints
				Posterior portion of intervertebral discs
				Cervical or thoracic nerve roots
Lateral Flexion	Tensile Stress		**Rotation**	Tensile Stress
	Lateral flexor muscles (Box 9.1)			Contralateral rotator muscles (Box 9.1)
	Brachial plexus			Facet joints
	Cervical nerve roots			Uncovertebral joints
	Facet joint capsules (contralateral)			Intertransverse ligaments
	Intertransverse ligaments (contralateral)			Alar ligaments
	Compression			**Compression**
	Intervertebral discs			Intervertebral discs
	Facet joints (ipsilateral)			Facet joints
	Nerve roots (ipsilateral)			Uncovertebral joints
	Laminae			
	Uncovertebral joints			

One of the peculiar aspects of whiplash injury is the delayed onset of symptoms. While many symptoms of pain and discomfort are immediately evident, some do not present for days or even weeks after the injury. The reason for delayed onset symptoms is not well understood, but could be related to tissue inflammation. However, inflammatory activity alone would not explain symptoms that occur weeks after an injury when initial inflammation has subsided.[12] Increased sensitivity of the neurological system that exaggerates symptoms is a likely explanation for delayed onset whiplash pain.[23-25] According to Melzack and Wall's gate theory, pain from one tissue may override sensations from others, which is common when multiple tissues are damaged.[26]

Whiplash is an acute injury, but its effects can linger, producing a chronic condition. Chronic symptoms include hypertonicity, muscle spasm, movement restrictions, and headaches. Current research suggests that *cervical facet joint dysfunction* may be a more frequent cause of chronic whiplash pain than tissue tearing of muscles or ligaments, as once believed.[21,22] Ligament damage can cause hypermobility and joint irritation. In some cases, muscular *atrophy* results from neurological damage or disuse. *Disc degeneration* or *osteoarthritis* can result from injuries to the joints. Many clients who have suffered WAD also have exaggerated sensitivity of soft tissues in the absence of any clearly evident mechanical damage. Heightened neurological activity after injury can have numerous detrimental effects and prolong the rehabilitation process. Keep in mind that although a client's symptoms may not appear related to an earlier whiplash injury, they could be residual effects from a previous WAD injury.

Box 9.4 Common WAD Symptoms in History & Palpation

History

- Dull, achy pain from muscle spasm or myofascial trigger points.
- Sharp pain in muscles from acute spasm, neurological sensitivity.
- Aching or stiffness that limits range of motion.
- Inflammation, heat, or redness, indicates acute swelling.
- Upper extremity neurological pain, paresthesia, or numbness, indicates nerve root or brachial plexus peripheral nerve damage.
- Sharp pain in tissues close to the spine, implicates facet joints, capsules, vertebral fractures, or ligament sprain.
- Dizziness, vertigo, or disorientation, indicates vascular disorders or cranial trauma (concussion).
- Problems with temporomandibular joint (TMJ) including bite problems or pain in muscles of mastication.
- Nausea resulting from vascular or neurological disorders.
- Mild to severe headache from injury to numerous structures.
- Breathing difficulties from damage to the phrenic nerve.

Palpation

- Local pain produced with pressure on muscles indicating muscular involvement.
- Hypertonicity of cervical muscles.
- Hyperesthesia, indicates increased central nervous system activity.
- Referred pain indicating trigger points.
- Palpable defect or disruption in continuity in muscle tissue indicating strain.
- Sharp, shooting, electrical-type pain or paresthesia implicating neurological structures.
- Palpable edema or heat from inflammatory activity.
- Misalignment of bony landmarks evidencing possible vertebral dislocations.
- Adhesions or scar tissue from chronic strain injury.

History

WAD clients generally report a head or neck trauma prior to the onset of symptoms. The symptoms may have appeared immediately or several weeks or even months later. Pain complaints are localized to the cervical region, but can radiate through the thoracic and lumbar regions or distally in upper extremities. The quality of the pain or symptoms varies based on the tissues involved. Some of the symptoms from whiplash injury are listed in Box 9.4. Ask about previous WAD injuries in the client's history.

Observation

WAD clients exhibit obvious movement limitations or postural alterations because of pain or physical inability. Limitations may be apparent in general movement, before they are evident in range-of-motion, resistance, or special tests. The client is also apt to show apprehension when attempting to perform various movements.

The client might be wearing a cervical collar, although these are primarily used only in severe cases. Signs of head or face trauma may also exist if the trauma is serious. While inflammatory activity is rarely visible, the practitioner may be able to palpate heat or swelling. In severe cases, redness due to inflammation is visible. If there is trauma to highly vascularized tissues, bruising may be evident. Bruising is usually purplish in the early stages of injury, changing to brown or greenish as time progresses.

Palpation

Tissues of the neck are expected to be tender and should be palpated with care and sensitivity. A list of possible findings during palpation with a WAD are included in Box 9.4. In many cases it is difficult or impossible to palpate the primary tissues injured. The longus colli is difficult to palpate safely and adverse pressure can be applied to other structures, such as the baroreceptors in the carotid sinus. It is not possible to palpate the alar ligaments because they are deep within the spinal canal. If the main injury is in one of these structures, the practitioner may not be able to reproduce the primary pain with palpation.

Range-of-Motion and Resistance Testing

Note that because WAD has a broad array of possible pathologies, it is important to apply biomechanical analysis to evaluate the nature of the problem. Evaluate motions most likely to produce pain at the end of the testing. Tests are performed with the client in a sitting position, unless noted otherwise.

AROM: Restrictions to active motion result from muscle spasm, pain avoidance, or a physical inability such as a vertebral displacement or facet joint dysfunction. Pain or restriction in extension may be due to stretching of the anterior longitudinal ligament, the anterior aspect of the annulus fibrosus, the anterior neck viscera, or stretching and eccentric contraction of the anterior cervical muscles.

Compression of the facet joints is apt to create pain. Compression of the posterior portion of the intervertebral discs or nerve roots may cause pain, paresthesia, burning, or numbness.

Pain or restriction in flexion may be due to stretching of the damaged facet joint capsules, the interspinous or posterior longitudinal ligaments, the ligamentum nuchae, or stretching and eccentric contraction of the posterior cervical muscles. Pain could also result from compression of the intervertebral discs or uncovertebral joints. For further information, active flexion may be evaluated in the supine position. If active flexion produces pain from the supine and not the sitting position, the anterior neck flexors may be involved.

Pain or restriction in lateral flexion may result from stretching the following tissues on the opposite side: nerves and nerve roots of the brachial plexus, facet joint capsules, intertransverse ligaments, and lateral flexor muscles. On the side of lateral flexion, there may be pain or restriction due to compressive stress on the cervical facet joints, nerve roots, laminae, intervertebral discs, uncovertebral joints, or concentric contraction of ipsilateral neck lateral flexors. Paresthesia, burning sensations, or numbness in the neck could result from compression or stretching of the nerves or nerve roots on either side.

Pain or restriction in rotation may occur from stretching the alar ligaments, facet joint capsules, or the rotators of the craniocervical region. Compression of the facet joints may elicit pain. The above motions may also produce vascular compression, including symptoms of: dizziness, vertigo, disorientation, ringing in the ears, blurred vision, or other sensory impairment caused by lack of blood flow to the brain.

PROM: The principles of evaluation during active movement listed above apply to passive movement as well. One exception involves pain that is generated during contraction of injured muscles. Passive movement does not require muscle contraction, thus pain from active muscle contraction would not be present here. For example, if the longus colli muscle were strained it would likely be painful in active flexion against resistance (i.e. gravity), but not in passive flexion. Pain would be felt in extension as the muscle is stretched.

MRT: Due to reactive muscle spasm, neck muscles may be painful with an MRT because of developed hypertonicity. Further evaluation will identify involved tissues. Myofascial trigger points may cause pain during an MRT of the cervical muscles. In a severe injury, pain could result from the muscles pulling on a damaged vertebrae and irritating either a fracture site or the facet joint.

Muscle weakness is a common result of muscle damage, joint dysfunction, or nerve compression or tension. Weakness may also be due to reflex muscular inhibition. Weakness with the MRT does not necessarily indicate muscle damage because there could be a neurological cause. See Table 2 for the muscles likely to be painful with resisted motions.

Differential Evaluation

Due to the potential tissue pathologies in whiplash, differential evaluation should consider all possible causes of tissue damage including muscle strain, ligament sprain, nerve compression or tension, cranial injury, vertebral subluxation or fracture, disc, pathology, or facet joint damage.

Suggestions for Treatment

Treatment options are highly varied because of the complexity of WAD. An effective treatment follows from accurate assessment. Once the primary tissue and injury are identified, treatment may progress that is consistent for that condition. Sprain, strain, disc pathology, and hypertonicity are dealt with in other sections of this chapter and chapter 4. Refer to these sections for discussion on preferred treatment options.

Generally with WAD, practitioners should proceed with gentle, myofascial approaches first. As the client is able to tolerate greater pressure levels, muscular dysfunction may be addressed with deeper techniques.[27] Caution is advised as there may be no immediate pain intolerance and excessive post-treatment soreness could result. Due to the potential damage of delicate structures in this area, referral to a physician for additional evaluation is strongly encouraged.

TORTICOLLIS

Torticollis literally means twisted neck. A person with torticollis exhibits **involuntary muscle contractions that lead to abnormal positions and/or tremors** or spasmodic movements of the neck and head.[28]

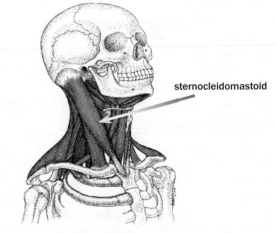

sternocleidomastoid

Figure 9.20 The sternocleidomastoid is the primary muscle affected in torticollis. (Mediclip image copyright, 1998 Williams & Wilkins. All rights reserved.)

Characteristics

Torticollis has several variations: congenital, acute or acquired, and spasmodic. *Congenital torticollis* presents in infants, occurring at birth or shortly after. The condition develops from a number of possible causes, such as malpositioning in the uterus or birthing trauma. Usually the **sternocleidomastoid** (SCM) muscle is affected, showing signs of shortening and sometimes fibrosis, scarring, or a palpable mass (Figure 9.20). Other causes of infant torticollis in addition to muscular dysfunction include *vertebral subluxation, scoliosis*, and *spinal cord abnormalities*. If the condition is primarily muscular, soft-tissue treatment within the first year generally resolves the problem. If left untreated, the condition is likely to become a permanent deformity and continue into adulthood.

The most common forms of torticollis are **acute** or **acquired** (sometimes called *wry neck*). These muscular conditions primarily involve the **SCM, trapezius, levator scapulae, splenius capitis, splenius cervicis**, or **scalenes** and appear in a broad spectrum of the population from children to adults. Acquired torticollis is caused by maintaining muscles in shortened positions for prolonged periods. Myofascial trigger points sometimes lead to the condition or may perpetuate it.[29] Awkward positions held for prolonged periods, such as poor sleeping postures, playing the violin, or holding a telephone between the head and shoulder can contribute to the condition. Acquired conditions develop initially with pain or slight spasm, then progress to more serious pain and symptoms.

An acute form might manifest from a head or neck injury such as *WAD* or *concussion*, and symptoms can appear immediately or be delayed. The condition sometimes has a structural component, for example if there was subluxation from impact. In children up to the age of ten, inflammation from *tonsillitis* or an *ear infection* can cause these symptoms. In older children and adults it is primarily a biomechanical problem.[30]

Spasmodic torticollis is the third type and there are several variations. This condition is also called *cervical dystonia* because it is a focal dystonia centralized in the cervical spine.[30, 31] Dystonia is a movement disorder characterized by involuntary muscle contractions that force the body into abnormal movements or postures. Current research suggests that this neurological condition may result from dysfunction in the **basal ganglia**, structures that assist in movement control deep in the brain [30].

Cervical dystonia was once thought to be psychological; thankfully those days appear to be over. The condition is considered *idiopathic* as its causes are uncertain. In some cases, trauma, such as to the head, is an initiating factor. It may be years before the condition appears. The condition can be entirely muscular or secondary to an underlying pathology, such as *neurological dysfunction* or infection. In other cases, it may be related to a family history of tremors, a reaction to a prescription medication, an eye condition, or a result of infection.[32] The condition

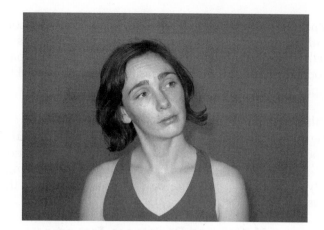

Figure 9.21 Characteristic postural distortion in torticollis.

may also be paired with other types of dystonia.

In some people there is a degree of neurological inhibition that is evident whereby touching the chin, face, or neck on the opposite side may decrease or alleviate the muscle spasm temporarily. Symptoms worsen with stress and can dissipate or disappear with sleep, only to recur several hours after waking. Significant pain can arise from muscle spasm and nerve impingement with any of the forms of torticollis. Torticollis can be confused with *epilepsy, muscular dystrophy*, or *Parkinson's disease*. Adults between the ages of thirty to fifty are most affected.

History

The practitioner should distinguish between the variations of torticollis based on information in the history. Pain may or may not be involved. Pain is similar among the varieties, although longevity varies. Congenital torticollis presents in infancy and is not necessarily painful. An adult who claims to have been born with the condition is assumed to have the congenital form. If a client asks for assistance in treating an infant with an apparent torticollis, it should be confirmed they have seen a physician for a diagnosis.

Clients with acute torticollis may have a history of traumatic injury, such as a car accident, but the condition could appear overnight. Spasmodic torticollis generally emerges gradually and becomes evident with difficulty in holding the head in a neutral position. Ask the client when he/she first became aware of the problem; family members might be the first to notice the condition. Ask the client about what time of day symptoms are worse.

Observation

The perpetual muscle spasms of torticollis frequently keep the client's head in a non-neutral position. Ordinarily, the head is laterally flexed toward the affected side, with the chin rotated to the opposite direction (Figure 9.21). In some cases the head may be held in forward flexion, hyperextension, or lateral flexion. Those with the congenital variation may have other postural distortions as well. Muscle spasm may be visible in the SCM. In spasmodic torticollis, tremors or spastic movements could be apparent.

Palpation

The muscles of the cervical region generally feel tight and produce pain. In some cases, especially if the condition has progressed for some time, a degree of fibrotic change may develop and there are palpable contractures in the muscles.

Range-of-Motion and Resistance Testing

AROM: Active motion is likely to be painful and limited. Motion is most limited in the direction opposite the contracted muscles. For example, if the individual has a spasm holding the head in a position of rotation to the left, active rotation to the right is limited. Pain and restriction are expected with further rotation to the affected side.

PROM: As with active motion, pain and movement limitation occur in the direction opposite that of the muscle contraction. A muscle spasm end feel presents when motion is attempted in this direction. Passive motion in the same direction as the contracted muscles may or may not produce pain or restriction.

MRT: Pain can develop with any MRT using the muscles of the neck and is likely felt when the primary actions of the affected muscles are engaged. There may also be weakness during manual resistance that is due to the muscle's chronic shortened state and the functional strength loss that ensues.

Differential Evaluation

Cerebral palsy, multiple sclerosis, muscle spasm, myofascial pain syndrome, myasthenia gravis, Parkinson's disease.

Suggestions for Treatment

Massage is helpful for managing torticollis, although the techniques used vary for the different types. For congenital torticollis, gentle massage and soft-tissue stretching techniques are helpful in relieving spasms. Acute/acquired torticollis is best treated with gentle and indirect methods such as muscle energy technique and positional release. These methods are preferred as direct pressure may be too intense for the client. As treatment progresses, other soft-tissue techniques such as effleurage, longitudinal stripping, stretching, and trigger point therapy can be employed within the client's tolerance level.

It is unclear what role massage plays in treating spasmodic torticollis. General relaxation massage may help by decreasing excessive activity in the central nervous system. Caution is advised because direct massage of the involved muscles could aggravate the problem in spasmodic torticollis and may not be beneficial (Rattray & Ludwig, 2000). Physical and occupational therapy are

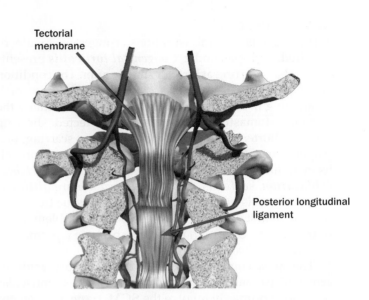

Figure 9.22 Anterior view of the deep suboccipital region with bodies of the vertebrae cut and removed. (3-D anatomy image courtesy of Primal Pictures Ltd. www.primalpictures.com.)

frequently used when the condition is in its early stages, with some forms of manual therapy appearing helpful. Oral medications and botulinum toxin (Botox) injections are used to halt chronic muscle spasm. Consult a physician to develop an appropriate coordinated treatment plan.

HERNIATED NUCLEUS PULPOSUS

The *herniated nucleus pulposus (HNP)* is often referred to as a *herniated disc*. The lay term for the condition is a *slipped disc* and is a misnomer. HNP can produce pain or neurological problems in the neck or upper extremities.

Characteristics

See herniated nucleus pulposus in Chapter 8 for a discussion of the anatomy and function of the *intervertebral disc*. Chapter 8 also explains the biomechanics and injury degrees in HNP.[34] Assessing the degree of herniation requires a diagnostic evaluation, such as an MRI; physical examination is not sufficient, although symptoms are identified during the process. Cervical disc herniations are relatively common and frequently appear in asymptomatic individuals; presence of a herniated disc does not necessarily imply a pathological problem.[35]

HNP usually occurs in a posterior-lateral direction. Due to the greater compressive load in the **lower cervical spine**, disc protrusions are more typical in that region. In addition the C6-7 **intervertebral foramina** are the smallest in the cervical region, creating less space for the nerve roots and increasing the chances of compression.[36] As the disc protrudes, it may press on nearby nerve roots. The nerve roots in the lower cervical spine feed the **brachial plexus**, and nerve compression symptoms can be felt down the upper extremity.

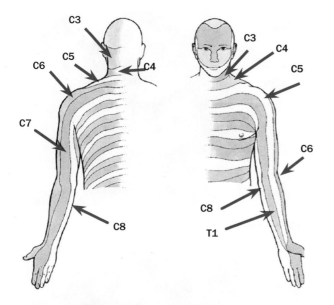

Figure 9.23 Dermatomes for cervical nerve roots. (Mediclip image copyright, 1998 Williams & Wilkins. All rights reserved.)

The **posterior longitudinal ligament** runs the length of the spinal canal and is directly posterior to the disc. In the upper region of the cervical spine this ligament is called the **tectorial membrane** (Figure 9.22). This structure generally prevents a straight protrusion of the disc. In cases where a straight posterior protrusion does happen, it can lead to upper *motor neuron lesions* or *quadriplegia*.[37] These disorders develop because the disc presses through the restraining ligament and directly on the dura mater and spinal cord, affecting innervation of structures not only in the upper extremity, but also below the level of the compression.

Certain positions of the neck increase the compressive load on the intervertebral discs and can contribute to either acute or *chronic herniations. Cervical lordosis* is lost with approximately 30⁰ of flexion, increasing pressure on the disc and vertebral structures.[38] This position is seen in *forward head posture* and other postural distortions. For every inch that the head moves forward from its normal posture, the compressive load on the lower neck is increased by the additional weight of the entire head.[2] Consequently, cervical disc herniations could result from long periods in a distorted posture.

In some cases the disc herniation is an acute injury with a sudden load placed upon the cervical spine. For example, herniations can result when an individual dives into a swimming pool and hits the head on the bottom. With the neck in partial flexion during the dive, the compressive load on the cervical spine is increased causing disc herniation.

The primary symptoms from HNP include pain, paresthesia, or weakness in the neck or upper extremities. Pain or paresthesia can skip areas throughout a dermatome or area of cutaneous innervation.[39] For example, pain or paresthesia from a cervical disc herniation could

be felt in the forearm and hand, but not in the upper arm. The location of symptoms felt from nerve root compression varies depending on the level of the protrusion in the cervical spine. Disc herniations are most common in the lower cervical spine and therefore incite symptoms affecting lower nerve roots of the brachial plexus. Pressure on a nerve root produces neurological symptoms in the dermatome associated with that nerve root (Figure 9.23). Motor weakness in the muscles supplied by fibers from these nerve roots may be apparent.

Pain is caused by pressure against the posterior longitudinal ligament, dura mater, or nerve roots. However, studies indicate that some people with herniated discs may not have associated pain.[35] Presence of a herniated disc does not determine disc protrusion as the source of pain. Evaluation of neck pain should be thorough in order to distinguish between the possible causes of pain.

History

The client with an HNP may complain of paresthesia, numbness, or sharp, electrical-type neck or upper extremity pain. Unilateral symptoms are more characteristic because the disc is more likely to protrude to one side. Symptoms can be bilateral and indicate a more serious problem due to a central protrusion on the spinal cord or protrusions on the nerve roots of both sides.

Certain positions or movements may aggravate or relieve symptoms. Clients with nerve compression frequently describe symptoms that are worse from sitting in poor postures or positions that cause increased neck flexion. Symptoms may dissipate as the individual moves around as long as the neck is not in a compromised position. Bed rest normally decreases pain because the compressive loads on the spine are reduced.

Observation

There are no distinct visual signs of an HNP. There may be visible postural distortions, such as the forward head posture. Apprehension about moving in certain directions could be apparent if the movements cause pain. In more severe cases, muscle atrophy may be visible in muscles innervated by the affected nerve root level.

Palpation

Tenderness and hypertonicity are usual in cervical muscles, but the pain is different from that felt from nerve compression. The transverse processes of the spine prevent the practitioner from pressing directly on the disc protrusion. Significant pressure or particular movements applied to the neck may contribute to the pressure on the affected nerve root and increase the client's symptoms.

Range-of-Motion and Resistance Testing

AROM: Pain or other neurological symptoms may be aggravated with active motion in any of the planes of movement because nerve roots are stretched against a protruding disc. Nerve root compression might develop due to narrowing of the intervertebral foramen during lateral flexion to the same side. Symptoms can also be aggravated from either flexion or hyperextension depending on the location of the disc protrusion. The location of nerve compression is not directly evident from motion that produces neurological symptoms.

An additional evaluation can be performed by abducting the shoulder as far as possible on the affected side, either actively or passively. Because this motion reduces tensile loads on the affected nerve root, the symptoms may decrease at the end of the movement. If the client has tightness in the pectoralis minor muscle or *pectoralis minor syndrome*, this movement can aggravate symptoms (this is the same position used in the Wright abduction test, see thoracic outlet syndrome).

PROM: Principles are the same as for active movement.

MRT: No significant pain or discomfort is likely with MRTs. In rare cases neurological pain is exacerbated during an MRT due to compensatory patterns that affect the involved vertebral segment. Muscles innervated by fibers from the affected nerve root may appear weak. Note that in many cases weakness is evident in the upper extremity muscles and not in those in the cervical region. See Table 2 at the end of the chapter for resisted muscle actions and assistance with which nerves and/or nerve roots might be affected.

Special Tests
Spurling Test
The client is seated on the treatment table with the head slightly laterally flexed to the affected side (Figure 9.24). The practitioner applies gentle pressure on the client's head in a straight downward (toward the floor) direction. If symptoms are aggravated on the affected side, it is a positive test for neural compression.

The Spurling test may be carried out in progressive stages with increased downward compression applied in each stage. The stages of increased pressure place a greater degree of potential compression on the nerve roots. If symptoms are aggravated during one of these stages it is not necessary to proceed to the others.

    Test Movement Stages
1. Compression with the head in a neutral position.
2. Compression with the head in partial extension and rotation to the affected side.
3. Compression with the head in lateral flexion to the affected side (as described above).

Explanation: Putting the head in the test position decreases the space near the intervertebral disc and the nerve root exiting the spine. When an axial load is applied, pressure is increased on the cervical vertebrae and discs causing them to protrude against adjacent structures. The stages help identify a disc protrusion's severity. If the protrusion is significant, symptoms are felt during compression with the head in neutral. If the protrusion is not

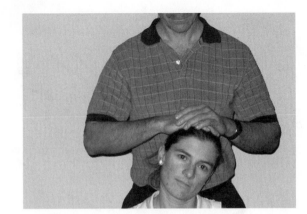

Figure 9.24 **Spurling test.**

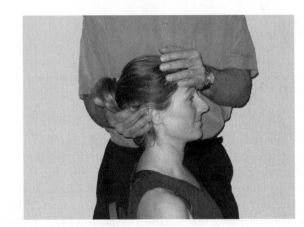

Figure 9.25 **Cervical distraction test.**

significant, symptoms may not be felt until compression is performed with the head in lateral flexion. The location of the protrusion may alter these results, so variations should be considered guidelines, not strict rules.

Cervical Distraction Test
The client is seated on the treatment table with the head in a neutral position. The practitioner's hands are placed in a position where a distraction force can be applied to the head and neck (Figure 9.25). Hands are placed on the occiput and underneath the chin or in other positions, such as behind the occiput and on the forehead. The hands can also be placed on each side of the head. The hands should not cover the client's ears, eyes, or face. If a hand is placed underneath the chin, make sure pressure is not applied to the throat or neck. Once hands are in position, apply a moderate distraction (lifting) force to the head and neck. If the radiating neurological symptoms are relieved, it indicates a problem involving pressure on the nerve roots.

Explanation: When a distraction force is applied to the neck, pressure is taken off the vertebral structures and the disc may no longer press against the affected nerve roots so there is a decrease in symptoms. Symptoms generally return once the force is removed and pressure returns to the area.

Slump test

See the description of the slump test in herniated nucleus pulposus, Chapter 8. The slump test is used to identify cervical disc pathology as well as lumbar pathologies. The primary goal is to determine where the symptoms are felt in the slump position. If they are felt in the upper extremity, then cervical nerve root involvement should be considered.

Differential Evaluation

Osteophytes, spinal tumors, spinal stenosis, cervical facet syndrome, arthritis, peripheral entrapment neuropathies, systemic neuropathies, cervical ligament sprain, cervical muscle strain.

Suggestions for Treatment

Numerous treatment strategies are advocated for treating cervical HNP. Treatments depend on the degree of herniation, which cannot be determined by physical examination alone. Where surgery was once considered almost essential for this condition, it is not as recommended now. Research shows that disc herniation problems can heal spontaneously without surgery or other invasive procedures.[40] Some rehabilitative exercises are suggested to encourage the disc to return to a normal position and away from affected nerve roots.[41] It is important to consult with a physician or other health professional for recommendations on treatment.

While massage is not absolutely contraindicated for disc herniations, treatment methods should be used cautiously. The transverse processes protect the nerve roots from further compression during most massage techniques, but symptoms could be aggravated by minor vertebral movements that result from pressure applied to the region. Massage is helpful to decrease muscle tension in the area and may reduce compressive loading on the disc. Massage should be performed carefully.

SPINAL LIGAMENT SPRAIN

Cervical muscles are smaller than other muscles and therefore less able to restrain movement or momentum of the head and neck. To compensate, there are numerous ligaments in the spine that limit movement between adjacent spinal segments. An overwhelming amount of force in a particular direction can damage these structures, causing a *spinal ligament sprain*. Forceful motions of the head and neck, such as occur in *whiplash*, are a frequent cause.

Characteristics

Ligaments are dense connective tissue structures composed of **elastin** and **collagen**. Elastin provides ligaments some degree of pliability, while collagen gives them tensile strength. Ligaments are designed to withstand tensile loads along the direction that their fibers run.[12] Because of the amount of elastin in cervical ligaments and their

BOX 9.5 CERVICAL LIGAMENTS & THEIR RESISTED ACTIONS	
Ligament	**Resisted Action**
Alar ligaments	Contralateral rotation
Anterior longitudinal ligament	Extension
Intertransverse ligaments	Lateral flexion
Ligamentum flavum	Flexion
Ligamentum nuchae	Flexion
Posterior longitudinal ligament	Flexion
Transverse ligament	Forward translation of the atlas

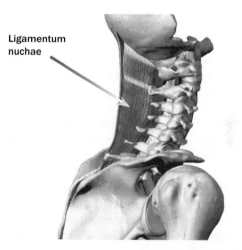

Ligamentum nuchae

Figure 9.26 Lateral view of the ligamentum nuchae. (3-D anatomy image courtesy of Primal Pictures Ltd. www.primalpictures.com.)

ability to elongate and recoil, researchers question how much force is necessary to cause a *sprain* to these ligaments. Spinal ligament sprains may not be as common as once thought, but remain a potential source of pain particularly with sudden force overload to the spine.

Ligaments throughout the spine have different anatomical characteristics depending on their location and primary function. Box 9.5 lists the primary ligaments in the cervical spine and the motions they are designed to resist. The **ligamentum nuchae** not only limits cervical flexion, but also provides a large surface area for cervical muscle attachments (Figure 9.26). It is located superficial to the spinous processes of the cervical vertebrae. The **supraspinous** and **interspinous ligaments** in the lumbar and thoracic region blend into the ligamentum nuchae in the cervical region. Also preventing excessive flexion of the spine is the **posterior longitudinal ligament**, located in the spinal canal on the posterior aspect of the vertebral bodies. The portion behind the top two cervical vertebrae is known as the **tectorial membrane** (Figure 9.22).

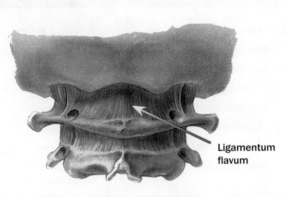

Figure 9.27 Posterior view of the suboccipital region showing the ligamentum flavum. (Mediclip image copyright, 1998 Williams & Wilkins. All rights reserved.)

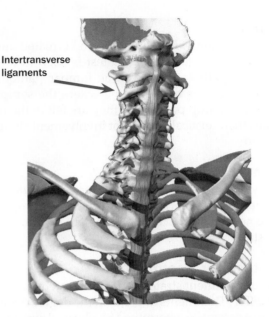

Figure 9.28 Anterior view of the intertransverse ligaments. (3-D anatomy image courtesy of Primal Pictures Ltd. www.primalpictures.com.)

The **ligamentum flavum** is located on the posterior aspect of the vertebral canal and is designed to hold the laminae of adjacent vertebrae together, elongating with flexion and shortening during extension (Figure 9.27). Its primary function is to prevent excessive flexion in the spine. This ligament has a high degree of elastin, making it capable of stretching and retracting without buckling and pressing on the dura mater or spinal cord. Its high degree of flexibility prevents it from being sprained as often as other spinal ligaments. On the anterior bodies of the vertebrae is the **anterior longitudinal ligament** that functions to prevent excessive extension of the spine (Figure 9.18).

The **alar ligaments** are located on each side of the dens on the axis and extend from the top of the dens to the occipital condyles. Their primary function is to prevent excessive contralateral rotation of the atlas and cranium (e.g. the left alar ligament limits rotation to the right) (Figure 9.19). The **transverse ligament** runs posterior to the dens and attaches to the inside of the vertebral arch of the atlas and functions to prevent forward translation of the atlas on the axis, which can severely damage the spinal cord and is often fatal (Figure 9.19). Between the transverse processes of adjacent vertebrae are the **intertransverse ligaments** which prevent lateral flexion to the opposite side (Figure 9.28).

An overwhelming sudden tensile load is the cause of a ligament sprain. Ligaments can be weakened by prolonged stress, making the ligament susceptible to injury from smaller loads. When evaluating an injury to the spine, determine whether the force of the injury could have caused tensile stress on particular spinal ligaments. For example, a sudden and forceful lateral flexion of the head and neck to the right could cause a sprain to the left intertransverse ligaments.

Cervical ligament sprains are more prevalent in people with systemic disorders such as *Ehlers-Danlos* or *Marfan syndromes*, because these conditions involve connective tissue weakness.[34] Women in the later stages of pregnancy experience a greater number of spinal ligament sprains due to increased ligamentous laxity resulting from elevated levels of the hormone relaxin. Forceful motions such as those that take place in *WAD* can cause cervical ligament sprains. Sprains are prone to reappear in areas where they have occurred previously. Joint hypermobility is often a precursor to sprain, so if there is hypermobility due to ligamentous laxity a sprain is more likely.

Identifying specific ligament sprains through physical examination is difficult due to the depth of the spinal ligaments and the abundance of soft tissues around the spine. A high-tech diagnostic procedure such as MRI is usually required although familiarity with characteristics of ligament sprains helps in the identification process.

Chapter 2 includes a comprehensive discussion of the physiology of ligament sprains as they pertain to all regions of the body. Chapter 4 contains details about assessing sprains including the history, observation, palpation, range-of-motion, and resistance testing of ligaments in any region of the body. The discussion in the section below is limited to specifics about cervical spinal ligaments, but the reader is encouraged to read these other sections for a more thorough understanding of the pathology and assessment of ligament sprains.

History

The client describes a sudden force load to the head or neck. Pain is likely felt close to the spine and is aggravated by movements that pull on the damaged fibers. The client may or may not remember the mechanics of the injury. Ask about previous sprains, injuries, accidents, or systemic disorders that cause laxity in the connective tissues.

Observation

There are rarely visual clues of a spinal ligament sprain. Inflammatory reactions in the sprained ligament are not visible due to the depth of the ligaments. If a sprain is severe, there may be associated vertebral dislocation which may be visually apparent and the spinous processes will appear misaligned. Misalignment needs to be investigated with high-tech diagnostic studies and cannot be confirmed by visual observation alone. Muscle spasm that results from the sprain may cause mobility and range-of-motion loss, which would be apparent during ROM evaluations.

Palpation

Spinal ligaments are difficult to palpate and some, such as the alar ligaments, are not palpable. The interspinous ligaments and the ligamentum nuchae are more superficial and palpation of these ligaments is apt to produce pain. There may be hypertonicity and tenderness in local muscles, due to reflex muscle splinting. Edema might be felt if the sprain is in a superficial ligament.

Range-of-Motion and Resistance Testing

AROM: Active motions increase pain when the motion is in the direction the ligament is designed to resist (Box 9.5). For example, active lateral flexion to the left is apt to create pain with a sprain to the right intertransverse ligaments. Motions that shorten or do not stress the damaged ligament either decrease pain or have no affect.
PROM: The same principles apply as for active motion.
MRT: There are no specific findings with most MRTs. However, there are fascial connections between the supraspinous ligaments and the parallel fibers of the erector spinae muscles. If the supraspinous ligaments are injured some pain may occur when these muscles are contracted during resisted spinal extension movements.

Differential Evaluation

Osteophytes, spinal tumors, spinal stenosis, cervical facet syndrome, cervical radiculopathy, muscle strain, myofascial trigger point pain, arthritis, peripheral entrapment neuropathies, systemic neuropathies.

Suggestions for Treatment

Deep friction massage is advocated for ligament sprains because it stimulates collagen production in the damaged tissues. The difficulty in accessing spinal ligaments makes this treatment approach questionable, except for the ligamentum nuchae. Rest from offending activities or stressful motion of the spine is necessary. In the majority of cases the ligaments heal without intervention.

Massage is effective in addressing corresponding muscle spasm and pain resulting from the injury. Overly aggressive stretching may irritate torn ligament fibers. In some cases muscle tightness may be protecting the region against excess movement during the healing process and initial stages of injury.

General Neuromuscular Disorders

In many cases, soft-tissue dysfunctions are not given a specific name. Adequate assessment is required to determine the tissues most likely involved and to take into account pathologies that may or may not have specific titles. Chapter 4 provides a discussion of the pathological processes of hypertonicity, myofascial trigger points, muscle strains, nerve compression and tension, tendinosis, tenosynovitis, ligament sprains, and osteoarthritis in any region of the body. Chapter 4 also includes the history, observation, palpation, relevant tests, and treatment suggestions sections for these conditions. The principles are the same for these conditions wherever they occur in the body.

Included in this section are specific tables and graphics for the cervical spine, including dermatomes, cutaneous innervation, trigger point referral patterns, and findings for MRTs. Tenosynovitis is not an issue in the cervical region as there are no tendons surrounded by a synovial sheath in this area. Tendinosis is also rare in the neck due to the structure and function of the muscles and tendons. Nerve compression and tension pathologies affect nerve roots and not peripheral nerves in the cervical spine.

Muscular hypertonicity and myofascial trigger points are one of the most common causes of neck pain. Muscular sources of neck pain can be overlooked in favor of joint disorders or other structural problems that are more easily identifiable with diagnostic testing procedures.[42, 43] A comprehensive approach to neck pain must consider pain that originates from muscular dysfunction.[29, 44] Muscular hypertonicity and myofascial trigger points develop in the neck especially as a result of postural stress. Myofascial trigger points can refer pain or characteristic neurological symptoms to the neck, shoulders, or upper extremity. Myofascial trigger point referral patterns for the major muscles in this region are shown in Figures 9.29 and 9.30.

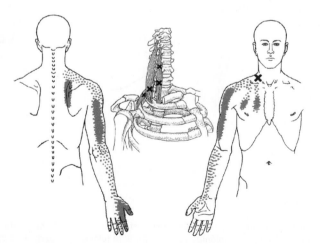

Figure 9.29 Myofascial trigger point referral pattern for the scalene muscles. (Mediclip image copyright, 1998 Williams & Wilkins. All rights reserved.)

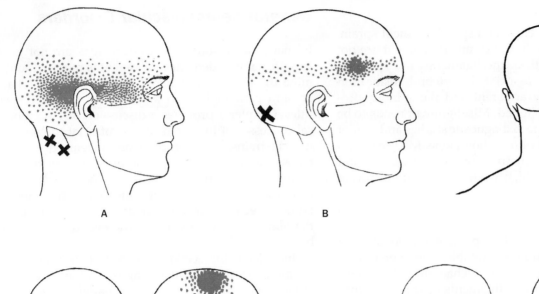

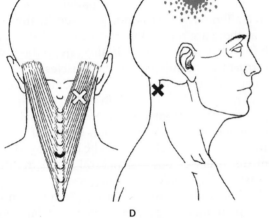

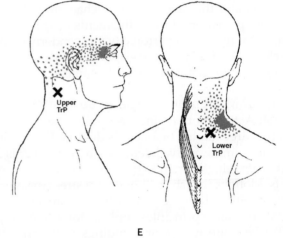

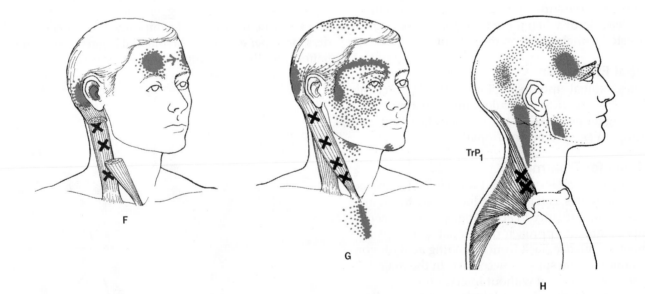

Figure 9.30 Myofascial trigger point referral patterns: Suboccipital muscles (A) Semispinalis-upper (B), Semispinalis-middle (C), Splenius capitis (D), Splenius cervicis (E), SCM (clavicular head) (F), SCM (sternal head) (G), Upper trapezius (H). (Images courtesy of Mediclip, copyright 1998 Williams & Wilkins. All rights reserved.)

TABLE 1 Joints, Associated Motions, Planes of Motion in Anatomical Position, Axis of Rotation, and Average ROM

Neck	Motion	Plane of Motion	Axis of Rotation	Avg. ROM (degrees)
	Flexion	Sagittal	Medial-lateral	45-50
	Extension	Sagittal	Medial-lateral	75-85
	Lateral flexion	Frontal	Anterior-posterior	40-45
	Rotation	Transverse	Superior-inferior	90

TABLE 2 Weakness with Manual Resistive Test and Possible Nerve Involvement

Muscle	Resisted Action	Possible Nerve Involvement if Action Weak
Iliocostalis cervicis	Extension	C4-T3
Interspinales cervicis	Extension	C3-C8
Intertransversarii cervicis	Lateral Flexion	C3-C8
Longissimus capitis	Extension	greater occipital (C3-C8)
Longissimus cervicis	Extension	C3-T3
Longus capitis	Flexion	C1-C3
Longus colli	Flexion	C2-C6
Obliquus capitis inferior	Rotation (Ipsilateral)	suboccipital (C1)
Obliquus capitis superior	Extension	suboccipital (C1)
Rectus capitis anterior	Flexion	C1-C2
Rectus capitis lateralis	Lateral Flexion	C1-C2
Rectus capitis posterior major	Extension	suboccipital (C1)
Rectus capitis posterior minor	Extension	suboccipital (C1)
Rotatores cervicis	Rotation (Contralateral)	C3-C8
Scalenus anterior	Flexion	C4-C6
Scalenus medius	Lateral Flexion	C3-C8
Scalenus posterior	Lateral Flexion	C6-C8
Semispinalis capitis	Extension	C2-T1
Semispinalis cervicis	Extension	C2-T5
Spinalis capitis	Extension	C3-T1
Spinalis cervicis	Extension	C4-C8
Splenius capitis	Extension	C3-C6
Splenius cervicis	Extension	C4-C8
Sternocleidomastoid	Rotation (Contralateral)	Accessory (XI), C2-C3
Trapezius (upper fibers)	Extension	Accessory (XI), C3-C4

Reference Table for Condition Assessment

This table lists a number of pathological conditions along the left-hand column. The top of the table lists common evaluation procedures. A ◆ in the box associated with a pathological condition and an evaluation procedure indicates that the procedure is commonly used to identify that pathology. A ● in the box associated with the condition and a range-of-motion or resistance test, indicates pain is likely with that test for that pathology. Conditions are listed alphabetically.

TABLE 3   REFERENCE TABLE FOR CONDITION ASSESSMENT

	AROM	PROM	MRT	Adson's maneuver	Allen test	Cervical distraction test	Military brace test	Slump test	Spurling test	Wright's abduction test
Cervical Facet Syndrome	●	●								
Herniated Nucleus Pulposus	●	●				◆		◆	◆	
Muscle Strains	●	●	●							
Muscular Hypertonicity	●	●								
Spinal Ligament Sprain	●	●								
Thoracic Outlet Syndrome	●	●		◆	◆		◆	◆		◆
Torticollis	●	●	●							
Whiplash	●	●	●			◆				

References

1. Berryman Reese N, Bandy WD. *Joint Range of Motion and Muscle Length Testing*. Philadelphia: W.B. Saunders Co.; 2002.
2. Liebenson Ce. *Rehabilitation of the Spine*. Baltimore: Williams & Wilkins; 1996.
3. Chaitow L, DeLany J. *Clinical Application of Neuromuscular Techniques*. Vol 1. Edinburgh: Churchill Livingstone; 2000.
4. Sheth RN, Belzberg AJ. Diagnosis and treatment of thoracic outlet syndrome. *Neurosurg Clin N Am*. Apr 2001;12(2):295-309.
5. Dawson D, Hallett M, Wilbourn A. *Entrapment Neuropathies*. 3rd ed. Philadelphia: Lippincott-Raven; 1999.
6. Kalra A, Thornburg M. Thoracic Outlet Syndrome. *eMedicine*. May 31, 2002. Available at: www.emedicine.com. Accessed January 17, 2005.
7. Chang AK, Bohan JS. Thoracic Outlet Syndrome. *eMedicine*. February 7, 2005. Available at: www.emedicine.com. Accessed April 20, 2005.
8. Alexandre A, Coro L, Azuelos A, Pellone M. Thoracic outlet syndrome due to hyperextension-hyperflexion cervical injury. *Acta Neurochir Suppl*. 2005;92:21-24.
9. Windsor RE. Cervical Facet Syndrome. *eMedicine*. 6-24-2005. Available at: www.emedicine.com. Accessed January 23, 2006.
10. Pearson AM, Ivancic PC, Ito S, Panjabi MM. Facet joint kinematics and injury mechanisms during simulated whiplash. *Spine*. Feb 15 2004;29(4):390-397.
11. Stemper BD, Yoganandan N, Gennarelli TA, Pintar FA. Localized cervical facet joint kinematics under physiological and whiplash loading. *J Neurosurg Spine*. Dec 2005;3(6):471-476.
12. White A, Panjabi M. *Clinical Biomechanics of the Spine*. 2nd ed. Philadelphia: Lippincott Williams & Wilkins; 1990.
13. Bogduk N, Aprill C. On the nature of neck pain, discography and cervical zygapophysial joint blocks. *Pain*. Aug 1993;54(2):213-217.
14. Kim KH, Choi SH, Kim TK, Shin SW, Kim CH, Kim JI. Cervical facet joint injections in the neck and shoulder pain. *J Korean Med Sci*. Aug 2005;20(4):659-662.
15. Palmieri F, Cassar-Pullicino VN, Dell'atti C, et al. Uncovertebral joint injury in cervical facet dislocation: the headphones sign. *Eur Radiol*. Dec 6 2005:1-4.
16. Aprill C, Bogduk N. The prevalence of cervical

zygapophyseal joint pain. A first approximation. *Spine.* Jul 1992;17(7):744-747.

17. Aprill C, Dwyer A, Bogduk N. Cervical zygapophyseal joint pain patterns. II: A clinical evaluation. *Spine.* Jun 1990;15(6):458-461.

18. Dwyer A, Aprill C, Bogduk N. Cervical zygapophyseal joint pain patterns. I: A study in normal volunteers. *Spine.* Jun 1990;15(6):453-457.

19. Spitzer WO, Skovron ML, Salmi LR, et al. Scientific monograph of the Quebec Task Force on Whiplash-Associated Disorders: redefining "whiplash" and its management. *Spine.* 1995;20(8 Suppl):1S-73S.

20. Chung YS, Han DH. Vertebrobasilar dissection: a possible role of whiplash injury in its pathogenesis. *Neurol Res.* Mar 2002;24(2):129-138.

21. Lord SM, Barnsley L, Wallis BJ, Bogduk N. Chronic cervical zygapophysial joint pain after whiplash. A placebo-controlled prevalence study. *Spine.* 1996;21(15):1737-1744; discussion 1744-1735.

22. Ketroser DB. Whiplash, chronic neck pain, and zygapophyseal joint disorders. *Minnesota Medicine.* 2000;83:51-54.

23. Curatolo M, Arendt-Nielsen L, Petersen-Felix S. Evidence, mechanisms, and clinical implications of central hypersensitivity in chronic pain after whiplash injury. *Clin J Pain.* Nov-Dec 2004;20(6):469-476.

24. Curatolo M, Petersen-Felix S, Arendt-Nielsen L, Giani C, Zbinden AM, Radanov BP. Central hypersensitivity in chronic pain after whiplash injury. *Clin J Pain.* Dec 2001;17(4):306-315.

25. Petersen-Felix S, Arendt-Nielsen L, Curatolo M. Chronic pain after whiplash injury- evidence for altered central sensory processing. *Journal of Whiplash & Related Disorders.* 2003;2(1):5-16.

26. Melzack R, Wall PD. *The Challenge of Pain.* New York: Basic Books, Inc.; 1983.

27. Alexander D. The importance of the Quebec task force on whiplash-associated disorders (WAD) for massage therapy. *Journal of Soft Tissue Manipulation.* 1996;3(4):4-12.

28. Smith DL, DeMario MC. Spasmodic torticollis: a case report and review of therapies. *J Am Board Fam Pract.* 1996;9(6):435-441.

29. Simons D, Travell J, Simons L. *Myofascial Pain and Dysfunction: The Trigger Point Manual.* Vol 1. 2nd ed. Baltimore: Williams & Wilkins; 1999.

30. Reynolds N, Ma J. Torticollis. *eMedicine.* July 1, 2004. Available at: www.emedicine.com. Accessed August 20, 2004.

31. Jankovic J, Leder S, Warner D, Schwartz K. Cervical dystonia: clinical findings and associated movement disorders. *Neurology.* Jul 1991;41(7):1088-1091.

32. Kahn ML, Davidson R, Drummond DS. Acquired torticollis in children. *Orthop Rev.* Aug 1991;20(8):667-674.

33. Adams M, Bogduk N, Burton K, Dolan P. *The Biomechanics of Back Pain.* Edinburgh: Churchill Livingstone; 2002.

34. Magee D. *Orthopedic Physical Assessment.* 3rd ed. Philadelphia: W.B. Saunders; 1997.

35. Boden SD, McCowin PR, Davis DO, Dina TS, Mark AS, Wiesel S. Abnormal magnetic-resonance scans of the cervical spine in asymptomatic subjects. A prospective investigation. *J Bone Joint Surg Am.* Sep 1990;72(8):1178-1184.

36. Ellenberg MR, Honet JC, Treanor WJ. Cervical radiculopathy. *Arch Phys Med Rehabil.* Mar 1994;75(3):342-352.

37. Wiederholt W. *Neurology for Non-Neurologists.* 4th ed. Philadelphia: W.B. Saunders; 2000.

38. Panjabi M, White A. *Biomechanics in the Musculoskeletal System.* New York: Churchill Livingstone; 2001.

39. Wisneski R, Garfin S, Rothman R, Lutz G. Lumbar disc disease. In: Herkowitz H, Garfin S, Balderston R, Eismont F, Bell G, Wiesel S, eds. *Rothman-Simeone: The Spine.* Vol 1. Philadelphia: W.B. Saunders Company; 1999:613-679.

40. Benoist M. The natural history of lumbar disc herniation and radiculopathy. *Joint Bone Spine.* 2002;69(2):155-160.

41. McKenzie R. Understanding centralisation. *J Orthop Sports Phys Ther.* Aug 1999;29(8):487-489.

42. Craton N, Matheson GO. Training and clinical competency in musculoskeletal medicine. Identifying the problem. *Sports Med.* 1993;15(5):328-337.

43. Freedman KB, Bernstein J. The adequacy of medical school education in musculoskeletal medicine. *J Bone Joint Surg Am.* 1998;80(10):1421-1427.

44. Waddell G. *The Back Pain Revolution.* Edinburgh: Churchill Livingstone; 1998.

10 Shoulder

Shoulder pain is the third most common musculoskeletal disorder, following low back and cervical spine pain.[1] The mechanics of the shoulder region are complex. Evaluation of shoulder pathologies must begin with a fundamental understanding of the motions of the shoulder region. That knowledge, along with awareness of common pathologies in the shoulder, allows the practitioner to apply effective evaluation and treatment strategies.

There are four articulations in the shoulder girdle: the scapulothoracic, sternoclavicular, acromioclavicular, and glenohumeral. Movement takes place mostly at the glenohumeral joint, with some contribution from the scapulothoracic articulation. The glenohumeral joint has the greatest range of motion of any joint in the body, allowing it to perform a wide variety of movements. Range-of-motion values are not calculated for scapulothoracic motions due to the difficulty in accurately measuring motion at that articulation. Motion at the sternoclavicular and acromioclavicular joints is minimal, so they are not calculated in clinical evaluation.

The shoulder's movement abilities are possible only at the expense of bony stability, requiring the soft tissues to play a more critical role in maintaining joint integrity. This increased responsibility for stabilization places the shoulder at risk for numerous soft-tissue injuries. Acute injuries result from incidents such as blows to the shoulder, falling on an outstretched arm, or forceful movements that dislocate or sublux the joint. Chronic injuries develop from the movement requirements in repetitive upper-extremity activities. Also problematic are activities requiring that the shoulder be held for a prolonged period in a position that impinges soft tissues. Shoulder problems and injuries are common in sports, recreation, and assorted occupations.

Movements and Motion Testing

SINGLE-PLANE MOVEMENTS

The primary joint in the shoulder complex is the glenohumeral; shoulder evaluations focus on this articulation. There are six primary single-plane movements at the glenohumeral joint: flexion, extension, medial rotation, lateral rotation, abduction, and adduction. Two accessory motions are sometimes evaluated in the glenohumeral joint: horizontal abduction (or horizontal extension) and horizontal adduction (or horizontal flexion). These two motions start with the arm abducted to 90^0 instead of in a neutral position. The associated motions, planes, axes of rotation, and range-of-motion values for the shoulder are listed in Table 2 at the end of the chapter.

The scapulothoracic articulation is a functional rather than anatomical joint, which is why it is referred to as an **articulation** rather than a **joint**. Range-of-motion values are not calculated for this articulation and there is no capsular pattern as there is no joint capsule. However, scapulothoracic motion is important in evaluating certain shoulder disorders. Motions at the scapulothoracic articulation include: elevation, depression, protraction, retraction, and upward/downward rotation. Due to the difficulty in measurements, range-of-motion tests are not provided for the motions at the scapulothoracic articulation.

Glenohumeral Joint

Flexion and **extension** occur in the **sagittal plane** (Figure 10.1). In flexion, the arm is raised from anatomical position straight forward and upward as far as possible. Extension is the return to anatomical position and any additional motion continuing in that direction. Average range of motion for glenohumeral flexion is 160^0 –180^0. A lesser range may still be considered normal because the shape of the acromion process can alter the available range in certain people. Average range of motion for glenohumeral extension is about 60^0.

Medial and **lateral rotations** are in the **transverse plane** (Figure 10.1). In medial rotation the humerus is rotated toward the midline of the body. It is easiest to observe medial and lateral rotation if the elbow is flexed. Medial rotation is stopped when the forearm contacts the abdomen and full evaluation requires the arm be placed behind the back. In lateral rotation the humerus is rotated away from the midline of the body. Medial rotation is measured from the neutral starting point (where the flexed forearm aims straight ahead) and average range of motion is about 90^0. Lateral rotation is measured from the same starting point as medial and average range is approximately 90^0.

Glenohumeral **abduction** and **adduction** occur in the **frontal plane** (Figure 10.1). In abduction, the arm is brought away from the mid-line of the body. Adduction is the return to anatomical position from any degree of abduction. Further glenohumeral adduction can be accomplished if the shoulder is slightly flexed so the arm is brought in front of the torso. Average range of motion in abduction is close to 180^0 and includes scapulothoracic as well as glenohumeral motion. Adduction is measured from anatomical position moving further into adduction. Once the arm is brought in front of the body average

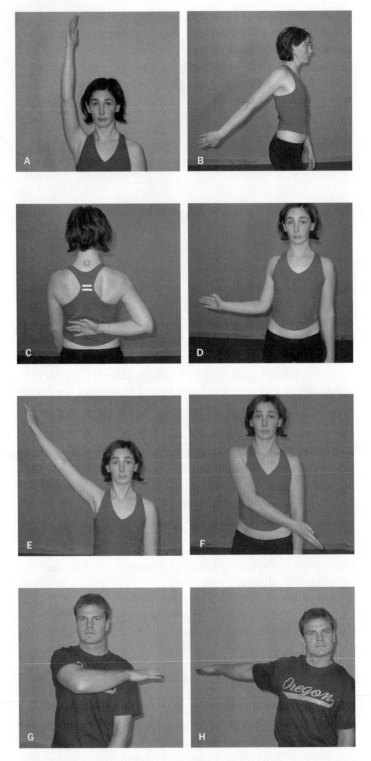

Figure 10.1 Shoulder flexion (A), extension (B), medial rotation (C), lateral rotation (D), abduction (E), adduction (F), horizontal adduction (G), and horizontal abduction (H).

range of motion in adduction is 50^0–75^0.

Horizontal adduction and **abduction** take place in the **transverse plane** (Figure 10.1). The starting point for evaluating horizontal abduction or horizontal adduction is with the arm in 90^0 of frontal plane abduction. From this position horizontal adduction occurs as the arm is brought across the chest. Horizontal abduction occurs when the arm moves from the starting point (90⁰ of abduction) in a posterior direction, as if reaching behind the body. Range of motion values are rarely calculated for horizontal abduction and adduction.

Scapulothoracic Articulation

Elevation and **depression** of the scapulothoracic articulation are in the **frontal plane**. These motions are translational (sliding) movements and therefore do not occur around an axis as in most other movements (Figure 10.2). Elevation is a superior movement of the scapula and is described as hiking the shoulder. In depression, the scapula moves in an inferior direction from an elevated or neutral position.

Protraction and retraction take place in multiple planes. Both movements are translational movements as the scapula slides around the thoracic rib cage. In protraction, the scapula moves in an anterior and lateral direction, as in reaching forward with the arm. Retraction is the reverse of protraction and occurs when the scapulae are pulled together in the back (Figure 10.2).

Upward and downward rotations are in the frontal plane. These are scapulothoracic motions around a single axis and are associated with abduction and adduction, respectively. The glenoid fossa of the scapula rotates upward during abduction of the shoulder and downward during adduction. Motion at the scapulothoracic articulation is difficult to isolate and measure and is therefore not included in range-of-motion evaluations or manual resistive tests. In some cases, scapulothoracic motion is evaluated in conjunction with overall glenohumeral mechanics (see the discussion of scapulohumeral rhythm in Frozen Shoulder Syndrome below).

Capsular Pattern

It is important to consider the role of the joint capsule when assessing joint function. Pathological problems in the capsule, such as *fibrosis* or *adhesion*, may be assessed with the joint's **capsular pattern**. The capsular pattern is a pattern of movement restriction that is characteristic to each individual joint. It is present in both active and passive motion. Capsular patterns are represented by a sequential listing of the movements from most likely to least likely limited. See the description of capsular pattern for the glenohumeral joint in Box 10.1.

RANGE-OF-MOTION & RESISTIVE TESTS

Results from single-plane movement analysis form the basis for further evaluation procedures. Movement testing should be performed in a certain order, allowing for an efficient evaluation and the least amount of accumulated discomfort or pain to develop. It is also general practice to leave movements known or expected to be painful to the end of the evaluation. When possible, the pain-free side is evaluated first.

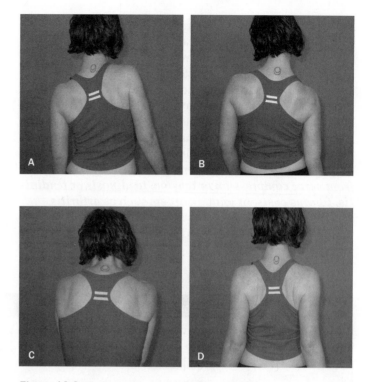

Figure 10.2 Right side scapulothoracic elevation (A), Right side depression (B), bilateral protraction (C), and bilateral retraction (D).

Box 10.1 Capsular Pattern for the Shoulder

Glenohumeral Joint
  Lateral rotation is limited first.
  Abduction is limited next.
  Medial rotation is last.

Active range-of-motion (AROM) movements are performed first to establish the client's movement abilities and pain symptoms. Passive range of motion (PROM) is performed next and manual resistive tests (MRT) follow. AROM results may make PROM assessment procedures unnecessary. If no pain occurs with active movement, pain is unlikely with passive movement. The practitioner should be familiar with the full step-by-step instructions and guidelines for how to interpret ROM and resistive test results explained in Chapter 3.

Active Range of Motion

Active range-of-motion evaluations are usually evaluated with the client in a standing position. When performing AROM evaluations, take into consideration the position of the shoulder to ensure the target tissues are engaged. For example, when the client actively abducts the shoulder from a standing position, the shoulder abductors are engaged concentrically. When the arm is returned to the body, the abductors work eccentrically even though the motion being engaged is shoulder adduction. A concentric contraction of the shoulder adductors requires a change in body position or in the way resistance is employed, such as when resistance is offered on the underside of the arm during the adduction movement.

Pain with active movement indicates problems in either the contractile or inert tissues associated with that movement. Factors prematurely limiting active movement in this region include *ligamentous or capsular damage, soft-tissue impingement, muscle tightness, pain from nerve compression or tension, tendinosis or tendinitis, fibrous cysts,* or joint disorders such as *arthritis*.

Compare AROM test results with those from PROM and manual resistive tests to identify possible reasons for

movement restriction. The primary muscles used to perform actions of the shoulder are listed in Box 10.2. Note that other muscles can contribute to the motion and subsequent dysfunction.

Passive Range of Motion

Passive motion tests are performed after active. Pain during passive movement predominantly implicates inert tissues. However, muscles and tendons that contract in the opposite direction are stretched at the end range of passive movement. The primary goal of passive movement is to have minimal or no muscular activity. If performing these movements with the client in an upright position does not adequately decrease muscular activity,

---

BOX 10.2 MUSCLE ACTIONS OF THE SHOULDER

Glenohumeral

Flexion
- Coracobrachialis
- Deltoid (anterior and middle portions)
- Pectoralis major (clavicular portion)
- Biceps brachii

Medial rotation
- Latissimus dorsi
- Pectoralis major
- Subscapularis
- Teres major
- Deltoid (anterior portion)

Abduction
- Deltoid (middle portion)
- Supraspinatus

Horizontal abduction
- Deltoid (posterior portion)

Extension
- Latissimus dorsi
- Deltoid (posterior portion)
- Teres major
- Triceps brachii (long head)

Lateral rotation
- Infraspinatus
- Teres minor
- Deltoid (posterior portion)

Adduction
- Latissimus dorsi
- Pectoralis major
- Teres minor
- Teres major
- Coracobrachialis

Horizontal adduction
- Pectoralis major
- Deltoid (anterior portion)

Scapular

Elevation
- Trapezius (upper)
- Levator scapulae
- Rhomboid (major & minor)

Protraction
- Serratus Anterior
- Pectoralis minor

Upward rotation
- Trapezius (upper & lower)
- Serratus anterior

Depression
- Trapezius (lower)

Retraction
- Trapezius (middle & lower)
- Rhomboid (major & minor)
- Levator scapulae

Downward rotation
- Rhomboid (major & minor)
- Levator scapulae

use a supine position.

PROM testing also evaluates end feel. Box 10.3 lists the normal end feel for motions of the glenohumeral joint. Review Chapter 3 for a discussion of normal and pathological end feel descriptions. Factors that could prematurely limit passive movement are the same as for active movement.

Manual Resistive Tests

A manual resistive test (MRT) produces pain when there is a mechanical disruption of tissue. Pain with an MRT indicates that one or more of the muscles and/or tendons performing that action are involved. Tendinosis and muscle strains are common in the shoulder region so these pathologies should be considered if there is pain with manual resistance.

Testing all of a muscle's actions is not necessary, as a muscle's secondary actions recruit other muscles and make the test results less accurate. Due to multiple actions of a muscle, some resisted actions isolate the muscle better than others; skill development in these procedures allows the practitioner to elicit more refined information.

Palpation during manual resistance elicits more information if the test alone does not create pain or discomfort. Refer to Box 10.2 for the list of primary muscles involved with each action. Table 1 at the end of the chapter lists actions commonly used for testing muscles in shoulder.

In some cases weakness is evident with MRTs. Factors that produce weakness include *lack of use, fatigue, reflex muscular inhibition,* or neurological pathology (*radiculopathy, peripheral neuropathy,* or a *systemic neurological disorder*). The nerves or nerve roots that may be involved are listed in Table 1 at the end of the chapter.

Shoulder

RESISTED FLEXION AND EXTENSION

For flexion, the client is standing or seated with the shoulder partially flexed. The client holds the arm in the flexed position as the practitioner attempts to pull it down into extension. The practitioner should ensure the hand is placed above the client's elbow so the elbow flexors are not recruited (Figure 10.3).

To test extension, the client is standing or seated with the arm in slight extension. The client holds the arm stationary as the practitioner attempts to push it into flexion. The practitioner should make sure the hand placed on the client's arm is above the elbow so the elbow extensors are not recruited (Figure 10.3).

RESISTED MEDIAL AND LATERAL ROTATION

To test medial rotation, the client is standing or seated with the elbow flexed to 90⁰. The client holds the arm stationary as the practitioner uses one hand to hold the client's elbow close to the torso and attempts to pull the client's forearm into lateral rotation with the other hand (Figure 10.3c).

To test lateral rotation, the client is standing or seated

GENERAL INSTRUCTIONS FOR ROM & RESISTIVE TESTS
Overall
• Determine motions possible at the joint to be tested.
• Select the motion to be evaluated.
• Determine the tissues involved in the motion.
• Leave motions expected to be painful to the last.
• Test the uninvolved side first.
• Ask about, note any reported pain or discomfort.
AROM
• Demonstrate the movement to be performed.
• Have the client perform the movement.
PROM
• Establish the joint's normal end feel.
• Have the client relax as much as possible.
• Use gentle and slow movements.
MRT
• Test one action at a time.
• Position should isolate the action/muscles involved.
• If pain is suspected, start in a mid-range position.
• Client uses a strong, but appropriate amount of effort.

Box 10.3 JOINT, ASSOCIATED MOTION, & NORMAL END FEEL

Glenohumeral	Flexion	Tissue stretch (soft)
	Extension	Tissue stretch (firm)
	Medial rotation	Tissue stretch (soft)
	Lateral rotation	Tissue stretch (firm)
	Abduction	Tissue stretch (soft)
	Adduction	Tissue stretch
	Horizontal abduction	Tissue stretch
	Horizontal adduction	Tissue stretch

with the elbow flexed to 90⁰. The client holds the arm stationary. The practitioner uses one hand to hold the client's elbow close to the torso and attempts to push the forearm into medial rotation with the other hand (Figure 10.3).

RESISTED ABDUCTION AND ADDUCTION

To test abduction, the client is standing or seated with the arm partially abducted. The client holds the arm in this position while the practitioner attempts to push it back to the client's torso. The practitioner should apply the pressure just above the client's elbow (Figure 10.3).

To test adduction, the client is standing or seated with the arm partially abducted. The client holds the arm in this position while the practitioner attempts to pull the arm into further abduction. The practitioner should apply pressure just above the client's elbow (Figure 10.3f).

RESISTED HORIZONTAL ADDUCTION AND ABDUCTION

To test horizontal adduction, the client is standing or

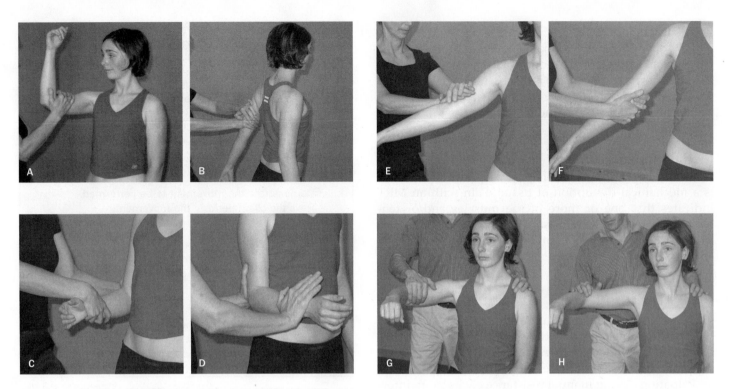

Figure 10.3 Resisted flexion (A), extension (B), medial rotation (C), lateral rotation (D), abduction (E), adduction (F), horizontal adduction (G), and horizontal abduction (H).

seated with the arm abducted to about 90⁰. The practitioner has one hand on the back of the client's opposite shoulder for stabilization and the other hand on the client's arm above the elbow. The client holds the position as the practitioner attempts to pull the arm into horizontal abduction (Figure 10.3).

For horizontal abduction the client is seated with the arm abducted to about 90⁰. The practitioner is standing behind the client with one hand on the client's opposite shoulder for stabilization and the other hand on the client's arm above the elbow. The client holds this position as the practitioner attempts to push the client's arm into horizontal adduction (Figure 10.3).

Structural and Postural Deviations

The following section covers structural or postural deviations unique to the shoulder. Under each condition there is a brief description of the condition's characteristics followed by likely HOPRS findings. If applicable, orthopedic tests are included in the special tests section. Sometimes there is no special orthopedic test listed for that condition. In that case, evaluation should focus on other portions of the assessment process, such as range-of-motion and resistance testing.

The glenohumeral joint is reliant on soft tissues to maintain stability and guide movement. Structural and postural deviations in this region can have an adverse effect on shoulder biomechanics. Many of the postural disorders mentioned below are precursors to more serious acute or chronic conditions in the shoulder region.

ELEVATED SHOULDER

Elevated shoulder **is a postural distortion stemming from hypertonicity in the shoulder and neck muscles**. While the condition does not always produce pain, the chronic tension in shoulder muscles frequently produces aching pain and may adversely affect shoulder mechanics.

Characteristics

Elevated shoulder can be a unilateral or bilateral problem. The distortion is generally caused by chronic tightness in the **levator scapulae** or **upper trapezius** muscles. In some cases the distortion is congenital, although this is not usual. Elevated shoulder typically results from chronic postural habits. An example is a person who spends time with a telephone cradled between the head and shoulder. In this position, the shoulder muscles are in constant isometric contraction and a pattern of hypertonicity results. Working at a desk for long periods also creates the pattern of chronic tension characteristic with elevated shoulders.

Biomechanical factors are not the only cause of elevated shoulder. Chronic psychological stress can manifest in particular **holding patterns** in the body. A common tension pattern resulting from chronic psychological stress is hypertonicity in the upper back and shoulder elevator muscles. Myofascial trigger points routinely develop in these muscles as a result of the chronic tension.[2]

History

The client is apt to report headache, shoulder, or neck pain. Though not always painful, the hypertonicity that

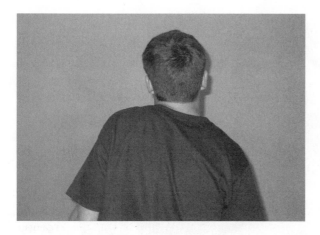

Figure 10.4 Elevated shoulder.

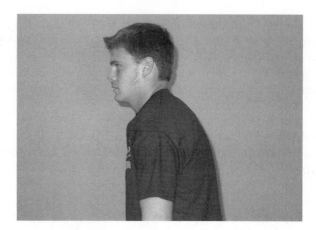

Figure 10.5 Slumped shoulders.

causes the distortion may produce aching pain. Ask about postural habits or ergonomic factors that might create tension in the shoulder region.

Observation
Elevated shoulder is visually apparent, particularly when only one shoulder is affected. When the client is viewed from the front or back, one shoulder is seen to be higher than the other (Figure 10.4). An anatomical grid chart is helpful as a reference. If both shoulders are affected, the shoulders will appear higher than they would naturally were there no excess tension in the affected muscles.

Palpation
The upper trapezius and levator scapulae muscles are apt to feel tight. If the problem is unilateral, the high side is likely to feel tighter than the opposite side. Specific deep palpation in the upper shoulder region may reveal the presence of myofascial trigger points. Common myofascial trigger point referral zones are listed in Figure 10.32-10.34 at the end of the chapter.

Range-of-Motion and Resistance Testing
AROM: Active elevation of the scapula may be limited on the affected side due to hypertonicity. Restriction in lateral flexion of the neck to the opposite side is likely due to muscular tightness.
PROM: There may be limitation in passive shoulder depression due to muscular tightness. Restriction is likely in active cervical lateral flexion to the opposite side.
MRT: Resisted shoulder elevation may elicit pain from hypertonicity or myofascial trigger points, but not always.

Suggestions for Treatment
The primary focus of treatment is postural retraining and neuromuscular re-education. Repetitive dysfunc-

tional patterns must be offset by repeated corrections that change the faulty biomechanics. Soft-tissue treatment, particularly massage and stretching, are helpful for hypertonicity and myofascial trigger points in the levator scapulae and upper trapezius muscles. Postural and ergonomic changes are required to treat the condition.

SLUMPED SHOULDERS

Slumped shoulders frequently coexist with an *upper thoracic kyphosis* and *forward head posture* (Chapter 9). The condition is common among those with sedentary lifestyles and is associated with poor posture. The altered position of the shoulders can lead to shoulder pathologies, as well as disorders of the upper thoracic vertebrae.

Characteristics
Postural balance in the shoulders is dependent on equalized tension between the anterior and posterior shoulder girdle muscles. When the medial rotators of the shoulder, particularly the **pectoralis major**, **latissimus dorsi**, **subscapularis**, and **teres major** are hypertonic they cause an increase in medial **rotation of the humerus and protraction of the scapulae which rolls the shoulder forward** in the slumped position (Figure 10.5). The rhomboids can become weakened from reciprocal inhibition leading to increased scapular protraction.[3]

The discussion of the *upper crossed syndrome* in Chapter 9 describes the neurological inhibition of the rhomboids. The same muscular dysfunction appearing in the upper crossed syndrome can occur with slumped shoulders. Along with shortening of the medial rotators of the shoulder there is typically muscular fatigue and myofascial trigger points that develop in the upper back. Fatigue from over-lengthening the **rhomboids** and **middle trapezius** causes pain similar to the pain of hypertonicity.

Slumped shoulders generally result from chronic postural distortions. The condition frequently affects individuals who work with their arms directly in front of them or sit for prolonged periods in poor postures. *Osteoporosis* or other causes of vertebral degeneration can also lead to the condition.

History
The client may report pain in the rhomboids and middle trapezius due to muscular fatigue and/or myofascial trigger points. There is rarely pain or discomfort felt in the internal rotators, except in palpation. Ask the client about postural stresses experienced through work. Ask the client if he or she has been diagnosed with osteoporosis or vertebral degeneration.

Observation
The posture can be viewed from several directions, but the lateral is most effective. From a lateral direction, the centerline of the glenohumeral joint is forward of the centerline of gravity in the body. Forward head posture and upper thoracic kyphosis are apt to accompany slumped shoulders. A reference, such as an anatomical grid chart, is helpful. Slumped shoulders are usually bilateral and the distortion appears similar on both sides.

Palpation
The upper chest muscles are hypertonic and tender. Tenderness in the upper back is expected as muscle fatigue and myofascial trigger points develop in the rhomboids and mid-trapezius muscles.

Range-of-Motion and Resistance Testing
AROM: Limitation in lateral rotation of the shoulder may be evident due to hypertonicity in the pectoralis major, which is also a medial rotator of the shoulder. There may be a sense of restriction to active retraction of the scapulae due to muscle tightness as well.
PROM: The same principles apply as for active motion.
MRT: Pain, discomfort, or muscle weakness is not likely with MRTs.

Suggestions for Treatment
Treatment should focus on the hypertonic muscles that have caused the postural distortion, including the pectoralis major, anterior deltoids, latissimus dorsi, and other medial rotators of the shoulder. Fascial elongation methods along with deep longitudinal stripping are helpful to encourage lengthening in these tissues. In addition, the upper back muscles should be treated for fatigue and tension.

It is difficult, if not impossible, to make lasting postural changes with soft-tissue work alone. Repetitive dysfunctional patterns should be offset by repeated corrections to change the faulty biomechanics. Postural retraining and neuromuscular re-education are necessary for improvement. Changes in ergonomics may be required as well.

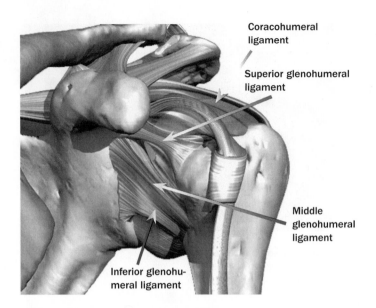

Figure 10.6 Anterior view of superior, middle, and inferior glenohumeral ligaments and coracohumeral ligament. (3-D anatomy image courtesy of Primal Pictures Ltd. www.primalpictures.com.)

Common Injury Conditions

FROZEN SHOULDER & ADHESIVE CAPSULITIS

The term *frozen shoulder* is used to refer to a set of symptoms in the shoulder involving pain and limited motion at the glenohumeral joint. Frozen shoulder is commonly used interchangeably with *adhesive capsulitis*. However, adhesive capsulitis refers to a discrete clinical pathology, whereas frozen shoulder refers to a variety of pathologies.[1] The pathologies that may be involved in frozen shoulder include not only adhesive capsulitis, but subacromial bursitis, calcific tendinitis, rotator cuff pathology, and other conditions limiting shoulder motion.[4] Primarily, frozen shoulder describes a functional limitation in range of motion associated with pain and stiffness. With improved diagnostics, the use of this term eventually may be abandoned for more accurate references.

The common element between frozen shoulder and adhesive capsulitis is pain and limited motion in the shoulder associated with inert tissues. Donatelli proposes a working definition of frozen shoulder as *glenohumeral stiffness resulting from a noncontractile element*.[1] Using Donatelli's definition, the term *frozen shoulder* is used here to refer to **glenohumeral stiffness and lost range of motion resulting from a noncontractile element in the shoulder that is not necessarily capsular in nature**.

Adhesive capsulitis **involves loss of active and passive motion due to adhesions within the glenohumeral joint capsule**.[5] There is a distinction between a stiff and painful shoulder without any capsular involvement (frozen shoulder) and that involving capsular adhesion (adhesive capsulitis).[6] While the anatomical tissues involved differ between frozen shoulder and adhesive capsulitis,

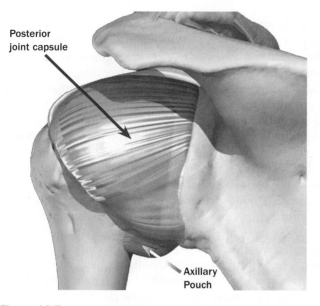

Figure 10.7 Posterior view of the shoulder showing the underside of the joint capsule, called the axillary recess or pouch (3-D anatomy image courtesy of Primal Pictures Ltd. www.primalpictures.com.)

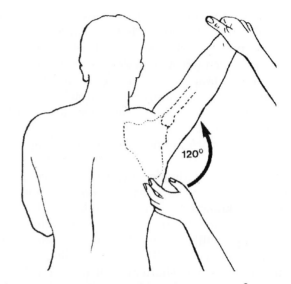

Figure 10.8 The scapulohumeral rhythm. For the 120^0 of abduction evident in the picture, approximately 80^0 has occurred at the glenohumeral joint and 40^0 at the scapulothoracic articulation. (Mediclip image copyright, 1998 Williams & Wilkins. All rights reserved.)

the symptoms, etiology, and clinical characteristics of the pathologies are virtually the same. In the discussion below, the term *frozen shoulder* is used unless there is a specific reference to adhesion within the glenohumeral joint capsule, in which case *adhesive capsulitis* is used.

Characteristics

The glenohumeral joint has the greatest range of motion of any joint in the body.[7] Consequently, a degree of slack or pliability in the joint capsule and surrounding soft tissues is necessary to allow full motion. If a full range of soft-tissue pliability is not available, limitation in joint range occurs and results in stiffness and pain. Pathological processes in a number of soft tissues of the shoulder can prevent full range of motion and produce the characteristic limitations of frozen shoulder, including *bursitis, calcific tendinitis, arthritis, myofascial trigger points, shortening of capsular tissues, adhesive capsulitis,* and other disorders.[8, 9]

Identifying frozen shoulder pathologies requires understanding the anatomical and biomechanical relationships in the glenohumeral joint and the supporting soft tissues. The **glenohumeral joint capsule** is composed of capsular and ligamentous fibers. On the anterior aspect of the capsule, the superior, middle, and inferior glenohumeral ligaments blend with the capsular fibers (Figure 10.6). On the superior side, stability is enhanced as the **coracohumeral ligament** blends with the capsular fibers (Figure 10.6). When the shoulder is in a neutral position the underside of the capsule, called the **axillary recess** or **axillary pouch**, is relaxed (Figure 10.7). During certain shoulder motions, especially abduction or lateral rotation, the axillary pouch is stretched and becomes taut.

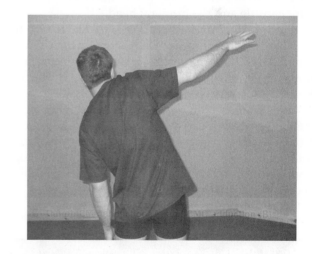

Figure 10.9 Evident compensation in abduction due to disturbance of the scapulohumeral rhythm.

There is a ratio of movement in the shoulder that occurs at the scapulothoracic articulation and at the glenohumeral joint in order to create full abduction, called the **scapulohumeral rhythm**.[10] The scapulohumeral rhythm is a 2:1 ratio of movement during abduction. This means that for every three degrees of shoulder abduction, two occur at the glenohumeral joint and one at the scapulothoracic articulation (Figure 10.8). The ratio is not exact all the way through abduction, but is a general guideline.

Conditions such as frozen shoulder can seriously alter the scapulohumeral rhythm. For example, in frozen shoulder glenohumeral abduction past about 40^0 is severely restricted or eliminated. All remaining movement in lifting the arm to the side is at the scapulothoracic articulation. Disturbance to the scapulohumeral rhythm produces characteristic compensations during shoulder abduction such as that shown in Figure 10.9.

In adhesive capsulitis, the main dysfunction involves the axillary pouch where adhesions form inside the capsule causing the inner walls of the pouch to adhere. In this state, the pouch can no longer fully stretch, causing pain and limited range of motion. Limitations are most likely in abduction and lateral rotation because these motions stretch the anterior/inferior portions of the capsule the most.[11]

Frozen shoulder is divided into two categories: primary and secondary.[5, 12] *Primary frozen shoulder* is idiopathic—its cause is unknown. There is some indication that it may be an autoimmune disorder but why the motion limitations develop is still unclear.[1] Pathological characteristics may include any of the following: shortening of the joint capsule; fibrosity and shortening of the coracohumeral ligament; subscapular bursitis; fibrosity within the rotator interval (portion of the glenohumeral joint capsule between the supraspinatus and subscapularis tendons); postural distortion in the shoulder; active myofascial trigger points in the shoulder muscles; or adhesions between rotator cuff muscles and articular inert tissues, such as the joint capsule and the humeral head.[13-17]

Secondary frozen shoulder results from another pathology, such as *rotator cuff tears, arthritis, bicipital tendinosis or tenosynovitis, surgery, shoulder separation, diabetes, or glenohumeral subluxation.*[4,12] The inciting trauma causes problems in the same tissues as primary frozen shoulder although there is more evidence of capsular adhesion in the secondary variation. In secondary frozen shoulder, scar tissue from the prior trauma can adhere the axillary folds of the joint capsule together. Some period of shoulder immobilization generally precedes the onset of symptoms.

Box 10.4 Stages of Frozen Shoulder

Stage One
Increasing pain
Gradual loss of joint volume
Lasting from 2 to 9 months

Stage Two
Diminished pain
More limited range of motion
Lasting from 4 to 12 months

Stage Three
Reduction of pain
Gradual restoration of motion
Lasting 12 months to years

The development of frozen shoulder and its resolution proceeds in stages. The stages are referred to as **pain, stiffness,** and **recovery**, or **stages one, two**, and **three**.[18] They are also described as freezing, frozen, and thawing, although there is obviously no thermal change accompanying this process (Box 10.4).[12] In both primary and secondary frozen shoulder, there is pain and limited movement. Due to the frequent involvement of the glenohumeral joint capsule or ligamentous tissues that are contiguous with it, motion limitations are characteristically in the capsular pattern of the shoulder.[1,11]

Women are affected more often than men, with more prevalence in people 40 to 70 years old. It is postulated that the hormonal changes that come with menopause may create tissue changes that make women susceptible to this condition.[1] Other metabolic and systemic factors may also play a role in the onset. There is an increased risk of developing frozen shoulder if the client is diabetic.[19, 20] Frozen shoulder can last as long as 18–24 months, and in some cases much longer.[18]

History
The client complains of pain during various shoulder motions, such as abduction, rotation, or flexion. The symptoms may interfere with daily activities, such as brushing teeth or hair, or dressing - all of which require lateral rotation in the glenohumeral region. Range of motion limitations are usually described as coming on gradually. Ask the client about systemic disorders such as diabetes, as they may be related to the onset of the condition. The condition happens with greater frequency in women who are in middle to later age. Ask the client about prior trauma, surgery, or injury to the shoulder that immediately preceded symptoms, which would indicate a secondary frozen shoulder.

Observation
When the shoulder is held in a neutral position there are no visible signs of frozen shoulder. Motion restrictions are visible during range-of-motion evaluation and extensive muscular compensation is evident. An alteration to the scapulohumeral rhythm is evident. The client often demonstrates apprehension when attempting to perform shoulder motions, particularly lateral rotation, abduction, or a combination of these motions.

Palpation
The inert soft tissues producing motion restriction are difficult to palpate due to their depth. Therefore it is unlikely to find pain with palpation as long as the shoulder is in a neutral position and the inert tissues are relaxed. The muscles around the shoulder may be hypertonic or tender as a result of lost motion, but not always. Because palpation in a neutral position rarely elicits pain in frozen shoulder, palpation may help distinguish this condition from other pathologies where damaged tissues are more easily palpable and do produce pain.

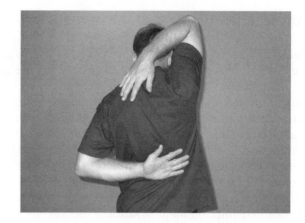

Figure 10.10 Apley scratch test.

Range-of-Motion and Resistance Testing

AROM: Pain and restricted range can follow the capsular pattern of the glenohumeral joint. Active motion has the greatest restriction in lateral rotation, second in abduction, and third in medial rotation. Compensating patterns are apparent as the client attempts active movements of the shoulder, particularly during abduction due to the disturbed scapulohumeral rhythm. Flexion may produce pain as well.

PROM: Because frozen shoulder primarily affects inert tissues and not contractile tissues, the same restrictions with active motion are observed with passive motion. The end-feel for lateral rotation, abduction, or medial rotation is tissue stretch, but occurs prior to the natural end range of motion and is commonly accompanied by severe pain.

MRT: Manual resistive tests are not likely to cause further discomfort. However, if they are performed in a position that stretches the joint capsule or other affected tissues, there may be pain even prior to the beginning of the test. For example, if the shoulder is laterally rotated there may be pain if a resisted lateral rotation is performed. Some weakness may be evident during MRTs and is due to reflex muscular inhibition.

Special Test

Apley Scratch Test

This test is used for evaluating range-of-motion limitations in the shoulder, but does not specifically assess frozen shoulder. However, the shoulder motions evaluated are relevant for frozen shoulder.

The client is standing and brings one arm as far as possible into abduction and lateral rotation as if scratching the upper back between the scapulae. The other arm is brought into adduction and medial rotation as if scratching the upper to mid-back (Figure 10.10). Position of the hands is observed and compared bilaterally. Each shoulder is tested in the upper position (abduction and lateral rotation) and the lower position (adduction and medial rotation). A person with frozen shoulder may have problems getting either shoulder into these positions. Problems with the abduction and lateral rotation are usually greater than adduction and medial rotation.

Explanation: Range-of-motion limitations are noted with inability to move the arm into the appropriate position, especially when compared to the unaffected side. For example, when comparing abduction and lateral rotation bilaterally, if the client is unable to reach down the back as far with the right arm as with the left, there is a limitation in range of motion on the right side. Because the motion being attempted in the right shoulder is abduction and lateral rotation, the restriction probably involves the adductors, medial rotators, or the glenohumeral joint capsule because these tissues all contribute to limiting abduction and lateral rotation.

Differential Evaluation

Subacromial bursitis, shoulder impingement, rotator cuff tears or tendinosis, calcific tendinitis, cervical neuropathy, brachial plexus compression, arthritis, subscapular bursitis, bicipital tendinosis or tenosynovitis, myofascial trigger point pain, thoracic outlet syndrome.

Suggestions for Treatment

Regardless of whether the condition is primary or secondary frozen shoulder, the affected inert tissues need to be lengthened and their mobility enhanced.[21] Massage can play a role in addressing soft-tissue restrictions, but is most effective when used in conjunction with other treatment methods such as ultrasound, which heats the deep capsular tissues and makes them more pliable.

Residual hypertonicity in muscles around the glenohumeral joint can be addressed with a variety of gliding, stripping, and static compression techniques. Stretching and movement should be encouraged in the direction of the motion restriction (abduction and lateral rotation). These motions must be done slowly and gradually. Stretching should be held just short of the pain or restriction barrier to encourage gradual tissue lengthening. Range-of-motion improvement is more effective when repeated regularly and it is essential for the client to perform some of these motions frequently on their own.[21-23] If conservative treatment is unsuccessful, surgery or joint manipulation under anesthesia may be performed by a physician in order to free the bound structures.

ROTATOR CUFF TEARS AND TENDINOSIS

Rotator cuff tears or *tendinosis* account for the largest percentage of soft-tissue shoulder disorders.[5] There is a close relationship and significant overlap between rotator cuff disorders and *shoulder impingement syndrome* because of the mechanics of the shoulder. For example, *supraspinatus tears* may result directly from subacromial impingement. The two conditions are distinguished here to better organize the information related to rotator cuff pathology. The various conditions caused by subacromial impingement (compressive stress) are addressed in the next Shoulder Impingement Syndrome section.

Characteristics

In many cases, rotator cuff injuries start as minor tendinosis or muscle overload and progress to more serious muscle damage as the fibers become fatigued and overused.[24] Tensile stress injuries can occur as chronic irritation from microtrauma or as an acute injury from overwhelming force. Severe injury may be avoided if early signs of dysfunction are addressed. Proper identification of the primary tissue(s) affected is essential when initiating treatment for these disorders.[25] To review the specific characteristics of muscle strains and tendinosis see Chapter 2.

The rotator cuff is composed of four muscles and their associated tendons: supraspinatus, infraspinatus, teres minor, and subscapularis (Figure 10.11). These muscles' primary function is to stabilize the glenohumeral joint. They also function to control and assist in shoulder movement. **When exposed to excessive or repetitive tensile loads greater than the muscle's strength, injuries develop and vary from minor tendinosis to complete rupture.**[26] All of the rotator cuff muscles are susceptible to injury, but damage occurs most often in the supraspinatus and least in the subscapularis.[1]

The **supraspinatus** is more susceptible to rotator cuff pathology because of its anatomical arrangement and the mechanical demands placed on it (Figure 10.12).[7] This muscle's primary function is to stabilize the **humeral head** and assist in producing glenohumeral abduction. The position of the distal muscle and tendon fibers underneath the **acromion process** makes the muscle susceptible to damage from impingement between the humeral head and the acromion process (see Shoulder Impingement Syndrome). In addition, the distal region of the tendon has less vascular supply, which increases its susceptibility to injury.[27]

Supraspinatus *strains* can be either partial-thickness tears, where the tear does not extend through the entire cross section of the muscle-tendon unit, or full-thickness tears. Tears result from excessive tensile loading, but can be aggravated by other factors such as *subacromial impingement*. Chronic compression causes degeneration of the fibers, which increases the risk of tearing from tensile loads. Recent studies of the mechanics of supraspi-

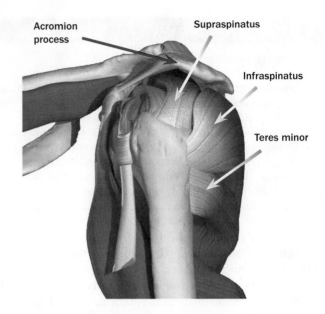

Figure 10.11 Lateral view of the left shoulder showing the rotator cuff tendons (subscapularis not visible in this view). (3-D anatomy image courtesy of Primal Pictures Ltd. www.primalpictures.com.)

natus tearing suggest that tears on the bursal (superior) side of the tendon are often a result of previous impingement. Those on the articular (inferior) side of the tendon are generally the result of excessive tensile loading and not necessarily caused by impingement.[28,29] There is also evidence that in rare cases the articular side of the tendon may be susceptible to impingement between the humeral head and the glenoid fossa.[30] In some cases, tensile loads on the supraspinatus are not overwhelming enough to produce fiber tearing, but do cause tendinosis, producing pain similar to a minor tear. Healing time may be extended, creating a chronic shoulder problem.

The **infraspinatus** and **teres minor** become dysfunctional due to tensile stress, not impingement (Figure 10.11). These muscle-tendon units can be eccentrically overloaded in any number of shoulder activities, such as throwing.[31] At the end of a throwing motion, the **infraspinatus** and **teres minor** muscles are under strong eccentric contraction to slow the momentum of the arm. Fiber fatigue can result from the continued stress. Pathology begins as a low-level tendinosis and if not properly addressed may end up as a full tear.[32] Tears are most likely to develop in the **musculotendinous junction**. Due to the accessibility of the muscles, these injuries are easier to identify than those that occur in the other two rotator cuff muscles.[33]

The **subscapularis** sustains few strains or tendon irritations due to its unique biomechanical characteristics (Figure 10.12). This muscle shares its main action with a number of other muscles, such as the **pectoralis major**, **latissimus dorsi**, **anterior deltoid**, and **teres major**, which prevent subscapularis overload. In addition, the glenohumeral joint capsule usually restricts lateral rotation before there is enough tensile load to cause a strain.

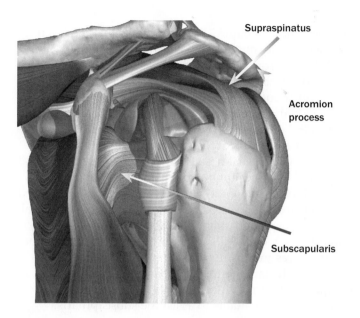

Supraspinatus

Acromion process

Subscapularis

Figure 10.12 Lateral view of the left shoulder showing the supraspinatus and subscapularis. (3-D anatomy image courtesy of Primal Pictures Ltd. www.primalpictures.com.)

In a forceful injury, such as a *shoulder dislocation*, strains to the subscapularis do take place. The subscapularis is a primary anterior support for the glenohumeral joint. It is assisted in this role by the **biceps brachii long head tendon**. Dislocations of the humeral head or bicipital tendon can create tensile forces strong enough to tear fibers and cause a strain.[34,35] Tendinosis is not likely with the subscapularis because the muscles that share actions with it generally prevent overuse.

Activities that can lead to subacromial compression primarily involve repetitive motions of the shoulder where the arm is brought into full flexion or abduction. Chronic periods of holding the shoulder in one of these positions could also lead to the fiber degeneration and tissue damage. Long periods of subacromial compression occur in occupations such as hairdressing, construction, or car mechanics. Various recreational activities such as swimming or throwing routinely cause rotator cuff damage. Tissue degeneration from previous stress or trauma followed by an acute injury can result in strains.

Pain from rotator cuff damage runs the gamut from mild aching in the shoulder to severe acute pain. The client may find it difficult to locate exactly where the pain is, but the pain is typically aggravated in abduction and forward flexion. Night pain is a common occurrence due to sleep positions where the humeral head may be jammed against the underside of the acromion process, especially with full-thickness tears of the supraspinatus.[36] The pain is worse when sleeping on the affected side.

Tendinosis or strain ordinarily affects individuals after age 40 due to the decreasing effectiveness of tissue repair.[37,38] Another reason may be pathological changes in the shape of the acromion process. See the discussion of the **hooked acromion** in the section on Shoulder

Impingement Syndrome for a discussion of acromion process changes resulting from age.

History

Rotator cuff tears can be acute or chronic. Tears frequently result from previous trauma, so ask the client about a history of repetitive motions or shoulder injuries. Find out if the client is engaged in sporting activities, such as baseball or swimming, or an occupation that requires overhead or throwing activities that cause muscle damage. Acute tears to the supraspinatus occur when the muscle-tendon unit is suddenly loaded. Ask the client about acute injuries, such as lifting something heavy or falling on an outstretched arm. Pain is often described as deep in the shoulder and the client will not be able to describe or point to its exact location.

If damage to the infraspinatus and teres minor is suspected, explore any recent activities that might cause sudden or repetitive eccentric forces on the posterior rotator cuff muscles. The client describes pain from infraspinatus and teres minor tearing in the posterior shoulder region and is able to reproduce pain by pressing on the damaged tissue.

The subscapularis may be torn in severe trauma, such as dislocation of the shoulder. When the client describes the initial onset, determine whether the forces creating the injury were particularly strong. The stronger the force, the more likely a subscapularis tear is involved. Pay particular attention to descriptions of forced lateral rotation, such as in a dislocation or subluxation, as this may indicate a subscapularis tear.

With tendinosis of any of the four rotator cuff muscles, the client reports gradual onset of pain as tissue damage may be minimal prior to becoming symptomatic. There is usually strong aching pain associated with activity that dissipates with rest.

Observation

There are no visible indicators of rotator cuff tears or tendinosis. While there may be an inflammatory response, the amount of tissue (including bone) over the injury site prevents it from being observable. Acute tears to the infraspinatus or teres minor are more visible as the muscles are superficial. Redness, swelling, or bruising may be visible if the tear is serious enough. Tears in the subscapularis, even when severe, rarely produce visible indicators due to the depth of the muscle and the overlying tissues. Inflammation may be evident in the region if the injury is severe enough.

Tendinosis is non-inflammatory and therefore produces no visible signs in any of the rotator cuff muscles. Keep in mind that in rare cases a true tendinitis (inflammation of the tendon) does appear, although usually at a low level and rarely visible.[39] Bone spurs or osteophytes that cause tissue tearing are visible with an x-ray.

Compensating patterns of movement or pain avoidance are normally evident. In ROM or MRT an individual shows visible apprehension when attempting to perform certain tests such as active or resisted abduction.

Palpation

Palpating tensile stress rotator cuff disorders is similar whether the pathology involves a tear or tendinosis. Tenderness and reproduction of the pain is expected when the site of tissue damage is palpated. Fibrosity and thickening may also be felt in the muscle or tendon. If there is an active inflammatory process, such as in a recent tear, excess heat may be felt. In addition, it is common for muscular hypertonicity to be present in the rotator cuff muscles and surrounding shoulder muscles.

If the injury involves a supraspinatus tear, palpation is difficult because the injury site is generally underneath the acromion process. However, in some cases the site of damage can be palpated by accessing the muscle in the supraspinous fossa or just inferior to the acromion process on the lateral aspect of the shoulder. When palpating the lateral acromial region, the practitioner may be able to determine whether the client has a hooked acromion, which is linked to an increased incidence of rotator cuff tears.[40] See Shoulder Impingement Syndrome for an explanation of the hooked acromion.

Injury to the infraspinatus or teres minor is relatively easy to identify with palpation. These muscle-tendon units are easily palpable on the posterior shoulder region. Note that tears and tendinosis primarily occur in the musculotendinous junction, so careful exploration of this region with palpation is important.[33]

Identification of tensile stress injury to the subscapularis is more difficult due to its inaccessibility. While tendinosis in the subscapularis is rare, the muscle should be investigated especially in more traumatic shoulder injuries as subscapularis tears frequently accompany serious injuries. Use caution when attempting to palpate the subscapularis as the brachial plexus and the vascular structures of the upper extremity lie very close to the distal end of the muscle.[41]

Range-of-Motion and Resistance Testing

AROM: With supraspinatus tears or tendinosis, pain is likely with active abduction, due to contraction of the muscle-tendon unit or from impingement. With impingement there may be pain with active flexion as well.[42]

If the injury is to other rotator cuff muscles, active motion without significant resistance and starting with the shoulder in a neutral position while the client is vertical is not likely to reproduce pain. For example, lateral rotation from a neutral position does not recruit enough muscle fibers to exaggerate pain sensations from a posterior rotator cuff tear or tendinosis in general.

The same would be true for medial rotation if the subscapularis were damaged. However, there may be pain at the far end of active motion in the opposite direction of the muscle's concentric action due to stretching the damaged fibers. Posterior rotator cuff tears or tendinosis, for instance, may be painful at the end of active medial rotation, where the muscles are stretched.

PROM: Pain from tears or tendinosis in the supraspinatus can occur in abduction or flexion due to compression of damaged tissues. Pain in the other rotator cuff muscles happens only at the end range of motion when they are stretched. For example with posterior rotator cuff muscle damage, pain occurs at the end of medial rotation .

MRT: Pain and weakness from stressing the tissue and reflex muscular inhibition appears from rotator cuff tears or tendinosis when the primary action of the injured muscle is tested. Resisted abduction is painful and weak for a supraspinatus injury. Resisted lateral rotation is painful and weak for tears/tendinosis in the infraspinatus and teres minor muscles. Resisted medial rotation is painful with damage to the subscapularis. Weakness in medial rotation may not be as evident due to the additional muscles available to assist the subscapularis.

Special Test
Drop-Arm Test

Of the four rotator cuff muscles, the supraspinatus muscle is most frequently injured. The drop-arm test assesses only the supraspinatus. It usually yields a positive result only when a tear is more serious (2nd or 3rd degree). Tendinosis is not likely to show up in this test.

The client is standing and raises the affected arm to 90° of abduction. Watch the pattern of movement as the arm is abducted. The client may have difficulty bringing the arm into position and visible apprehension or discomfort may be evident with the movement. In addition, movement may not be smooth and coordinated. The client may drop the arm due to their inability to hold it in the abducted position.

If the client is able to hold the arm in the abducted position, the client should attempt to slowly lower the arm back down. A positive test is when the client is unable to smoothly lower the arm or there is significant pain with the action. In some cases the practitioner may place a slight resistance load on the arm and the additional load causes the arm to drop to the client's side (Figure 10.13).

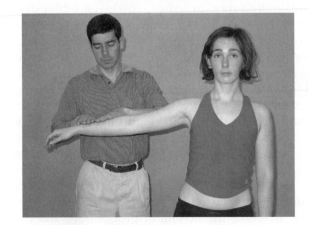

Figure 10.13 Drop-arm test.

Explanation: The supraspinatus plays a critical role in abducting the humerus. It must hold the head of the humerus close to the glenoid fossa so the deltoid can generate the power of abduction. When there is a sudden pain sensation in this region, the body's neurological system may shut off motor signals through **reflex muscular inhibition**. A load is placed on the supraspinatus from holding the arm in abduction, causing pain and producing an immediate reflex muscular inhibition. The arm has either a pattern of erratic movement or may completely drop as a result.

Differential Evaluation

Subacromial bursitis, shoulder impingement, calcific tendinitis, suprascapular neuropathy, bicipital tendinosis, cervical radiculopathy, myofascial trigger point referrals, acromioclavicular joint injury, frozen shoulder/adhesive capsulitis, glenohumeral subluxation.

Suggestions for Treatment

Rotator cuff tears and tendinosis are treated according to their severity and whether the injury is acute or chronic. These injuries should be treated with the same guidelines as other muscle strains or tendinosis. The primary focus is on reducing tissue dysfunction at the injury site to either encourage collagen production or facilitate healthy scar tissue repair. To accomplish this, deep transverse friction massage is performed. There will be difficulty accessing portions of the supraspinatus and subscapularis muscles due to their anatomical locations.

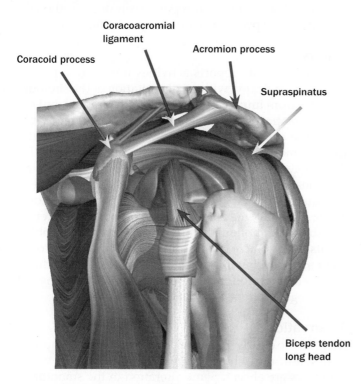

Figure 10.14 Lateral view of the left shoulder showing coracoacromial arch and soft tissues vulnerable to impingement. (3-D anatomy image courtesy of Primal Pictures Ltd. www.primalpictures.com.)

In addition, treatment includes lengthening affected muscles using deep longitudinal stripping, pin-and-stretch techniques, or passive or facilitated stretching. Practitioners should address hypertonic and compensating muscles, depending on when the injury happened. Grade 3 strains should be referred to another health professional, although massage may be helpful once the initial injury has had time, generally several weeks, for initial healing.

SHOULDER IMPINGEMENT SYNDROME

Shoulder impingement syndrome **involves compression of non-neural soft tissues between the head of the humerus and the underside of the coracoacromial arch.** Impingement may lead to tissue degeneration and is subsequently associated with a number of other shoulder disorders, such as *tendinosis, rotator cuff tears, calcific tendinitis, bone spurs,* and *subacromial bursitis.*

Characteristics

Soft-tissue impingement occurs in the shoulder as tissues are compressed underneath the **coracoacromial arch**. The arch is composed of the **acromion process, coracoacromial ligament**, and **coracoid process** (Figure 10.14).[43] Tissues vulnerable to compression under the arch include the upper margin of the **glenohumeral joint capsule, coracohumeral ligament, supraspinatus** muscle-tendon unit, long head of the **biceps brachii tendon**, and the **subacromial bursa**.

Impingement can result purely from the structure of the coracoacromial arch, but also results from a combination of coracoacromial architecture along with repetitive motions, especially those involving flexion and internal rotation of the humerus.[44] In some cases **bone spurs** or **osteophytes** develop on the underside of the acromion process and serve to further decrease the subacromial space and impinge tissues.[40] The space where the supraspinatus emerges from under the acromion process is also called the **supraspinatus outlet**.[45] Myofascial trigger points or hypertonic muscles in the shoulder region can also cause dysfunctional biomechanical relationships and lead to impingement problems.[8]

Shoulder impingement syndrome is described in terms of Neer's progressive stages (Box 10.6).[46] Stage 1 is more common in patients younger than 25 years. This stage is characterized by acute inflammation, edema, and hemorrhage in the affected tissues. Repeated overhead use of the upper extremity is usually involved. Stage 2 occurs more often in patients between 25 and 40 years old. There is progressive degeneration in the rotator cuff structures that involves fibrosis and tendon degeneration. Stage 3 generally affects patients older than 40 years. Tears of the supraspinatus and long head of the biceps tendon may develop. In addition, bone spurs and osteophytes may grow along the underside of the acromion and further contribute to subacromial impingement.

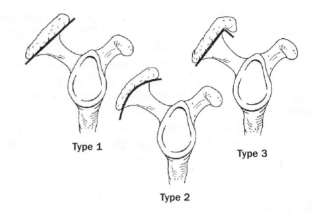

Figure 10.15 Acromion process types (Reproduced with permission from Magee D. Orthopedic Physical Assessment. 3rd ed. Philadelphia: W.B. Saunders; 1997.)

A further classification of impingement pathologies divides the conditions into primary or secondary categories. While both categories involve clients who perform repetitive overhead motion or constant overhead positions, primary impingement is caused by the architecture of the subacromial region.[43,47] Secondary impingement comes from underlying instability in the glenohumeral joint and faulty biomechanics, but does not necessarily involve decreases in the subacromial space.[48,49]

Primary impingement is directly related to the variations in shape of the acromion process and the corresponding subacromial space. Cadaveric studies indicate three variations in the shape of the acromion process (Figure 10.15).[40,50] **Type 1** acromion is present in approximately 17% of the population and has as a flat undersurface. **Type 2** has a curved undersurface and occurs in approximately 43% of the population. **Type 3** is referred to as a **hooked acromion** and is present in approximately 40% of the population. The hooked acromion is associated with a greater incidence of impingement and rotator cuff pathology.[40, 51] One study noted that in over 800 shoulder specimens the hooking of the acromion was not found in anyone under 30 years of age.[52] Apparently, hooking of the acromion results from calcification of the attachment of the coracoacromial ligament.

Secondary impingement also involves compression of structures under the coracoacromial arch, which is created by alterations in shoulder biomechanics. Instability in the glenohumeral joint leads to hypermobility of the humeral head during shoulder activities. As a result, structures in the subacromial region are more likely to be compressed during motion. Several biomechanical factors lead to secondary impingement including rotator cuff muscle weakness, posterior capsule tightness, and dysfunctional coordination of scapulothoracic muscles.[53,54]

Subacromial impingement results from repetitive overhead motions of the arm or long periods with the arm held overhead. In recreational activities impingement syndrome is common in swimmers and those involved in throwing activities. Occupational stresses, such as those mentioned in the Rotator Cuff Tears section, are also a cause of impingement.

Pain is ordinarily reported in the lateral or anterior region of the glenohumeral joint. The pain is associated with motions that increase soft-tissue compression, such as flexion, abduction, or medial rotation when the shoulder is flexed. Night pain is common because of tissue compression while sleeping in certain positions for long periods.[55] The client often reports pain deep in the joint and difficulty specifying the location of pain.

History

The client usually reports activities involving repetitive abduction or flexion with medial rotation of the shoulder. The pain from impingement is generally gradual, but certain traumatic injuries can alter glenohumeral mechanics and cause symptoms to come on acutely. Weakness that accompanies pain in certain movements is typical. The client may report an inability to lift the arm into certain positions when additional resistance is placed upon it.

Inquire about the client's age at the onset of symptoms. A young client may be able to perform more repetitive shoulder motions before an impingement problem results. Due to acromion process morphology, the older client may develop impingement with less activity due to a hooked acromion, bone spurs, osteophytes, or overall tissue degeneration.

Observation

There are no clearly observable signs of shoulder impingement syndrome. While there may be inflammation, visible indicators are absent. Some alteration in the smoothness of movement can take place during range-of-motion evaluation. There may also be visible apprehension when attempting to perform abduction or flexion.

During ROM evaluation, disturbances to the scapulohumeral rhythm are frequently visible (see Frozen Shoulder above). Compensating patterns of motion are evident as the client attempts to avoid pain during actions such as flexion and abduction. Postural distortions such as upper thoracic kyphosis and a medially rotated glenohumeral joint should be noted as they change glenohumeral mechanics and could lead to impingement.[53]

Palpation

It is difficult to produce the pain of the primary complaint because impingement occurs under the acromion process. However, if the impingement affects the distal supraspinatus tendon or the subacromial bursa, tenderness is common inferior to the acromion process on the lateral shoulder. Excess edema or other palpable signs of inflammation such as heat are normally not identifiable because of the depth of the tissues.

If the primary region of impingement is under the coracoacromial ligament, the biceps brachii long head tendon is usually affected. In this case, palpating the anterior shoulder region, particularly if performed with the shoulder in flexion, may reproduce pain.

Range-of-Motion and Resistance Testing

AROM: Pain increases with motions that further compress the tissues under the coracoacromial arch. These motions include abduction and flexion. Active movements recruiting the supraspinatus elicit pain and limitation. Pain avoidance may accompany a lack of coordination. Compare AROM findings in these positions with the passive tests to identify any increased role of contractile tissues.

PROM: As with active motion, pain is elicited during abduction or flexion. Pain is likely to be increased with medial rotation when the shoulder is already in flexion (see the Hawkins-Kennedy test below). Other motions of the shoulder are generally not painful especially if performed from a neutral (anatomical) position.

MRT: Resisted abduction and flexion may be painful. Because elbow flexion is a primary action of the biceps brachii, resisted elbow flexion might also reproduce the primary pain if the biceps tendon is affected. Weakness in abduction or flexion is common due to reflex muscular inhibition. Pain is not likely in other resisted motions if performed from a neutral position.

Special Tests

Hawkins-Kennedy Impingement Test

The client is standing facing the practitioner. The practitioner brings the client's shoulder and elbow into 90° of flexion. From this point the humerus is medially rotated (passively) until the end range of motion is met (Figure 10.16). If this movement reproduces the client's primary discomfort, there is a good chance that tissue is impinged under the coracoacromial arch.

Explanation: When the humerus is brought into 90° of flexion some of the anterior tissues, such as the biceps

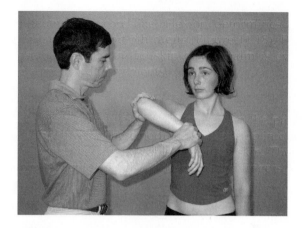

Figure 10.16 Hawkins-Kennedy Impingement test.

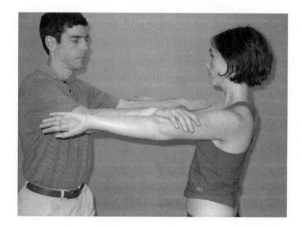

Figure 10.17 Empty can test.

brachii long head and the anterior-superior margin of the glenohumeral joint capsule, are compressed under the coracoacromial arch. As the humerus is medially rotated from the flexed position, those tissues as well as the supraspinatus tendon and coracohumeral ligament are compressed under the arch and pain is expected. This test does not determine the exact tissues affected because numerous tissues can be compressed in the final position.

Empty Can Test

The empty can test is usually performed bilaterally, even when one shoulder is symptomatic. The non-affected side is used for comparison. If pain is reproduced at any of the point during the test, continuing the test is unnecessary.

The client faces the practitioner. From this position the client brings both arms into 45° of horizontal adduction. The client is asked about pain or discomfort as the position is held. With the arms in partial horizontal adduction, the client is instructed to medially rotate the arms, as if emptying cans held in the hands (Figure 10.17). At the end of this motion the practitioner asks about pain or discomfort. The client holds the arms in the final position

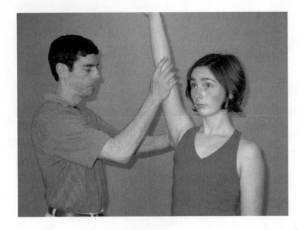

Figure 10.18 Neer impingement test.

while the practitioner attempts to push both arms down with moderate effort. Pain that reproduces the primary complaint is a positive result.

Explanation: The final positioning of the glenohumeral joint is similar to that used in the Hawkins-Kennedy impingement sign described above (flexion with medial rotation). However, the final step of the test engages the supraspinatus in a resisted isometric contraction. The practitioner should evaluate pain at each point in the test. Pain could indicate impingement of soft tissues under the coracoacromial arch. If pain is most exaggerated with the final step, it is a good indication that the supraspinatus is the primary tissue involved because it is engaged in resisted contraction.[56]

Neer Impingement Test

The client faces the practitioner. The practitioner slowly brings the client's arm into full forward flexion (Figure 10.18). The practitioner watches for signs of apprehension and asks about pain or discomfort during the movement. Pain that reproduces the primary discomfort is a positive test and indicative of soft-tissue impingement under the coracoacromial arch.

Explanation: When the humerus is brought into full flexion, the anterior and superior soft tissues under the coracoacromial arch are vulnerable to compression. Pain is likely caused by impingement of the long head of the biceps brachii, the anterior-superior portion of the glenohumeral joint capsule, and/or the coracohumeral ligament.[57] This is a passive positional test and does not recruit any particular muscle-tendon unit so specific information about muscle involvement is not evident.

Differential Evaluation

Subacromial bursitis, rotator cuff tears, rotator cuff tendinosis, calcific tendinitis, suprascapular neuropathy, frozen shoulder/adhesive capsulitis, acromioclavicular joint injury, bicipital tendinosis, brachial plexus pathology, cervical disc radiculopathy, myofascial trigger point pain, thoracic outlet syndrome, labral damage.

Suggestions for Treatment

This condition involves soft-tissue impingement under the coracoacromial arch. To best address the condition compression of the tissues must be reduced. If the problem is sufficiently advanced, surgery may be an appropriate choice in reshaping the acromion process.[58] In some cases, the pathology can be addressed with conservative treatments that focus on correcting dysfunctional biomechanics, such as reducing or eliminating offending activities.[53, 59] Myofascial trigger points or hypertonic muscles should be addressed with massage and stretching. Treating the surrounding muscles may be helpful in addressing this complaint.

SUBACROMIAL BURSITIS

Due to its location the **subacromial bursa** can be compressed under the coracoacromial arch from acute trauma or repetitive stress, causing *subacromial bursitis* (see also Shoulder Impingement Syndrome).[60, 61]

Characteristics

To prevent compression of soft tissues against the bone, there is a **bursa** under the **acromion**. The bursa is sometimes described as two separate bursae because it covers such a large region and may have a small division in it. The upper portion under the acromion process is the **subacromial bursa** (Figure 10.19). The more distal portion, under the deltoid muscle, is called the **subdeltoid bursa**. When the arm is fully abducted the bursa moves up under the acromion process.

Pressure on the bursa is a primary cause of bursitis, but inflammation can also result from autoimmune diseases such as *rheumatoid arthritis*, infection, *gout*, *calcific deposits*, or other systemic disorders.[61] The symptoms and patterns of pain are the same as for shoulder impingement. Pain is commonly reported in the lateral or anterior region of the glenohumeral joint. The pain is associated with motions that increase soft-tissue compression, such as flexion, abduction, or medial rotation when the arm is flexed. Night pain is characteristic because of tissue compression while sleeping.[55] The client often reports pain deep in the joint and difficulty identifying a specific location of pain.

In many cases the client demonstrates a **painful arc** during abduction, with pain only appearing in a portion of the movement.[62] Pain begins shortly after initiating abduction and continues to about 135°. After this point, no pain is generally experienced during the remainder of abduction (Figure 10.20). The arc of pain takes place because irritated tissue, in this case the bursa, is compressed as the client abducts the shoulder. After a certain amount of abduction, the irritated tissue moves proximally under the acromion process and is no longer compressed. The painful arc is frequently indicative of a problem in the subacromial bursa, but other soft tissues demonstrate the same painful arc as they move under the acromion process. For example, the painful arc occurs with *rotator cuff tears*, *tendinosis*, and *calcific tendinitis*.[50]

Subacromial bursitis can develop from repetitive compressive activities or from an impact trauma with a high compressive load. Similar to *shoulder impingement*, subacromial bursitis results from repetitive overhead motions of the arm or long periods with the arm held overhead. People involved in swimming or throwing activities also experience the condition, as well as those in certain occupations (see Shoulder Impingement above).

History

Subacromial bursitis pain is typically described as a dull shoulder ache. The client usually reports activities involving repetitive abduction or flexion with medial rotation of the shoulder. Pain is primarily gradual, but certain traumatic injuries can alter glenohumeral mechanics and cause symptoms to come on acutely. Identify the presence of any systemic disorders, infectious conditions, or autoimmune pathologies that could initiate inflammation of the bursa.

Ask about symptoms indicating infection or swelling in other regions of the body, which would also suggest a systemic infection that could have acutely inflamed the bursa. Weakness that accompanies pain in certain movements is likely. Ask about the client's age at the onset of symptoms. A young client may be able to perform more repetitive shoulder motions before developing bursitis. Subacromial bursitis is more typical as the client ages.

Observation

Swelling in the subacromial bursa is not visible because it is deep to the bony structure of the shoulder girdle. Alterations in smooth movement or facial apprehension signs may be evident during active and passive motion evaluation. Limitations to smooth movement are most apparent during abduction.

Palpation

If subacromial bursitis is the only presenting pathology, palpation may not elicit tenderness because the acromion process prevents access. If the portion of the bursa causing the problem is more distal (the subdeltoid portion), pain will be elicited with palpation inferior to the lateral edge of the acromion process near the greater tubercle of the humerus. The surrounding muscles may be tender, but not always. It is typical for surrounding shoulder muscles to be hypertonic. Local tenderness could exist from systemic disorders.

Range-of-Motion and Resistance Testing

AROM: Pain is expected with motion that further compresses the bursa. The bursa is likely to be irritated by abduction, but also by flexion. There may be weakness or lack of smoothness in these motions, caused by reflex muscular inhibition. Watch for the presence of a painful arc during active abduction of the arm.

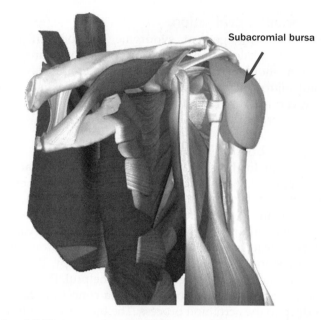

Figure 10.19 Anterior/lateral view of the left shoulder showing the subacromial bursa. A portion lies under the acromion process. (3-D anatomy image courtesy of Primal Pictures Ltd. www.primalpictures.com.)

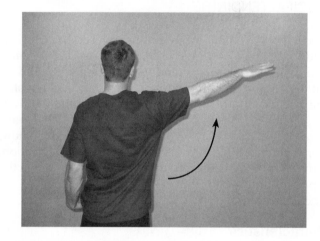

Figure 10.20 Painful arc demonstration. Pain begins with abduction, continues through about 135°, then subsides.

PROM: Pain occurs in both abduction and forward flexion and is usually the same as that felt during active movement. A painful arc may be present in PROM as well.

MRT: Typically, there is no increase in pain with an MRT. Unless the bursa is being compressed at the point where the test is performed, there is no additional compression by muscular contractions. The lack of pain during an MRT is one helpful way to differentiate bursitis from other muscle-tendon pathologies, such as *supraspinatus impingement* or *rotator cuff tears* and *tendinosis*. Weakness during resisted abduction or flexion may result from reflex muscular inhibition if the bursa is being compressed in the starting position.

Differential Evaluation

Shoulder impingement syndrome, rotator cuff tears, tendinosis, calcific tendinitis, suprascapular neuropathy, frozen shoulder/adhesive capsulitis, acromioclavicular joint injury, bicipital tendinosis, brachial plexus pathology, cervical disc radiculopathy, myofascial trigger point pain, thoracic outlet syndrome, labral damage.

Suggestions for Treatment

Treatment for bursitis requires reducing the inflammation and alleviating additional pressure on the bursa. Traditional treatments for bursitis include oral anti-inflammatory medication or corticosteroid injection. Massage cannot directly treat the inflamed bursa. Various soft-tissue techniques are used to relax the shoulder girdle muscles and are an effective adjunct therapy. Reducing hypertonicity in shoulder muscles is helpful. Pressing on the inflamed bursa is normally not a concern because it is deep to the acromion process. The bursa's depth is also a reason that topical thermal treatments, such as moist heat, are helpful for decreasing muscle tension but not contraindicated in treatment (as ultrasound would be).

CALCIFIC TENDINITIS

Tendinitis is usually an inflammatory condition in the tendon that results from chronic overuse. *Calcific tendinitis* is different and is **a tendon condition produced by the deposit of calcium hydroxyapatite crystals** (crystalline calcium phosphate). This condition is different from the calcium deposits that occur in tendons that have degenerated due to age or injury. Tendons in the elbow, hip, knee, and ankle may also be affected by calcification. In the shoulder, calcific tendinitis occurs most often in the **supraspinatus tendon**, but can develop in any of the rotator cuff tendons.[63, 64, 65]

Characteristics

There is controversy about what produces calcific tendinitis. The condition previously was thought to be a result of age or tissue degeneration. However, the calcium deposits of calcific tendinitis (phosphates) are different from the calcium salts found in *degenerative calcification*. Although the etiology has not been determined, there are several generally accepted aspects of the condition. The deposits do not appear to be caused by trauma or systemic disease.[63] For example, they are seldom related to *rotator cuff tears*. While it is conceivable that calcification could be involved in impingement, many researchers see no correlation.[63,65, 66]

Calcium deposits disappear and reabsorb just as readily as they appear. The fact that the calcification can spontaneously heal strengthens the argument that it is not related to a degenerative process. In addition, these calcium deposits are found in healthy tissue and in people younger than would be expected with degenerative calcification. The disorder is most common in clients

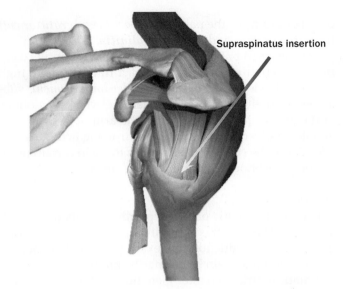

Figure 10.21 Superior view of the left shoulder. Calcific tendinitis affects the supraspinatus tendon most. (3-D anatomy image courtesy of Primal Pictures Ltd. www.primalpictures.com.)

between 30 and 60 years of age and affects women more than men.[63,67] An X-ray is usually necessary to identify calcific tendinitis.

Calcium deposits are usually located 1-2 cm proximal to the **supraspinatus insertion** (Figure 10.21). Due to location of the supraspinatus beneath the **acromion process**, calcific tendinitis can be mistaken for *supraspinatus tendinitis/tendinosis*, which involve tears or impingement. There are 4 phases to calcific tendinitis. In the **formative phase**, the deposit develops and enlarges. The condition then proceeds through a **resting phase**, where the deposit may or may not produce pain but can produce mechanical dysfunction if big enough. The **resorptive phase** involves inflammation that works to break the deposit down. This phase can be quite painful. Finally, in the **postcalcific phase** the deposit is fully reabsorbed and the tendon heals.[68]

Pain with calcific tendinitis varies across a spectrum from no pain to severe pain. The deposits are found in asymptomatic people and those with shoulder pain not related to the calcification. Calcium deposits present in 3-20% of people without shoulder pain and 7% of people with shoulder pain.[63] When the condition produces pain, the symptoms resemble *shoulder impingement syndrome* and can result in intense pain. Pain can come on rapidly, sometimes within 24-48 hours, which can help distinguish the condition from impingement pain, rotator cuff disorders, and *frozen shoulder*.[69] Night pain from sleeping positions is common. Rest may or may not provide pain relief. Shoulder position can also be unrelated to pain, although pain may increase when the arm is raised above the shoulder. Some clients report an inability to find a pain-free position, even with the arm motionless.[69,70]

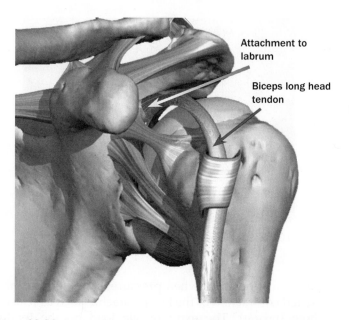

Figure 10.22 Anterior view of the left shoulder. Biceps long head tendon turns across the top of the humerus and attaches to the supraglenoid tubercle (not visible). (3-D anatomy image courtesy of Primal Pictures Ltd. www.primalpictures.com.)

History
The client usually reports sharp pain in the shoulder region that came on suddenly. Pain is often described as similar to a toothache in its deep, throbbing nature. In addition to pain, limited shoulder motion is commonly reported. The pain pattern is different from that of overuse tendinitis/tendinosis, which comes on gradually instead of suddenly. Clients report pain during activity as well as at rest. Ask about positions that produce or relieve pain. Failure to identify consistent positions that decrease pain is indicative of the condition.

Observation
There are no specific findings with observation. Visible apprehension and movement guarding are common during range-of-motion evaluations due to pain avoidance. Motions of the shoulder, especially in abduction or flexion are often irregular due to pain or altered biomechanics. Reflex muscular inhibition can cause enough weakness to make movements visibly uncoordinated.

Palpation
Pain with palpation in the region of the greater tuberosity of the humerus is likely to be severe and mimic the client's pain. There may be residual tenderness in surrounding muscles, along with hypertonicity. While this condition is described as a tendinitis, swelling is rarely evident so palpable indicators of inflammation are absent.[69]

Range-of-Motion and Resistance Testing
AROM: Pain may be present with compression of irritated tissues and is most probable in abduction or flexion. When pain is present, a painful arc during abduction of the shoulder is possible (see discussion in the Subacromial Bursitis section). Motion, if painful, may be erratic due to pain. However, calcific tendinitis is not always painful with motion, so lack of pain with ROM evaluation does not indicate absence of the condition.
PROM: The same principles apply as for active motion.
MRT: Resisted abduction of the shoulder may or may not produce pain as the affected tendon is recruited. There may be pain in other resisted actions where the affected tendon is not recruited.

Differential Evaluation
Rotator cuff tears, tendinosis, shoulder impingement syndrome, frozen shoulder/adhesive capsulitis, glenoid labrum injuries, bicipital tendinosis, labral damage, cervical disc pathology, thoracic outlet syndrome.

Suggestions for Treatment
A clear treatment protocol for calcific tendinitis has not been established. In most cases it is treated with conservative measures including stretching, rest and shoulder slings, along with anti-inflammatory medications. Treatments are used to relieve stress on the supraspinatus tendon. Breaking up the calcification is also performed by extracorporeal shock wave therapy, similar to treatments for kidney stones and bone spurs.[67]

Consult the client's physician for appropriate guidance about any possible use of massage. Massage could be contraindicated as it could damage fibers. Soft-tissue therapy may have a possible role in the final resorptive phase to break up calcification in the tissue, but no research documents this use and pain may prevent this treatment.

BICIPITAL TENDINOSIS

When *tendinosis* develops in the anterior shoulder region, it usually affects the long head of the biceps brachii. Either the **long or short heads of the biceps are susceptible to the collagen degeneration process** of tendinosis, but the long head is more vulnerable because of increased friction in the bicipital groove.[71]

Characteristics
The **biceps long head tendon** makes a right-angled turn as it courses across the top of the **humerus** before attaching to the **supraglenoid tubercle** of the scapula (Figure 10.22). The tendon is at a mechanical disadvantage because the sharp turn increases friction between bone and tendon. The tendon is surrounded by a **synovial sheath** to reduce friction against the sides of the **bicipital groove**. Friction between the tendon and its sheath can cause *tenosynovitis*, as well as tendinosis. On the anterior humerus, the upper portion of the tendon is pressed firmly into the **bicipital groove** where it plays a fundamental role in maintaining the position of the humeral head and preventing dislocation.[72, 73] While tendinosis can

affect any region of the tendon, it is most apt to occur in the upper portion of the long head.

Repetitive motions involving flexion of the shoulder, elbow, or supination of the forearm can cause chronic tendon overload. These movements are primary actions of the biceps brachii. Bicipital tendinosis characteristically results from occupational activities. For example, repeated supination from using a screwdriver or resisting the torque of a rotary power drill could overwhelm the tendon. Cumulative stress of the tendon leads to collagen degeneration within the tendon fibers (tendinosis). Despite the fact that overuse problems of the biceps tendon infrequently demonstrate inflammatory activity, the term *tendinitis* is still used.[74]

Bicipital tendinosis or tenosynovitis could also result from impingement of the tendon under the **coracoacromial arch**.[74, 75] In this case, the presentation of pain is similar to that of rotator cuff tears or tendinosis and the condition may be perceived as a rotator cuff or impingement pathology. Misdiagnosis of bicipital tendinosis can result and is not unusual. Tendinosis and tenosynovitis are rarely a result of acute trauma and the onset of symptoms is gradual.

Additional problems can occur at the attachment site of the biceps brachii long head at the supraglenoid tubercle of the scapula. The tendon has fibrous attachments to the superior margin of the glenoid labrum. Consistent tensile loads sufficient to produce tendinosis may also cause tearing or damage to the glenoid labrum and cause a *SLAP lesion*. See the discussion of SLAP lesions in the Glenoid Labrum Injuries section below.

History

The client reports diffuse, aching pain in the anterior shoulder region which may radiate to the elbow. Pain can be aggravated by elbow flexion or forearm supination with significant resistance. Pain is worse during overhead motions of the upper extremity or when lifting or pulling heavy objects. It is common for the client to report repetitive elbow or shoulder activity prior symptom onset. Pay close attention to the description of the activity to determine if the biceps brachii is involved. Rest from offending activity usually relieves symptoms. Pain might be felt at the onset of an activity but then subsides during the activity, only to recur later when activity ceases.

Observation

There are no visual factors to identify bicipital tendinosis. Although the condition is frequently described as *tendinitis*, inflammation is rare.[39] Even in the event of an inflammatory tendinitis, visible inflammation is not common. There may be observable patterns of movement restriction caused by pain avoidance, especially during active flexion of the shoulder.

Palpation

There is tenderness over the long head of the biceps bra-

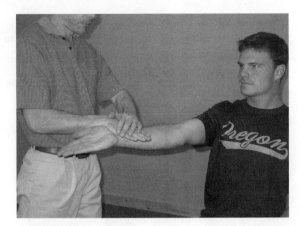

Figure 10.23 Speed's test.

chii, which increases when pressure is applied during a resisted contraction of the biceps brachii (such as resisted elbow flexion). The extra tensile load on the tendon makes it more sensitive to palpation. Hypertonicity may be present in nearby shoulder muscles. Myofascial trigger points sometimes develop in response to the tissue dysfunction and may elicit characteristic referral patterns when palpated.

Range-of-Motion and Resistance Testing

AROM: If pain is elicited in active flexion of the shoulder it is usually due to impingement of the tendon under the coracoacromial arch and not from the load on the tendon. Pain is unlikely with active elbow flexion or forearm supination because the amount of tension on the tendon during active movement without additional resistance is not sufficient to stress the tendon. As the biceps brachii is stretched at the far end of active elbow and shoulder extension, there may be pain.

PROM: As with active motion, shoulder flexion can produce pain due to impingement. Pain may occur at the end of passive shoulder extension from stretching of the muscle-tendon unit and pulling the long head of the biceps against the anterior humeral head.

MRT: Pain and/or weakness may be evident during resisted shoulder flexion, elbow flexion, supination, or combinations of these motions. Elbow flexion and supination are better motions to evaluate during manual resistive tests as they more effectively isolate the long head of the biceps brachii. The short head contributes more to shoulder flexion.[7]

Special Test
Speed's Test

The client stands with 90^0 of shoulder flexion, the elbow fully extended, and the forearm supinated. The client attempts to hold the position as the practitioner applies downward pressure (Figure 10.23). If pain is reproduced during contraction and resistance, it is a positive test.

Another variation is also used. Once the client's arm is in the position above, the practitioner pushes the client's arm toward the floor while the client slowly releases the contraction. Pain felt during the eccentric movement is a positive test. The resisted eccentric contraction is more challenging than the static muscle resistance, so the tests are performed in above order.

Explanation: The starting position is such that when pressure is applied by the practitioner, all three actions of the biceps brachii are engaged simultaneously and the increased load reproduces the client's symptoms.[76] In the second variation, the client slowly allows the arm to be lowered (moving in extension). This engages an eccentric contraction in the biceps brachii. In addition to the eccentric contraction, the tendon from the long head of the biceps brachii slides in the bicipital groove as the shoulder moves in extension. If there is tendinosis or tenosynovitis in the tendon, this movement against the humerus with the tendon under tensile load causes the primary pain to be reproduced.

Differential Evaluation
Shoulder impingement syndrome, subacromial bursitis, upper extremity nerve entrapments, acromioclavicular joint pathology, rotator cuff disorders, glenoid labrum damage, frozen shoulder/adhesive capsulitis, arthritis.

Suggestions for Treatment
Treatment for bicipital tendinosis follows the same protocol as for other tendinosis conditions. Massage is particularly helpful. Emphasis is placed on reducing tension on the affected muscle-tendon unit through stripping and broadening techniques as well as general effleurage and superficial sweeping cross-fiber techniques.

The primary tissue dysfunction of collagen degeneration must be addressed, which is best treated with deep friction massage. However due to the position of the bicipital tendon, transverse friction to the tendon should be avoided. There is a possibility that the tendon could be subluxed from the bicipital groove if too much pressure is applied in a transverse direction, especially if there is weakness in the transverse humeral ligament.[55] Pressure and movement, regardless of the direction, stimulate collagen production, so deep longitudinal friction is safest and just as effective.[77]

SHOULDER SEPARATION

Shoulder separation is an informal term for **a sprain to the ligaments of the acromioclavicular or coracoclavicular joints**. This condition is not the same as a *shoulder dislocation*, which involves the translation of the humerus (see Glenohumeral Dislocation below). Shoulder separations are common injuries in contact sports, occupational activities, and automobile accidents.

Characteristics
In a shoulder separation, the injury occurs at the **acromioclavicular joint (AC joint)**, which is where the **acromion** and the **clavicle** meet. The primary causes of separations involve the shoulder being struck by a falling object or the individual falling directly on the shoulder.[78] In the injury, the stabilizing ligaments of the AC joint are sprained. The **acromioclavicular (AC) ligament** stabilizes the AC joint and the **conoid** and **trapezoid ligaments** stabilize the **clavicle** and the **coracoid process** of the **scapula** (Figures

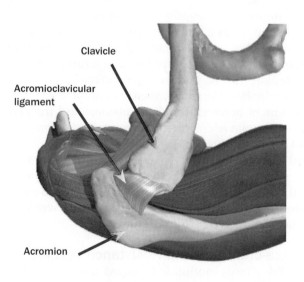

Figure 10.24 Superior view of the left acromioclavicular joint. (3-D anatomy image courtesy of Primal Pictures Ltd. www.primalpictures.com.)

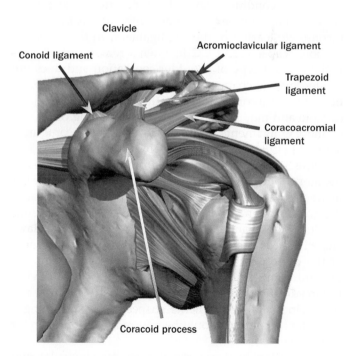

Figure 10.25 Anterior shoulder view. (3-D anatomy image courtesy of Primal Pictures Ltd. www.primalpictures.com.)

Box 10.7 Shoulder Separation Types

Type 1

AC ligament not completely torn

Joint capsule intact

CC ligaments intact

No structural changes

Type 2

AC ligament completely torn

Joint capsule torn

CC ligaments possibly stretched or torn

Collarbone may be misaligned

Type 3

AC ligament completely torn

Joint capsule torn

CC ligaments significantly damaged

Distal clavicle forced inferiorly

Deltoid and trapezius possibly torn

10.24, 10.25). The conoid and trapezoid are sometimes referred to as one structure called the **coracoclavicular (CC) ligament(s)**. It is the AC ligament that is usually injured in a shoulder separation, but more severe injuries affect the coracoclavicular ligament complex as well.

The severity of the injury ranges from mild to a severe, deforming condition. Shoulder separations are categorized into three types.[79, 80] **Type 1** separations involve an incomplete tearing of the AC ligament. In these sprains the joint capsule and CC ligaments remain intact. This is the mildest type of shoulder separation and does not create physical changes in the structures. **Type 2** separations involve a complete tear of the AC ligament and joint capsule and may also involve some stretching or tearing of the CC ligaments. The collarbone may become misaligned in this type and more pain results.

Type 3 separations involve a complete tear of the AC ligament, joint capsule, and significant damage to the CC ligaments. These sprains are the most serious and cause the greatest pain and loss of stability. Type 3 separations produce significant alteration in the position of the **clavicle**, which can displace and cause tearing or detachment of the **deltoid** or **trapezius**, causing obvious structural disfiguration.[80] In these severe injuries, the distal clavicle is forced inferiorly so that it approximates the first rib, producing a bulge.[81] Clients suspected of sustaining a shoulder separation should be referred to a physician for further evaluation.

In addition to damaging the acromioclavicular and coracoclavicular ligaments, falls or impacts to this region can cause a sprain and/or dislocation to the **sternoclavic-**

ular joint. *Sternoclavicular sprains* are not as common, but can be serious because a dislocation of the proximal end of the clavicle may cause it to press on or rupture the trachea or jugular vein.[82] Sprains or dislocations at the sternoclavicular joint are considered a separate pathology and are not called shoulder separations.

If the clavicular disruption has compressed the **brachial plexus,** the client may report symptoms such as pain, numbness, paresthesia, or weakness in the upper extremity. In these cases, an acute traction injury to the brachial plexus might be suspected when in fact a shoulder separation has caused acute *brachial plexus compression*.

History

A client with shoulder separation reports a sudden traumatic injury to the lateral shoulder region, which may include falling on the shoulder or a strong blow to the area. Sharp, intense pain is experienced at the time of injury and ligament damage causes subsequent tenderness. The client reports pain during various movements of the shoulder. Night pain develops due to the client's sleeping position.[79]

Observation

Due to ligament tearing, visible swelling may be observed. If the trauma is severe enough, capillaries are ruptured and bruising results. In Type 2 and 3 separations there is dislocation of the distal clavicle. Clavicular dislocation appears as a pronounced bump or divot at the AC joint compared to the other side.[81] Movement restrictions and apprehension due to pain are observable during range-of-motion testing.

Palpation

The AC joint is painful with palpation. The level of tenderness depends on severity of the injury. A Type 1 injury is not as tender as a Type 3 injury. The distal clavicle might be somewhat mobile when palpated as a result of ligament damage. For comparison, determine the mobility present at the AC joint in the unaffected shoulder when it is palpated. Generally, there is only a slight degree of movement between the distal clavicle and the acromion when the clavicle is pressed. Excess movement will exist as long as fibrous scar tissue has not had time to develop and bind the clavicle into a new position. For example, if the shoulder separation was two years prior there could still be a partial clavicular dislocation, but no movement when the distal clavicle is pressed because scar tissue has adhered the clavicle into position.

Range-of-Motion and Resistance Testing

AROM: Active motion is expected to be painful in flexion, abduction, or horizontal adduction. These motions place stress on the AC joint as well as the CC ligaments. Movement restriction and decreased range of motion occur due to pain avoidance.

PROM: Same principles apply as for active movement.

MRT: Pain or weakness is not usually evident during resisted movement of the shoulder if the test is performed in a position close to neutral for the shoulder. However, due to muscle attachments on the clavicle, such as the deltoid, trapezius, or pectoralis major, resisted motions that involve these muscles may be painful as they pull the clavicle and stress the damaged ligaments. In addition, because Type 3 sprains may cause a tear or detachment of the trapezius or deltoid muscle, resisted motions that recruit these muscles are weak and painful.

Special Test
Cross Over Test
The client is standing or seated. The practitioner brings the client's arm into full horizontal adduction to evaluate pain reproduction (Figure 10.26). If the primary complaint is reproduced, it is a positive test. To minimize the client's discomfort the test can be performed passively. Because horizontal adduction stresses the ligaments of the distal clavicular region, and ligaments are inert tissues, it does not matter if the action is performed actively or passively. There may be benefit in performing the test passively so no accessory muscle activity is involved and the client's pain is reduced.

Explanation: When the arm is brought across the chest in horizontal adduction, the distal clavicle is pressed against the acromion process and pushes against the edge of the acromion. If the ligaments are intact, they prevent accessory motion at the articulation. With damage to the AC or CC ligaments, there is tensile stress on the resisting ligaments and pain results.

Differential Evaluation
Glenoid labrum injury, subacromial bursitis, shoulder impingement, rotator cuff pathology, clavicular fracture, glenohumeral subluxation or dislocation, humeral or scapular fracture.

Suggestions for Treatment
Physical therapy is a common course of treatment to reestablish stability in the acromioclavicular complex. The clavicle should be in the proper position when the ligaments start the rebuilding process and scar tissue develops. An arm sling is generally used for this purpose.[83] In some cases the clavicle heals in a slightly different position. The altered position rarely causes long-term functional impairment and is primarily a cosmetic issue because there is an enlarged bump at the AC joint from the protruding distal end of the clavicle.

Deep friction massage is helpful to encourage collagen rebuilding in the damaged ligament fibers. However if the tear is severe, friction should not be performed until well after the initial inflammatory phase (up to 72 hours post-injury). If the injury is more severe, a longer period of delay is warranted and consultation with a physician is recommended. Massage and stretching are useful to prevent spasm of the surrounding muscles or the devel-

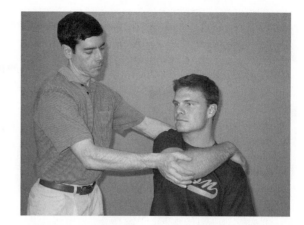

Figure 10.26 Cross over test.

opment of capsular adhesions due to the long periods of relative immobility that may be necessary to encourage ligament rebuilding.

GLENOHUMERAL DISLOCATION/ SUBLUXATION

Due to its range of motion, the **glenohumeral joint** is dislocated more than other joints.[84] **The joint can be completely forced out of the joint capsule, partially translated, or forced out with an immediate return to position.** *Glenohumeral (shoulder) dislocations* are common injuries in contact sports, occupational activities, and automobile/motorcycle accidents.

Characteristics
The bony contact surface between the head of the **humerus** and the **glenoid fossa** is minimal because the humeral head is larger and the glenoid fossa is relatively flat, although it is described as a ball-and-socket joint (Figure 10.27). A true ball-and-socket joint, such as the iliofemoral, has more stability due to the amount of bony contact between the femoral head and the deeper socket of the acetabulum. In the glenohumeral joint, the socket is shallower, but is deepened by the **glenoid labrum** surrounding the rim of the glenoid fossa. The ligaments, labrum, and joint capsule play a primary role in maintaining stability of the humerus for shoulder motion.

When the head of the humerus is forced out of the glenoid fossa and stays out, the injury is called a *glenohumeral dislocation*. A *subluxation* is when the joint is partially dislocated and the humeral head does not fully move out of the fossa or when the humeral head moves out of the fossa and then returns.[84] Dislocations and subluxations can result from chronic instability or traumatic injury. The majority of dislocations initially result from traumatic forces, which can then lead to instability and repeated dislocation or subluxation in the future.

If instability is present in the glenohumeral joint, strong forces are not needed to dislocate the shoulder . The client

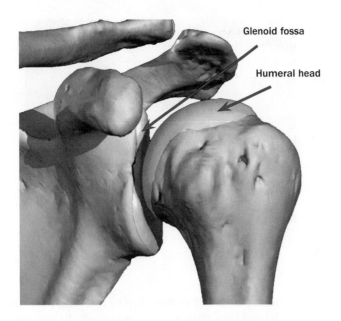

Glenoid fossa

Humeral head

Figure 10.27 Anterior view of the glenohumeral joint; glenoid labrum not shown. (3-D anatomy image courtesy of Primal Pictures Ltd. www.primalpictures.com.)

with a history of instability or subluxation/dislocation is more susceptible to dislocation. These problems are often recurrent, especially in athletes or adolescents, and young athletes in particular.[85] Once the ligaments in the region are stretched from prior injury, the joint is vulnerable to dislocation or subluxation. Shoulder instability involves a range of disorders from mild laxity and hypermobility to severe dislocation; it can create disability and lifelong physical impairment.[86, 87] Instability can occur in a single direction, such as anterior instability, or be in several directions, which is described as multi-directional instability. *Anterior instability* is the most common and accounts for close to 95% of all shoulder instabilities.[5]

Instability can also result from repetitive shoulder motions that place tensile stress on the shoulder's ligaments or joint capsule. In particular, repeated throwing motions produce instability from the constant tensile stress on tissues.[86, 88] Once instability develops it leads to a continuum of problems such as subluxation, *impingement, rotator cuff pathology*, and eventually *dislocation*.[89] Repeated subluxations or dislocations can be a precursor to *tendinosis, arthritis, nerve injuries of the brachial plexus, fractures, bone spurs,* or *labral damage*.[87, 90-92]

Systemic diseases, such as *Ehlers-Danlos* or *Marfan syndromes*, can cause wide-scale ligamentous laxity.[93, 94] *Laxity* allows the humeral head to be passively translated (as opposed to the normal motions of rolling) within the glenoid fossa, but the motion does not cause pain or impair function. Laxity can make an individual susceptible to subluxation or dislocation.[95]

The direction of subluxation or dislocation is related to the forces applied to the glenohumeral joint. The largest number of dislocations are anterior and occur with a combination of abduction and lateral rotation of the

humerus, which is also likely to cause a *Bankart lesion*.[85, 96] A Bankart lesion is an avulsion of the glenohumeral joint capsule and labrum from the inferior glenoid rim (see Glenoid Labrum Injuries next).[97, 98]

Subluxations are not usually as painful as dislocations, but the level of pain depends on the status of the humeral head. There may or may not be pain if the humeral head returns to position after being forced out of the joint. In some cases subluxations are not painful at all.[90] If the humeral head is in a partially dislocated position, it may be painful due to additional pressure on the edge of the glenoid labrum. If there is a suspicion of a dislocation, the client should be immediately referred to a physician who can properly reduce the dislocation in order to prevent damage to neurovascular structures.[84] Clients with suspected subluxation may also need referral to a physician who can diagnose the level of injury.

Clients who have experienced a glenohumeral subluxation will report a movement or impact that caused sudden pain and a significant decrease in range of motion. Muscle spasm immediately after the incident will continue to limit range of motion. If the joint has moved back into position, pain gradually subsides, but muscle spasm may linger. If the client suffers a dislocation, there will be very sharp immediate pain with a complete inability to use the arm. Due to pain, the arm is usually held close to the side in an effort to prevent movement. *Muscle spasm* accompanies the dislocation and is likely to remain for some time after the dislocation has been reduced (put back in position).

History

The client reports a sudden force to the shoulder that causes severe pain, and which is followed by the inability to move the arm. When possible, identify the mechanics of the injury to determine whether the trauma involved motions that produce dislocations or subluxations (abduction and lateral rotation in particular). The client is likely to hold the arm in an adducted and internally rotated position in an effort to avoid pain. Ask about the level of pain associated with the injury. The client may report self-reducing (replacing) the dislocated joint, especially if it is a recurring injury. Ask about a history of dislocation or subluxation. If there was no acute trauma, ask about any history of systemic conditions that result in ligamentous laxity or repetitious activities that would produce instability.

Observation

A client with a glenohumeral dislocation holds the arm close to the body to prevent further movement that might increase pain. In addition, a **sulcus** or indentation may be visible just below the edge of the acromion process indicating a shift in the position of the humeral head (Figure 10.28). The sulcus is only visible if the shoulder remains dislocated. If there is sufficient trauma associated with the dislocation or subluxation, there may observable signs of inflammation such as redness and edema.

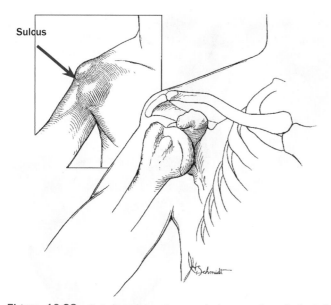

Figure 10.28 Anterior dislocation producing a sulcus (indentation) indicating the dropped position of the humeral head. (Mediclip image copyright, 1998 Williams & Wilkins. All rights reserved.)

With a complete dislocation, motion is not possible. With subluxation there is likely to be visible apprehension (called the **apprehension sign**) when the shoulder is moved close to the position(s) of vulnerability, usually abduction and lateral rotation. When the arm is moved into a vulnerable position, the proprioceptors recognize the position as one in which the shoulder may again move out of position.[55] Pay particular attention to the client's facial expressions during range-of-motion evaluations.

Palpation
Significant tenderness with palpation around the shoulder joint is due to muscle spasm and inflammation. The affected ligaments and joint capsule are too deep to easily palpate. If the humeral head is dislocated, the sulcus just below the acromion process is identifiable as a soft spot and indentation just above the curve of the humeral head. The displacement of the humeral head may also be recognizable with palpation depending on its position. If the humerus is only partially out of the glenoid fossa, its positional alteration may not be easily palpable.

Range-of-Motion and Resistance Testing
AROM: A soft-tissue therapist **should not attempt ROM** testing with a client presenting signs of a dislocation. In a dislocation, active motion is not possible due to the humeral head being out of the glenoid fossa. The client holds the arm close to the body to prevent intentional or unintentional movement of the glenohumeral joint. With subluxation, active movement may be possible in all directions, but is often limited by pain or apprehension.[99]
PROM: Passive movement should not be attempted with a dislocation. If the client expresses apprehension at any

attempt to move the joint, then consider it an important indicator that the joint may be dislocated. If there is a suspicion of a dislocation, the client should be immediately referred to a physician who can properly reduce the dislocation in order to prevent damage to neurovascular structures.[84] If there is subluxation, be very cautious and slow in the application of passive range-of-motion evaluation and watch for signs of apprehension. Visible apprehension helps identify the motions and directions of movement that are particularly vulnerable. Subluxations should also be referred to a physician.

MRT: Muscle contractions are not functional if the shoulder is dislocated. With subluxation, resisted contractions may be weak due to neurological inhibition or pain avoidance. Ordinarily there is no specific damage to the muscle-tendon unit and pain does not present with resisted movements. Pain and/or weakness are elicited in the subscapularis if the subluxation or dislocation is severe, because subscapularis fibers are frequently torn along with the anterior capsular structures in an anterior dislocation.[84] Soft-tissue therapists should not attempt MRT testing of clients presenting signs of dislocation.

Differential Evaluation
Glenoid labrum damage, severe rotator cuff tears, clavicular fracture, subacromial impingement, neurovascular damage, biceps tendon subluxation.

Suggestions for Treatment
If the shoulder is dislocated, the individual should see a physician who is trained to reduce the dislocation (replace the humerus). No attempt to reduce the dislocation should be made by practitioners without the scope of practice or training to do so. Severe damage to neurovascular structures may occur if reduction is done improperly.

Proper identification of a subluxation or dislocation is important, especially if the injury was severe enough to cause damage to the joint capsule or labrum. The client with a suspected dislocation or subluxation should be referred to a physician for additional evaluation. In these cases surgery may be necessary in order to reconnect the structures that have pulled away from their attachment sites or to tighten up the loose joint capsule.

Following reduction of a dislocation or subluxation, general massage may be helpful to alleviate the corresponding reflexive muscle spasm in the shoulder complex, which can lead to other biomechanical disturbances.

GLENOID LABRUM INJURIES

Glenoid labrum injuries were not well understood or addressed prior to the advent of arthroscopy and magnetic resonance imaging (MRI). In the last 20 years advances in evaluation have shown the important role the labrum plays in shoulder stability. While injury to the labrum was known to occur with *dislocation* and *subluxation*, it is now clear that the damage to the labrum can develop

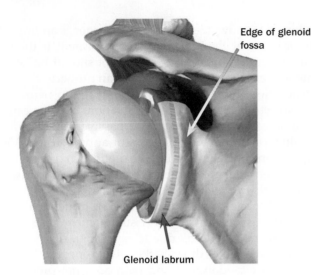

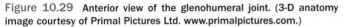

Figure 10.29 Anterior view of the glenohumeral joint. (3-D anatomy image courtesy of Primal Pictures Ltd. www.primalpictures.com.)

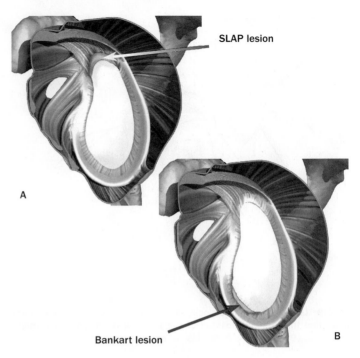

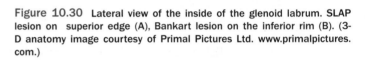

Figure 10.30 Lateral view of the inside of the glenoid labrum. SLAP lesion on superior edge (A), Bankart lesion on the inferior rim (B). (3-D anatomy image courtesy of Primal Pictures Ltd. www.primalpictures.com.)

from a number of causes and treatment is necessary for proper shoulder function.

Characteristics

In order to increase stability in the glenohumeral joint without compromising range of motion, a fibrocartilaginous ring called the **glenoid labrum** surrounds the **glenoid fossa**, creating more depth to the fossa and allowing the humeral head to more fully insert into the glenoid cavity (Figure 10.29). The glenoid labrum attaches to the glenoid fossa and has fibrous continuity with other stabilizing tissues in the joint including the **glenohumeral ligaments, the long head of the biceps brachii**, **glenohumeral joint capsule**, and the **long head of the triceps brachii**.

Injuries to the labrum include cracking, chipping or, most frequently, tearing and develop in different regions of the labrum. Tears to the rim of the labrum result from falling on an outstretched arm and driving the humeral head against the opposite side of the labrum. A subluxation, dislocation, or impact to the shoulder can also produce labrum damage, as can sudden tensile stress that might occur when lifting something heavy. While acute injuries are the most common cause of glenoid labrum injury, chronic tensile forces on the capsulolabral complex can also produce minor degrees of tearing or separation.[100] Athletes, such as those involved in throwing, experience this type of repetitive use labrum injury.

Damage usually occurs in the superior or inferior aspects.[101] A primary site of labral damage is the upper rim of the labrum where the tendon from the long head of the biceps brachii attaches. While the bony attachment for the biceps tendon is the **supraglenoid tubercle**, the tendon also has fibrous attachment to the superior portion of the glenoid labrum (Figure 10.22).[102] If the biceps brachii is forcefully contracted, the tendon can pull the **superior rim of the labrum** strongly enough to tear away from the glenoid fossa.[44] This injury is called a *SLAP*

lesion because the direction of the tear is along the superior labrum, from anterior to posterior (Figure 10.30).[103]

Another common cause of SLAP lesions occurs at the end of the throwing motion, when the biceps brachii suddenly contracts eccentrically to slow the rapid motion of elbow extension.[102] The sudden contraction pulls on the biceps attachment site, creating a SLAP lesion. Snyder classifies SLAP lesions into four categories (see Box 10.8).[103]

Another common injury of the glenoid labrum is the *Bankart lesion,* which occurs on the **anterior** or **inferior side of the labrum**. The Bankart lesion develops when the inferior glenohumeral ligament or capsular fibers tear away from the anterior or inferior margin of the glenoid labrum (Figure 10.30).[97, 104] Similar to a SLAP lesion, the injury may involve minor tearing or fraying of the ligament and labrum or a more serious **bucket-handle tear** with fragments of the labrum extending into the joint. Unlike the SLAP lesion, the biceps brachii tendon is not involved. Rather, it is the ligaments and joint capsule that create the tensile stress and pull on the joint capsule and labrum. Bankart lesions are often caused by forceful abduction with lateral rotation of the shoulder, such as occurs in throwing. Dislocations produce more Bankart lesions than SLAP lesions.

Pain develops from irritation of the richly innervated structures in the shoulder, such as the **glenohumeral joint capsule**. Damage to these tissues along with the labrum is common.[100] Consequently, it may be difficult to pinpoint the exact source of pain. Symptoms are similar to other shoulder injuries, making evaluation challenging.

If labral damage is suspected, the client should be referred to a physician for evaluation. MRI or arthroscopy are considered most accurate in determining the degree, location, and severity of labral injuries because the tissues are deep and inaccessible to physical examination.[105] Physical examination is important in evaluating these conditions, but great care should be taken to not stress already damaged tissue.[105, 106] Ligamentous damage often coincides with labral injury and shoulder instability is likely to result from ligament damage. Decreased stability makes the glenohumeral joint more susceptible to dislocation or subluxation.

History

A client with a labral tear is likely to report an acute injury, such as impact to the shoulder or falling on an outstretched arm. The injury can also occur in the midst of normal shoulder activities such as throwing. The client usually describes unspecific but deep pain in the shoulder, but pain is not always felt. The lack of extensive innervation to the glenoid labrum means that a fair amount of tissue damage can occur before pain is felt. Overhead activities tend to produce more pain than other movements. Night pain occurs due to sleeping position.

The client may describe popping, catching, clicking, or grinding sensations during various movements, due to portions of torn labral tissue impairing smooth glenohumeral movement. There will also be range-of-motion loss, shoulder instability, and loss of strength.

Observation

Due to the depth of the glenoid labrum, there are no visible signs of the injury. Swelling will also be too deep to be visible. To avoid pain, the client may be apprehensive in performing various shoulder motions. If motion is possible, it is common to observe lack of continuity throughout the motion as pain and tissue damage cause alterations in biomechanical function. Clients with significant shoulder instability or an acute injury to the shoulder that implicates labral damage should be referred for diagnosis.

Palpation

Because the labrum is difficult to palpate directly and has little innervation, palpation is not particularly helpful in identifying damage. Pain in the shoulder region during palpation is more likely an indicator of damage to other soft tissues and not the labrum, and may be present with or without a labral tear. With a labral tear or other injury to the joint complex there will be tenderness due to reflex muscle spasm. If the shoulder is lightly palpated during range-of-motion evaluations, clicking or locking sensations are sometimes palpable as well as audible.

Range-of-Motion and Resistance Testing

AROM: Pain may be felt with active motion in several directions. There is no correlation between pain with a

---

Box 10.8 Snyder Classification of SLAP Lesions
Type 1
Superior portion of labrum frayed
Labrum & biceps attachment intact
Type 2
Superior labrum frayed
Superior labrum detached from glenoid fossa
Instability in biceps tendon attachment
Type 3
Bucket-handle tear of superior labrum
Tear does not extend into biceps tendon
Portion of torn labrum hangs into joint cavity
Type 4
Bucket-handle tear goes into biceps tendon
Portion of torn labrum hangs into joint cavity

---

particular motion and a specific labral injury. Popping or clicking can be felt with certain motions if a damaged fragment of labrum is in the joint space. Clients with suspected labral damage or shoulder instability should be referred to a physician for diagnosis.

PROM: Principles are the same as for active movement. Use caution performing PROM evaluation with suspected internal joint injuries such as labral damage.

MRT: Pain may be felt with resisted contractions of the biceps brachii muscle with a SLAP lesion. The contraction of the biceps pulls on the damaged portion of the superior labrum. Pain is not likely in other motions, as other shoulder muscles do not attach to the damaged labrum. There may be weakness in other resisted motions due to reflex muscular inhibition.

Special Test

While there are several special orthopedic tests used to identify labral damage, none are considered highly accurate. High-tech diagnostic evaluation, such as MRI, is necessary to identify labral damage. In some cases Speed's test, which stresses the biceps brachii tendon, can produce pain when a SLAP lesion is present.

Differential Evaluation

Glenohumeral subluxation, subacromial impingement, biceps tendon pathology without labral damage, calcific tendinitis, brachial plexus injury, cervical radiculopathy, rotator cuff injury, acromioclavicular joint injury, shoulder dislocation/subluxation.

Suggestions for Treatment

Because damage to the glenoid labrum is an internal joint disorder, there is little that massage can do to benefit this condition. It is most appropriately treated with other approaches such as physical therapy if the labral tear is minor. In more severe injuries, surgery is warranted. Because surgery may be required, the massage practitioner should refer clients suspected of having labral damage to a physician for evaluation and treatment. Massage may be beneficial as part of a coordinated treatment plan that addresses hypertonicity in surrounding muscles and increasing balance in tissues.

GENERAL NEUROMUSCULAR DISORDERS

In many cases, soft-tissue dysfunctions are not given a specific name. Adequate assessment is required to determine the tissues most likely involved and to take into account pathologies that may or may not have specific titles. Chapter 4 provides a discussion of the pathological processes of hypertonicity, myofascial trigger points, muscle strains, nerve compression and tension, tendinosis, tenosynovitis, ligament sprains, and osteoarthritis in any region of the body. Chapter 4 also includes the history, observation, palpation, relevant tests, and treatment suggestions sections for these conditions. The principles are the same for these conditions wherever they occur in the body.

Included in this section are specific tables and graphics for the shoulder, including dermatomes, cutaneous innervation, trigger point referral patterns, and findings for MRTs. Tenosynovitis is rare in the shoulder as the biceps brachii is the only tendon in this region surrounded by a synovial sheath. Nerve compression or tension pathologies produce symptoms in the shoulder from either a cervical radiculopathy (spinal nerve root compression) or a peripheral neuropathy (peripheral upper extremity nerve injury). Some of the locations in the shoulder where peripheral neuropathies occur are discussed in Chapter 9 as discrete nerve compression pathologies, such as the variations of thoracic outlet syndrome. Other regions of

BOX 10.9 REGIONS OF POSSIBLE NERVE ENTRAPMENT

Radial Nerve
　Axillary region

Branches of the Brachial Plexus
　Between the clavicle & first rib
　Under the pectoralis minor

Axillary Nerve
　Quadrilateral space

Suprascapular Nerve
　Suprascapular notch
　Spinoglenoid notch

Note: With a traumatic blow, any of the nerves in the axillary region may be affected.

common nerve compression are listed in Box 10.9.

Sensory symptoms from a cervical radiculopathy may be felt in the proximal upper extremity and are experienced within the dermatome associated with that nerve root (Figure 10.31). Sensory symptoms of peripheral neuropathy are felt in the region of cutaneous innervation for the nerve affected (Figure 10.32). Radiculopathies or peripheral neuropathies can cause motor dysfunction and produce weakness in the muscles innervated by the affected nerve (Box 10.10).

Muscular hypertonicity develops in the shoulder as a result of repetitive motion or postural stress. Myofascial trigger points can develop in the affected muscle(s) due to chronic muscular tension or trauma and refer pain or characteristic neurological sensations to various areas of the shoulder, neck, back, or arm. Common myofascial trigger point referral patterns for the major muscles in this region are shown in Figures 10.33-10.35.

BOX: 10.10 INNERVATION OF THE SHOULDER MUSCLES

Dorsal Scapular Nerve	Lateral Pectoral Nerve	Thoracodorsal Nerve	Accessory Nerve
Levator scapulae	Pectoralis major (clavicular head)	Latissimus dorsi	Trapezius
Rhomboid major & minor	Pectoralis minor		
		Musculocutaneous nerve	Suprascapular Nerve
Long Thoracic Nerve	Medial Pectoral Nerve	Biceps brachii	Supraspinatus
Serratus anterior	Pectoralis major (sternal head)	Brachialis	Infraspinatus
	Pectoralis minor	Coracobrachialis	
	Subscapular Nerve	Axillary Nerve	
	Subscapularis	Teres minor	
	Teres Major	Deltoid	

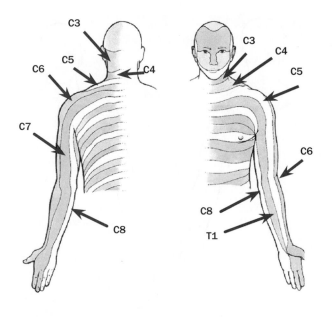

Figure 10.31: Dermatomes of the neck and upper extremity. (Mediclip image copyright, 1998 Williams & Wilkins. All Rights Reserved.)

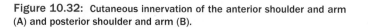

Figure 10.32: Cutaneous innervation of the anterior shoulder and arm (A) and posterior shoulder and arm (B).

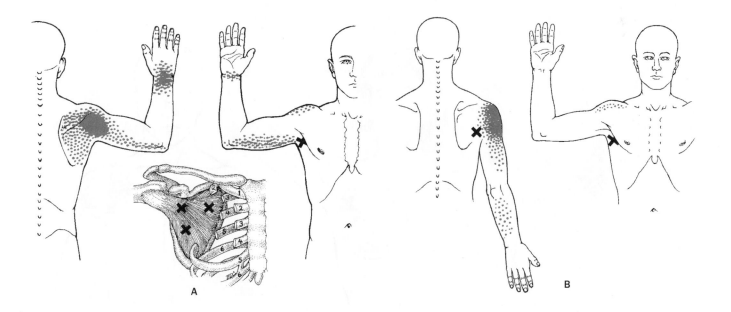

Figure 10.33 Myofascial trigger point referral patterns: Subscapularis (A), Teres major (B), (Images courtesy of Mediclip, copyright 1998 Williams & Wilkins. All rights reserved.)

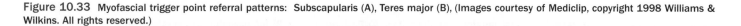

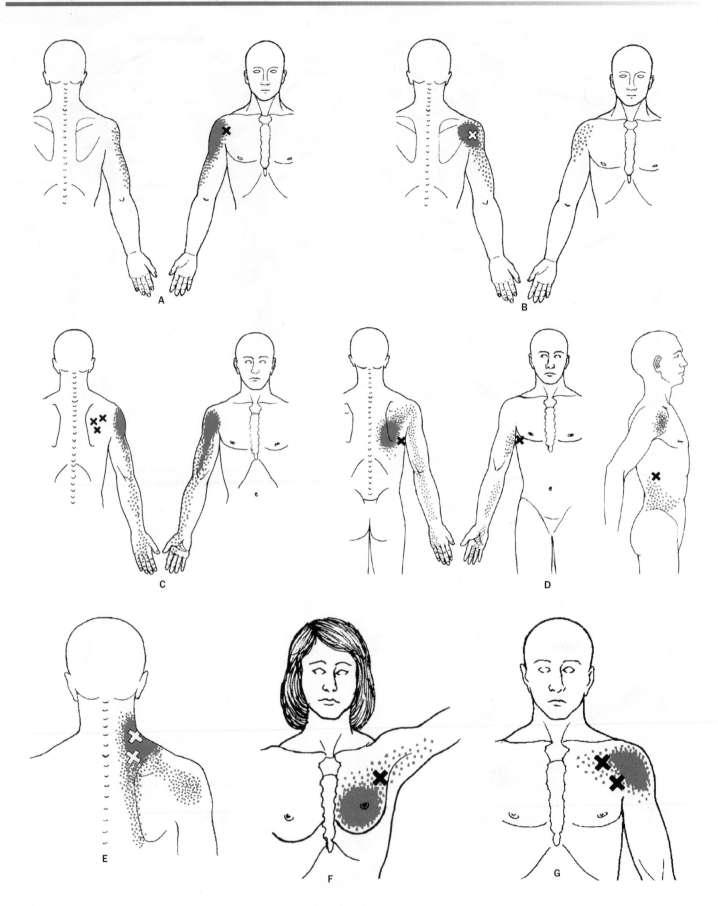

Figure 10.34 Myofascial trigger point referral patterns: Anterior deltoid (A), Posterior deltoid (B), Infraspinatus (C), Latissimus dorsi (D), Levator scapulae (E), Pectoralis major (F) & (G). (Images courtesy of Mediclip, copyright 1998 Williams & Wilkins. All rights reserved.)

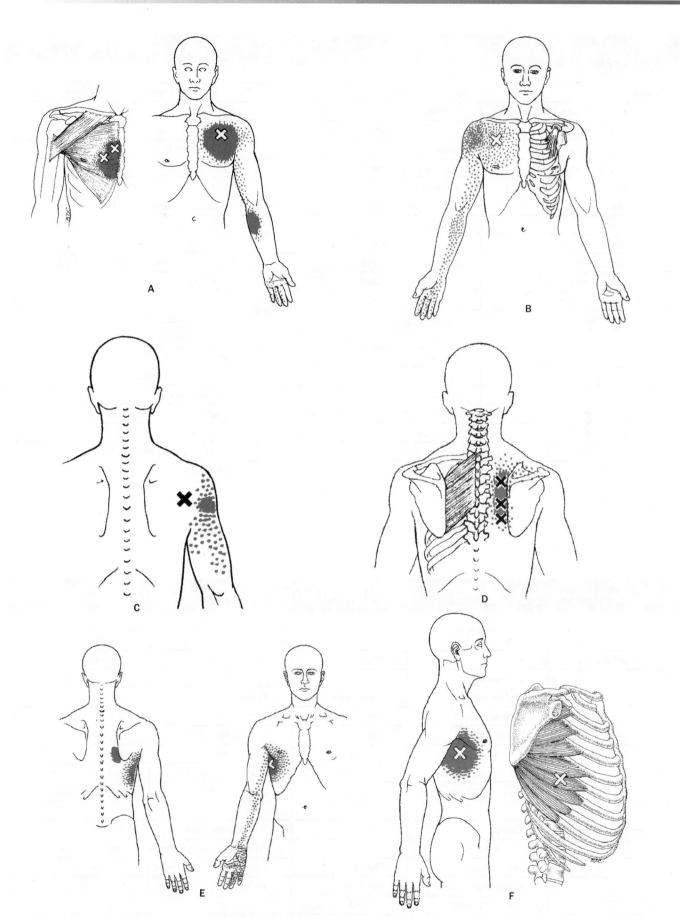

Figure 10.35 Myofascial trigger point referral patterns: Pectoralis major (A), Pectoralis minor (B), Teres minor (C), Rhomboid major and minor (D), Serratus anterior (E) & (F).– (Images courtesy of Mediclip, copyright 1998 Williams & Wilkins. All rights reserved).

TABLE 1 WEAKNESS WITH MANUAL RESISTIVE TEST AND POSSIBLE NERVE INVOLVEMENT

Muscle	Resisted Action	Possible Nerve Involvement if Action Weak
Coracobrachialis	Flexion	Musculocutaneous (C5-C7)
Deltoid (anterior)	Flexion & medial rotation	Axillary (C5-C6)
Deltoid (middle	Abduction	Axillary (C5-C6)
Deltoid (posterior)	Extension & lateral rotation	Axillary (C5-C6)
Infraspinatus	Lateral rotation	Suprascapular (C5-C6)
Latissimus dorsi	Extension, medial rotation	Thoracodorsal (C6-C8)
Levator scapulae	Scapular elevation	C3-C4 spinal nerves, dorsal scapular (C5)
Pectoralis major	Horizontal adduction	Medial and lateral pectorals (C5-T1)
Pectoralis minor	Scapular protraction	Medial and lateral pectoral (C5-T1)
Rhomboid major	Scapular retraction	Dorsal scapular (C5)
Rhomboid minor	Scapular retraction	Dorsal scapular (C5)
Serratus anterior	Scapular protraction	Long thoracic (C5-C7)
Subscapularis	Internal rotation	Subscapular (C5-C6)
Supraspinatus	Abduction	Suprascapular (C5-C6)
Teres major	Medial rotation	Subscapular (C5-C6)
Teres minor	Lateral rotation	Axillary (C5-C6)
Trapezius (lower)	Scapular retraction & upward rotation	Accessory (X1) and C3-C4
Trapezius (middle)	Scapular retraction	Accessory (X1) and C3-C4
Trapezius (upper)	Scapular elevation	Accessory (X1) and C3-C4

TABLE 2 JOINTS, ASSOCIATED MOTIONS, PLANES OF MOTION IN ANATOMICAL POSITION, AXIS OF ROTATION, AND AVERAGE ROM

Joint/Articulation	Motion	Plane of Motion	Axis of Rotation	Avg. ROM (degrees)
Glenohumeral	Flexion	Sagittal	Medial-lateral	160-180
	Extension	Sagittal	Medial-lateral	60
	Medial rotation	Transverse	Superior-inferior	90
	Lateral rotation	Transverse	Superior-inferior	90
	Abduction	Frontal	Anterior-posterior	120
	Adduction	Frontal	Anterior-posterior	45 (with flexion)
	Horizontal abduction	Transverse	Superior-inferior	Not calculated
	Horizontal adduction	Transverse	Superior-inferior	Not calculated
Scapulothoracic	Elevation	Frontal	Translational (no axis)	Not calculated
	Depression	Frontal	Translational (no axis)	Not calculated
	Protraction	Multiple	Translational (no axis)	Not calculated
	Retraction	Multiple	Translational (no axis)	Not calculated
	Upward rotation	Frontal		Not calculated
	Downward rotation	Frontal		Not calculated

Reference Table for Condition Assessment

This table lists a number of pathological conditions along the left-hand column. The top of the table lists common evaluation procedures. A ◆ in the box associated with a pathological condition and an evaluation procedure indicates that the procedure is commonly used to identify that pathology. A ● in the box associated with the condition and a range-of-motion or resistance test, indicates that pain is likely with that test for that pathology. Conditions are listed alphabetically.

TABLE 3   REFERENCE TABLE FOR CONDITION ASSESSMENT

	AROM	PROM	MRT	Apley scratch test	Drop arm test	Hawkins-Kennedy sign	Empty can test	Neer impingement test	Speed's test	Cross over test
Elevated Shoulder	●	●	●							
Slumped Shoulder	●	●								
Frozen Shoulder/Adhesive Capsulitis	●	●	●	◆						
Rotator Cuff Tears & Tendinosis	●	●	●		◆					
Shoulder Impingement Syndrome	●	●	●			◆	◆	◆		
Subacromial Bursitis	●	●								
Calcific Tendinitis	●	●	●							
Bicipital Tendinosis	●	●	●						◆	
Shoulder Separation	●	●	●							◆
Glenohumeral Dislocation/Subluxation										
Glenoid Labrum Injury	●	●	●							

References

1. Donatelli R. *Physical Therapy of the Shoulder*. 3rd. ed. Philadelphia: Churchill Livingstone; 1997.
2. Travell JS, D. *Myofascial Pain and Dysfunction: The Trigger Point Manual*. Vol 1. 1st ed. Baltimore: Williams & Wilkins; 1983.
3. Chaitow L, DeLany J. *Clinical Application of Neuromuscular Techniques*. Vol 1. Edinburgh: Churchill Livingstone; 2000.
4. Pearsall AW. Adhesive Capsulitis. *eMedicine*. 7-30-2002. Available at: www.emedicine.com. Accessed January 23, 2005.
5. Malone T, McPoil T, Nitz A. *Orthopedic and Sports Physical Therapy*. 3rd ed. St. Louis: Mosby; 1997.
6. Neviaser RJ, Neviaser TJ. The frozen shoulder. Diagnosis and management. *Clin Orthop*. Oct 1987(223):59-64.
7. Neumann DA. *Kinesiology of the Musculoskeletal System*. St. Louis: Mosby; 2002.
8. Simons D, Travell J, Simons L. *Myofascial Pain and Dysfunction: The Trigger Point Manual*. Vol 1. 2nd ed. Baltimore: Williams & Wilkins; 1999.
9. Pearsall AW, Speer KP. Frozen shoulder syndrome: diagnostic and treatment strategies in the primary care setting. *Med Sci Sports Exerc*. Apr 1998;30(4 Suppl):S33-39.
10. McQuade KJ, Smidt GL. Dynamic scapulohumeral rhythm: the effects of external resistance during elevation of the arm in the scapular plane. *J Orthop Sports Phys Ther*. Feb 1998;27(2):125-133.
11. Cyriax J. *Textbook of Orthopaedic Medicine Volume One: Diagnosis of Soft Tissue Lesions*. Vol 1. 8th ed. London: Bailliere Tindall; 1982.
12. Sandor R. Adhesive capsulitis - optimal treatment of 'frozen shoulder'. *Physician Sportsmed*. 2000;28(9):23-29.
13. Simons DG. Review of enigmatic MTrPs as a common cause of enigmatic musculoskeletal pain and dysfunction. *J Electromyogr Kinesiol*.

2004;14(1):95-107.

14. Simotas AC, Tsairis P. Adhesive capsulitis of the glenohumeral joint with an unusual neuropathic presentation - A case report. *Amer J Phys Med Rehabil*. 1999;78(6):577-581.

15. Pollock RG, Duralde XA, Flatow EL, Bigliani LU. The use of arthroscopy in the treatment of resistant frozen shoulder. *Clin Orthop*. Jul 1994(304):30-36.

16. Ozaki J, Nakagawa Y, Sakurai G, Tamai S. Recalcitrant chronic adhesive capsulitis of the shoulder. Role of contracture of the coracohumeral ligament and rotator interval in pathogenesis and treatment. *J Bone Joint Surg Am*. Dec 1989;71(10):1511-1515.

17. DePalma AF. *Surgery of the Shoulder*. Philadelphia: JB Lippincott; 1983.

18. Reeves B. The natural history of the frozen shoulder syndrome. *Scand J Rheumatol*. 1975;4(4):193-196.

19. Balci N, Balci MK, Tuzuner S. Shoulder adhesive capsulitis and shoulder range of motion in type II diabetes mellitus: association with diabetic complications. *J Diabetes Complications*. May-Jun 1999;13(3):135-140.

20. Kordella T. Frozen shoulder & diabetes. Frozen shoulder affects 20 percent of people with diabetes. Proper treatment can help you work through it. *Diabetes Forecast*. Aug 2002;55(8):60-64.

21. Miller MD, Wirth MA, Rockwood CAJ. Thawing the frozen shoulder: the 'patient' patient. *Orthopedics*. 1996;19(10):849-853.

22. Diercks RL, Stevens M. Gentle thawing of the frozen shoulder: a prospective study of supervised neglect versus intensive physical therapy in seventy-seven patients with frozen shoulder syndrome followed up for two years. *J Shoulder Elbow Surg*. Sep-Oct 2004;13(5):499-502.

23. Bulgen DY, Binder AI, Hazleman BL, Dutton J, Roberts S. Frozen shoulder: prospective clinical study with an evaluation of three treatment regimens. *Ann Rheum Dis*. 1984;43(3):353-360.

24. Jobe FW, Kvitne RS, Giangarra CE. Shoulder pain in the overhand or throwing athlete. The relationship of anterior instability and rotator cuff impingement. *Orthop Rev*. Sep 1989;18(9):963-975.

25. Lowe W. Orthopedic assessment skills in bodywork care of rotator cuff injury. *Journal of Bodywork and Movement Therapies*. 1997;1(2):81-86.

26. Riley GP, Harrall RL, Constant CR, Chard MD, Cawston TE, Hazleman BL. Tendon Degeneration and Chronic Shoulder Pain - Changes in the Collagen Composition of the Human Rotator Cuff Tendons in Rotator Cuff Tendinitis. *Ann Rheum Dis*. 1994;53(6):359-366.

27. Lohr JF, Uhthoff HK. The microvascular pattern of the supraspinatus tendon. *Clin Orthop*. 1990(254):35-38.

28. Uhthoff HK, Sarkar K. Classification and definition of tendinopathies. *Clin Sports Med*. Oct 1991;10(4):707-720.

29. Fukuda H, Hamada K, Yamanaka K. Pathology and pathogenesis of bursal-side rotator cuff tears viewed from en bloc histologic sections. *Clin Orthop*. May 1990(254):75-80.

30. Edelson G, Teitz C. Internal impingement in the shoulder. *J Shoulder Elbow Surg*. Jul-Aug 2000;9(4):308-315.

31. Meister K. Injuries to the shoulder in the throwing athlete. Part one: Biomechanics/pathophysiology/classification of injury. *Am J Sports Med*. Mar-Apr 2000;28(2):265-275.

32. Mehta S, Gimbel JA, Soslowsky LJ. Etiologic and pathogenetic factors for rotator cuff tendinopathy. *Clin Sports Med*. Oct 2003;22(4):791-812.

33. Garrett WE. Muscle strain injuries. *Am J Sports Med*. 1996;24(6 Suppl):S2-8.

34. Bennett WF. Arthroscopic repair of anterosuperior (supraspinatus/subscapularis) rotator cuff tears: a prospective cohort with 2- to 4-year follow-up. Classification of biceps subluxation/instability. *Arthroscopy*. Jan 2003;19(1):21-33.

35. Neviaser RJ, Neviaser TJ, Neviaser JS. Anterior dislocation of the shoulder and rotator cuff rupture. *Clin Orthop*. 1993(291):103-106.

36. Blevins FT. Rotator cuff pathology in athletes. *Sports Med*. Sep 1997;24(3):205-220.

37. Arcuni SE. Rotator cuff pathology and subacromial impingement. *Nurse Pract*. May 2000;25(5):58, 61, 65-56 passim.

38. Neer CS, 2nd, Craig EV, Fukuda H. Cuff-tear arthropathy. *J Bone Joint Surg Am*. 1983;65(9):1232-1244.

39. Khan KM, Cook JL, Taunton JE, Bonar F. Overuse tendinosis, not tendinitis - Part 1: A new paradigm for a difficult clinical problem. *Physician Sportsmed*. 2000;28(5):38+.

40. Bigliani LU, Ticker JB, Flatow EL, Soslowsky LJ, Mow VC. The relationship of acromial architecture to rotator cuff disease. *Clin Sports Med*. Oct 1991;10(4):823-838.

41. Moore K, Dalley A. *Clinically Oriented Anatomy*. 4th ed. Philadelphia: Lippincott Williams & Wilkins; 1999.

42. Kim TK, McFarland EG. Internal impingement of the shoulder in flexion. *Clin Orthop*. Apr 2004(421):112-119.

43. Wolin P, Tarbet J. Rotator cuff injury: addressing overhead overuse. *Physician Sportsmed*. 1997;25(6).

44. Fleisig GS, Andrews JR, Dillman CJ, Escamilla RF. Kinetics of baseball pitching with implications about injury mechanisms. *Am J Sports Med*. Mar-Apr 1995;23(2):233-239.

45. Rockwood CA, Matsen FA. *The Shoulder*. Philadelphia: WB Saunders; 1990.

46. Neer CS, 2nd. Impingement lesions. *Clin Orthop*.

1983(173):70-77.

47. Neer CS, 2nd. Anterior acromioplasty for the chronic impingement syndrome in the shoulder: a preliminary report. *J Bone Joint Surg Am.* Jan 1972;54(1):41-50.

48. Allegrucci M, Whitney SL, Irrgang JJ. Clinical implications of secondary impingement of the shoulder in freestyle swimmers. *J Orthop Sports Phys Ther.* Dec 1994;20(6):307-318.

49. Belling Sorensen AK, Jorgensen U. Secondary impingement in the shoulder. An improved terminology in impingement. *Scand J Med Sci Sports.* 2000;10(5):266-278.

50. Magee D. *Orthopedic Physical Assessment.* 3rd ed. Philadelphia: W.B. Saunders; 1997.

51. Epstein RE, Schweitzer ME, Frieman BG, Fenlin JM, Jr., Mitchell DG. Hooked acromion: prevalence on MR images of painful shoulders. *Radiology.* May 1993;187(2):479-481.

52. Edelson JG. The 'hooked' acromion revisited. *J Bone Joint Surg Br.* Mar 1995;77(2):284-287.

53. Depalma MJ, Johnson EW. Detecting and treating shoulder impingement syndrome. *Physician Sportsmed.* 2003;31(7).

54. Kamkar A, Irrgang JJ, Whitney SL. Nonoperative management of secondary shoulder impingement syndrome. *J Orthop Sports Phys Ther.* May 1993;17(5):212-224.

55. Ellenbecker TS. *Clinical Examination of the Shoulder.* St. Louis: Elsevier Saunders; 2004.

56. Holtby R, Razmjou H. Validity of the supraspinatus test as a single clinical test in diagnosing patients with rotator cuff pathology. *J Orthop Sports Phys Ther.* Apr 2004;34(4):194-200.

57. Neviaser RJ, Neviaser TJ. Observations on impingement. *Clin Orthop.* 1990(254):60-63.

58. Rockwood CA, Lyons FR. Shoulder impingement syndrome: diagnosis, radiographic evaluation, and treatment with a modified Neer acromioplasty. *J Bone Joint Surg Am.* 1993;75(3):409-424.

59. Ingber RS. Shoulder impingement in tennis/racquetball players treated with subscapularis myofascial treatments. *Arch Phys Med Rehabil.* 2000;81(5):679-682.

60. Rattray F, Ludwig L. *Clinical Massage Therapy: Understanding, Assessing and Treating over 70 Conditions.* Toronto: Talus Incorporated; 2000.

61. Salzman KL, Lillegard WA, Butcher JD. Upper extremity bursitis. *Am Fam Physician.* 1997;56(7):1797-1806, 1811-1792.

62. Kessel L, Watson M. The painful arc syndrome. Clinical classification as a guide to management. *J Bone Joint Surg Br.* May 1977;59(2):166-172.

63. Woodward A. Calcifying Tendonitis. *eMedicine* [web site]. July 2, 2004. Available at: www.emedicine.com. Accessed January 31, 2005.

64. Hurt G, Baker CL, Jr. Calcific tendinitis of the

shoulder. *Orthop Clin North Am.* Oct 2003;34(4):567-575.

65. Loew M, Sabo D, Wehrle M, Mau H. Relationship between calcifying tendinitis and subacromial impingement: a prospective radiography and magnetic resonance imaging study. *J Shoulder Elbow Surg.* 1996;5(4):314-319.

66. Maier M, Stabler A, Schmitz C, et al. On the impact of calcified deposits within the rotator cuff tendons in shoulders of patients with shoulder pain and dysfunction. *Arch Orthop Trauma Surg.* Jul 2001;121(7):371-378.

67. Cosentino R, De Stefano R, Selvi E, et al. Extracorporeal shock wave therapy for chronic calcific tendinitis of the shoulder: single blind study. *Ann Rheum Dis.* Mar 2003;62(3):248-250.

68. Uhthoff HK, Loehr JW. Calcific Tendinopathy of the Rotator Cuff: Pathogenesis, Diagnosis, and Management. *J Am Acad Orthop Surg.* 1997;5(4):183-191.

69. Wolf WB. Calcific tendinitis of the shoulder. *Physician Sportsmed.* 1999;27(9).

70. Wainner RS, Hasz M. Management of acute calcific tendinitis of the shoulder. *J Orthop Sports Phys Ther.* Mar 1998;27(3):231-237.

71. Pfahler M, Branner S, Refior HJ. The role of the bicipital groove in tendopathy of the long biceps tendon. *J Shoulder Elbow Surg.* 1999;8(5):419-424.

72. Rodosky MW, Harner CD, Fu FH. The role of the long head of the biceps muscle and superior glenoid labrum in anterior stability of the shoulder. *Am J Sports Med.* 1994;22(1):121-130.

73. Post M, Benca P. Primary tendinitis of the long head of the biceps. *Clin Orthop.* 1989(246):117-125.

74. Patton WC, McCluskey GM, 3rd. Biceps tendinitis and subluxation. *Clin Sports Med.* Jul 2001;20(3):505-529.

75. Curtis AS, Snyder SJ. Evaluation and treatment of biceps tendon pathology. *Orthop Clin North Am.* Jan 1993;24(1):33-43.

76. Holtby R, Razmjou H. Accuracy of the Speed's and Yergason's tests in detecting biceps pathology and SLAP lesions: comparison with arthroscopic findings. *Arthroscopy.* Mar 2004;20(3):231-236.

77. Gehlsen GM, Ganion LR, Helfst R. Fibroblast responses to variation in soft tissue mobilization pressure. *Med Sci Sport Exercise.* 1999;31(4):531-535.

78. Shaw MB, McInerney JJ, Dias JJ, Evans PA. Acromioclavicular joint sprains: the post-injury recovery interval. *Injury.* Jun 2003;34(6):438-442.

79. Lemos MJ. The evaluation and treatment of the injured acromioclavicular joint in athletes. *Am J Sports Med.* 1998;26(1):137-144.

80. Kim J. Acromioclavicular Injury. *eMedicine* [web page]. 5-16-2003. Available at: www.emedicine.com. Accessed February 2, 2005.

81. Fink EP. Injuries to the Acromioclavicular Joint.

In: J. T, Shephard R, eds. *Current Therapy in Sports Medicine*. 3rd ed. St. Louis: Mosby; 1995:174-177.

82. Marker LB, Klareskov B. Posterior sternoclavicular dislocation: an American football injury. *Br J Sports Med*. Mar 1996;30(1):71-72.

83. Turnbull JR. Acromioclavicular joint disorders. *Med Sci Sports Exerc*. 1998;30(4 Suppl):S26-32.

84. Wilk K. The Shoulder. In: Malone TR, McPoil T, Nitz AJ, eds. *Orthopedic & Sports Physical Therapy*. 3rd ed. St. Louis: Mosby; 1997.

85. Hayes K, Callanan M, Walton J, Paxinos A, Murrell GA. Shoulder instability: management and rehabilitation. *J Orthop Sports Phys Ther*. Oct 2002;32(10):497-509.

86. Cooper J. Throwing Injuries. In: Donatelli R, ed. *Physical Therapy of the Shoulder*. 3rd ed. New York: Churchill Livingstone; 1997.

87. Mahaffey BL, Smith PA. Shoulder instability in young athletes. *Am Fam Physician*. May 15 1999;59(10):2773-2782, 2787.

88. Zarins B, Rowe CR. Current concepts in the diagnosis and treatment of shoulder instability in athletes. *Med Sci Sports Exerc*. Oct 1984;16(5):444-448.

89. Jobe FW, Pink M. Classification and treatment of shoulder dysfunction in the overhead athlete. *J Orthop Sports Phys Ther*. Aug 1993;18(2):427-432.

90. Warren RF. Subluxation of the shoulder in athletes. *Clin Sports Med*. Jul 1983;2(2):339-354.

91. Dalton SE, Snyder SJ. Glenohumeral instability. *Baillieres Clin Rheumatol*. Dec 1989;3(3):511-534.

92. Cleeman E, Flatow EL. Shoulder dislocations in the young patient. *Orthop Clin North Am*. Apr 2000;31(2):217-229.

93. Aldridge JM, 3rd, Perry JJ, Osbahr DC, Speer KP. Thermal capsulorraphy of bilateral glenohumeral joints in a pediatric patient with Ehlers-Danlos syndrome. *Arthroscopy*. May-Jun 2003;19(5):E41.

94. Giampietro PF, Raggio C, Davis JG. Marfan syndrome: orthopedic and genetic review. *Curr Opin Pediatr*. Feb 2002;14(1):35-41.

95. Matsen FA, 3rd, Zuckerman JD. Anterior glenohumeral instability. *Clin Sports Med*. 1983;2(2):319-338.

96. Walton J, Paxinos A, Tzannes A, Callanan M, Hayes K, Murrell GA. The unstable shoulder in the adolescent athlete. *Am J Sports Med*. Sep-Oct 2002;30(5):758-767.

97. Rowe C. Anterior Glenohumeral Subluxation/Dislocation: The Bankart Procedure. In: Torg JS, Shephard R, eds. *Current Therapy in Sports Medicine*. 3rd ed. St. Louis: Mosby; 1995:222-227.

98. Baker CL, Uribe JW, Whitman C. Arthroscopic evaluation of acute initial anterior shoulder dislocations. *Am J Sports Med*. Jan-Feb 1990;18(1):25-28.

99. Aronen JG. Anterior shoulder dislocations in sports. *Sports Med*. May-Jun 1986;3(3):224-234.

100. Yahara M. Shoulder. In: Richardson JK, Iglarsh ZA, eds. *Clinical Orthopaedic Physical Therapy*. Philadelphia: W.B. Saunders Company; 1994.

101. Terry GC, Friedman SJ, Uhl TL. Arthroscopically treated tears of the glenoid labrum. Factors influencing outcome. *Am J Sports Med*. Jul-Aug 1994;22(4):504-512.

102. Andrews JR, Carson WG, Jr., McLeod WD. Glenoid labrum tears related to the long head of the biceps. *Am J Sports Med*. Sep-Oct 1985;13(5):337-341.

103. Snyder SJ, Karzel RP, Del Pizzo W, Ferkel RD, Friedman MJ. SLAP lesions of the shoulder. *Arthroscopy*. 1990;6(4):274-279.

104. Novotny JE, Nichols CE, Beynnon BD. Kinematics of the glenohumeral joint with Bankart lesion and repair. *J Orthop Res*. Jan 1998;16(1):116-121.

105. Nam EK, Snyder SJ. The diagnosis and treatment of superior labrum, anterior and posterior (SLAP) lesions. *Am J Sports Med*. Sep-Oct 2003;31(5):798-810.

106. Liu SH, Henry MH, Nuccion S, Shapiro MS, Dorey F. Diagnosis of glenoid labral tears. A comparison between magnetic resonance imaging and clinical examinations. *Am J Sports Med*. Mar-Apr 1996;24(2):149-154.

11 Elbow, Forearm, Wrist, & Hand

The elbow, forearm, wrist, and hand make up a complex unit. Numerous articulations, muscles, bones, tendons, and ligaments work together to form a kinetic chain capable of performing multiple functions. Due to the degree of involvement of the upper extremity in daily functions, injuries and pain conditions are common and many result from overuse. Due to the number of articulations in this region, assessing movement and muscle action is challenging, especially in the hand.

The hands and fingers are designed for precise manipulation of objects, but not for the repetitive motion stress to which they are frequently subjected. These types of motions lead to a number of the repetitive stress injuries that afflict the upper extremity. The small size of the bones, muscles, tendons, and ligaments in the wrist and hand also make them vulnerable to high force loads, such as those which occur when falling on an outstretched hand.

Peripheral nerve compression pathologies affect the distal upper extremity more than other areas of the body. Identifying entrapment syndromes requires thoughtful and thorough evaluation of various motor and sensory symptoms. A variety of nerve compression causes should be considered. Immediately assuming the presence of high-profile conditions, such as carpal tunnel syndrome, may lead to inaccurately identifying the condition and overlooking less well-known pathologies.

Movements and Motion Testing

SINGLE-PLANE MOVEMENTS

There are numerous joints and motions to evaluate in the distal upper extremity. Flexion and extension occur at the elbow while pronation and supination occur at the proximal and distal radioulnar joints. While there are eight individual carpal bones at the wrist, the majority of movement occurs between the proximal row of carpal bones and the radius. This articulation is called the radiocarpal joint. There are four primary movements at the wrist: flexion, extension, radial deviation (also called abduction), and ulnar deviation (also called adduction).

Actions of the hand require a high degree of specific movement in the thumb and fingers. There are four primary motions at the thumb and fingers: flexion, extension, abduction, and adduction. These motions occur at the numerous finger and thumb joints although the interphalangeal joints only allow flexion and extension. Oddly enough, while these motions are named the same for the thumb and fingers, they occur in different planes. See the discussion of this naming anomaly for thumb motions in Box 11.1. The associated motions, planes, axes of rotation, and range-of-motion values for this region are listed in Table 1 at the end of the chapter.

Elbow

Elbow **flexion** and **extension** occur in the **sagittal plane** at the **humeroulnar** and **humeroradial joints** (Figure 11.1). Flexion occurs as the forearm is brought toward the upper arm from anatomical position. The forearm is in full extension in anatomical position. Average range of motion for elbow flexion is about 150⁰. Range-of-motion values are not calculated for elbow extension because end range is at full extension.

Forearm

In the forearm, **pronation** and **supination** occur in the **transverse plane** at the **proximal** and **distal radioulnar joints** (Figure 11.2). From anatomical position, pronation takes place as the forearm rotates in a medial direction and supination is rotation laterally. Although the majority of motion is at the proximal radioulnar joint, there is movement in the distal radioulnar joint as well. Average range of motion for each movement is 80⁰.

Wrist

Flexion, extension, radial deviation, and **ulnar deviation** occur at the **radiocarpal joint**, with some accessory motion at the **carpal bones** of the wrist. **Flexion** and **extension** occur in the **sagittal plane** (Figure 11.3). Flexion occurs as the palm is brought toward the anterior surface of the forearm. Average range of motion is 80⁰ for flexion and 70⁰ for hyperextension.

Radial deviation (abduction) and **ulnar deviation**

(adduction) occur in the **frontal plane** (Figure 11.4). From anatomical position, ulnar deviation takes place when the ulnar side of the hand is moved in a medial direction. With radial deviation the radial side of the hand is moved laterally. Average range of motion for radial deviation is 20⁰; ulnar deviation is 30⁰.

Thumb

Thumb movement is at the **carpometacarpal (CMC), metacarpophalangeal (MCP)** and **interphalangeal (IP) joints.** At the CMC, MCP, and IP joints, **flexion** and **extension** occur in the **frontal plane** (Figure 11.5). In CMC and MCP flexion, the thumb is brought across the

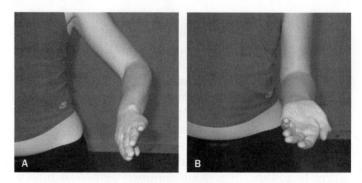

Figure 11.2 Forearm pronation (A) and supination (B).

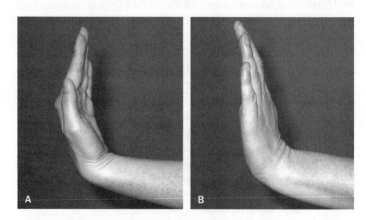

Figure 11.3 Wrist flexion (A) and extension (B).

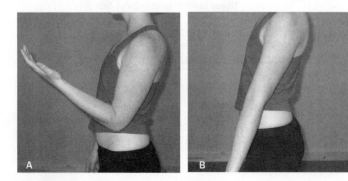

Figure 11.1 Elbow flexion (A) and extension (B).

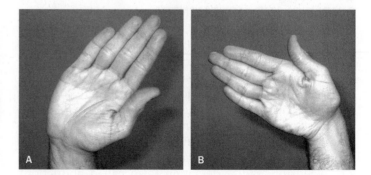

Figure 11.4 Wrist radial deviation (A) and ulnar deviation (B).

palm, which requires a slight degree of abduction as well. In extension, the thumb moves in a lateral direction from anatomical position. Average range of motion for flexion is approximately 15^0; 20^0 for extension.

In IP flexion, the tip of the thumb is brought toward the anterior surface of the palm. Extension is the return to anatomical position. Average range of motion for IP flexion at the thumb is 80^0. Values are not calculated for extension; further movement is generally not available.

Abduction and **adduction** at the CMC and MCP joints occur in the **sagittal plane** (Figure 11.6). Abduction occurs from anatomical position as the thumb moves anterior from the palm. Adduction is the return of the thumb from an abducted position. Average range of motion for abduction is 70^0. Further adduction, when the thumb moves past the hand, is minimal so values are not calculated.

Fingers

In the **metacarpophalangeal (MCP), proximal interphalangeal (PIP)**, and **distal interphalangeal (DIP)** joints, **flexion** and **extension** occur in the **sagittal plane** (Figure 11.7). Movement at the MCP joint occurs as the finger is brought toward the anterior surface of the palm from anatomical position. Returning the finger to anatomical position is extension in the MCP; hyperextension is movement past full extension. Average range of motion for MCP flexion is 90^0; hyperextension is approximately 30^0 with more passive motion possible than active.

Movement at the PIP and DIP joints occurs as the tip of the finger is brought toward the anterior surface of the palm in flexion. The finger is in full extension in anatomical position and ordinarily there is no additional range of extension available. Average range of motion for finger flexion at the PIP joint is 100^0; average range of motion at the DIP joint is 85^0–90^0.

Abduction and **adduction** at the MCP joint is in the **frontal plane** (Figure 11.8). Abduction is different for the four fingers because finger abduction is movement away from the midline of the hand versus the midline of the body.[4] Adduction is the return to anatomical position. No

Box 11.1 Clinical Notes

Motion of the Thumb

Terminology for the motions of the thumb is inconsistent and erroneous in some texts. Frontal plane motion in the thumb is called either abduction/adduction or extension/flexion, depending on the source. The reason for this lack of consistency concerns both anatomy and biomechanics.

The orientation of the carpometacarpal (CMC) joint of the thumb is almost perpendicular to that of the fingers. As a result, the motions of the thumb are opposite those of the fingers. Thumb movement terms should be based on anatomical structure not similarity with the motions of the fingers. Sagittal plane movement of the fingers is flexion/extension and in the thumb it is abduction/adduction. Frontal plane movement of the fingers is abduction/adduction and flexion/extension in the thumb.

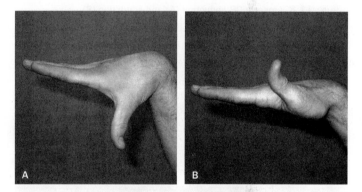

Figure 11.6 Thumb CMC abduction (A) and CMC adduction (B).

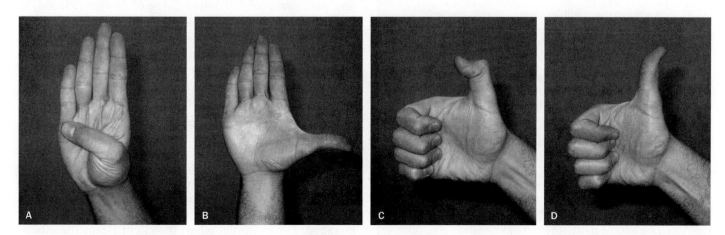

Figure 11.5 Thumb CMC flexion (A) CMC extension (B) IP flexion (C) and IP extension (D).

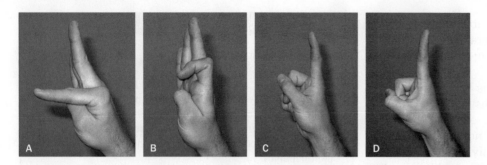

Figure 11.7 Finger MCP flexion (A), PIP flexion (B), DIP flexion (C), and MCP, PIP, and DIP extension (D).

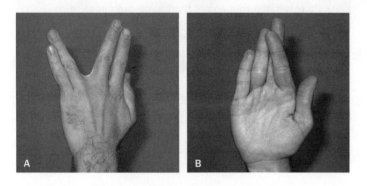

Figure 11.8 Finger MCP abduction (A) and adduction (B).

range-of-motion values for adduction or abduction are usually calculated at the MCP joint.

Capsular patterns

Range-of-motion testing in the elbow, forearm, wrist, and hand requires evaluation at several articulations. It is important to consider the role of the joint capsule when assessing joint function. Pathological problems in the capsule, such as fibrosis, may be visible with the joint's capsular pattern. The capsular pattern is a pattern of movement restriction that is characteristic to each individual joint. It is present in both active and passive motion. Capsular patterns are represented by a sequential listing of the movements from most likely to least likely limited. See Box 11.2 for the capsular patterns in this region.

RANGE-OF-MOTION & RESISTIVE TESTS

Results from single-plane movement analysis form the basis for further evaluation procedures. Movement testing should be performed in a certain order, allowing for an efficient evaluation and the least amount of accumulated discomfort or pain to develop. It is also general practice to leave movements known or expected to be painful to the end of the evaluation. When possible, the pain-free side is evaluated first.

Active range-of-motion (AROM) movements are performed first to establish the client's movement abilities and pain symptoms. Passive range of motion (PROM) is performed next and manual resistive tests (MRT) follow. AROM results may make PROM assessment procedures unnecessary. If no pain occurs with active movement, pain is unlikely with passive movement. The practitioner should be familiar with the full step-by-step instructions and guidelines for how to interpret (ROM) and resistive test results explained in Chapter 3.

Active Range of Motion

Active motions are usually evaluated with the client in a vertical (either seated or standing) position. When performing AROM evaluations, take into consideration the position of the limb to ensure the target tissues are engaged. For example, when the client flexes the elbow (by lifting the forearm toward the upper arm), the elbow

---

BOX 11.2 CAPSULAR PATTERNS FOR DISTAL UPPER EXTREMITY

Elbow

Flexion more limited than extension

Forearm Radioulnar joints

Pronation and supination usually equally limited

Wrist

Flexion and extension equally limited

Possible slight limitation in radial and ulnar deviation

Thumb CMC joint

Abduction most limited

Extension limited after abduction

Thumb MCP & IP joints

Flexion more limited than extension

Fingers MCP, PIP, & DIP joints

Flexion limited most, followed by extension

BOX 11.3 MUSCLE ACTIONS OF THE ELBOW, FOREARM, & WRIST

Elbow	**Flexion**	**Extension**
	Brachialis	Triceps brachii
	Biceps brachii	Anconeus
	Brachioradialis	
	Pronator teres	
	Extensor carpi radialis longus	
	Flexor carpi radialis	
	Flexor carpi ulnaris	

Forearm	**Pronation**	**Supination**
	Pronator teres	Biceps brachii
	Pronator quadratus	Supinator

Wrist	**Flexion**	**Extension**
	Flexor carpi radialis	Extensor carpi radialis longus
	Flexor carpi ulnaris	Extensor carpi radialis brevis
	Palmaris longus	Extensor carpi ulnaris
	Flexor digitorum superficialis	Extensor digitorum
	Flexor digitorum profundus	

Wrist	**Radial Deviation**	**Ulnar Deviation**
	Extensor carpi radialis longus	Extensor carpi ulnaris
	Extensor carpi radialis brevis	Flexor carpi ulnaris
	Extensor pollicis longus	
	Extensor pollicis brevis	
	Flexor carpi radialis	
	Abductor pollicis longus	

flexors are engaged concentrically. When the elbow returns to anatomical position it is not the elbow extensors that are responsible for the action, but the elbow flexors as they employ an eccentric contraction. Engaging the elbow extensors requires a change in body position or in the way resistance to the movement is offered.

Pain with active movement indicates problems in either the contractile or inert tissues associated with that movement. Factors prematurely limiting active movement in this region include *ligamentous or capsular damage, muscle contractures*, pain from *nerve compression or tension, tendinosis, tenosynovitis, fibrous cysts,* or *joint disorders* such as *arthritis*.

Compare AROM test results with those from PROM and manual resistive tests to identify possible reasons for movement restriction. The muscles used to perform actions of the elbow, forearm, wrist, and hand are listed in Box 11.3. Note that other muscles can contribute to the motion and subsequent dysfunction.

GENERAL INSTRUCTIONS FOR ROM & RESISTIVE TESTS

Overall
- Determine motions possible at the joint to be tested.
- Select the motion to be evaluated.
- Determine the tissues involved in the motion.
- Leave motions expected to be painful to the last.
- Test the uninvolved side first.
- Ask about, note any reported pain or discomfort.

AROM
- Demonstrate the movement to be performed.
- Have the client perform the movement.

PROM
- Establish the joint's normal end feel.
- Have the client relax as much as possible.
- Use gentle and slow movements.

MRT
- Test one action at a time.
- Position should isolate the action/ muscles involved.
- If pain is suspected, start in a mid-range position.
- Client uses a strong, but appropriate amount of effort.

Box 11.4 Muscle Actions of the Thumb

Thumb (CMC)	**Flexion**	**Extension**
	Flexor pollicis longus	Extensor pollicis brevis
	Opponens pollicis	Extensor pollicis longus
	Flexor pollicis brevis	Abductor pollicis longus
	Adductor pollicis	
Thumb (CMC)	**Abduction**	**Adduction**
	Abductor pollicis longus	Adductor pollicis
	Abductor pollicis brevis	Extensor pollicis longus
	Extensor pollicis brevis	First dorsal interosseous
	Opponens pollics	
	Palmaris longus	
Thumb (MCP)	**Flexion**	**Extension**
	Adductor pollicis	Extensor pollicis longus
	Flexor pollicis longus	Extensor pollicis brevis
	Flexor pollicis brevis	
	Abductor pollicis brevis	
Thumb (MCP)	**Abduction**	**Adduction**
	Abductor pollicis brevis	Adductor pollicis
Thumb (IP)	**Flexion**	**Extension**
	Flexor pollicis longus	Extensor pollicis longus
		Abductor pollicis brevis

Passive Range of Motion

Passive motion is performed after active. Pain during passive movement predominantly implicates inert tissues. However, muscles and tendons that contract in the opposite direction are stretched at the end range of passive movement.

PROM testing also evaluates end feel. Box 11.6 lists the primary joint locations and their normal end feel. Review Chapter 3 for a discussion of normal and pathological end feel descriptions. Factors that could prematurely limit passive movement are the same as for active movement.

Manual Resistive Tests

A manual resistive test (MRT) produces pain when there is a mechanical disruption of tissue. Pain with an MRT indicates that one or more of the muscles and/or tendons performing that action are involved. Testing all of a muscle's actions is not necessary, as a muscle's secondary actions recruit other muscles and make the test results less accurate. Palpation elicits more information if the test alone does not produce pain or discomfort. Refer to

Box 11.3-5 for the list of primary muscles involved with each action. Table 2 at the end of the chapter lists actions commonly used for testing muscles in the elbow, forearm, wrist, and hand.

In some cases weakness is evident with MRTs. Factors that produce weakness include lack of use, *fatigue, reflex muscular inhibition*, and possibly a neurological pathology (*radiculopathy, peripheral neuropathy*, or a *systemic neurological disorder*). The nerves or nerve roots that may be involved are listed in Table 1 at the end of the chapter.

Elbow

Resisted Flexion and Extension

To test flexion, the client is standing or seated with the elbow flexed to 90^0. The practitioner places one hand on the posterior distal end of the client's humerus. The other hand is placed at the distal forearm. The client holds this position as the practitioner attempts to push the client's forearm into extension (Figure 11.9).

To test extension, the client is prone on the treatment

Box 11.5 Muscle Actions of the Fingers

Finger (MCP)	Flexion	Extension
	Flexor digitorum superficialis	Extensor digitorum
	Flexor digitorum profundus	Extensor indicis
	Lumbricales	
	Palmar interossei	
	Dorsal interossei	

Finger (MCP)	Abduction	Adduction
	Dorsal interossei	Palmar interossei
	Extensor digitorum	Extensor indicis

Finger (PIP & DIP)	Flexion	Extension
	Flexor digitorum profundus	Extensor digitorum
	Flexor digitorum superficialis (PIP only)	Extensor indicis
		Lumbricales
		Palmar interossei
		Dorsal interossei

Box 11.6 Joints, Associated Motion, & Normal End Feel

Joint	Motion	End Feel
Elbow	Flexion	Soft-tissue approximation
	Extension	Bone to bone
Forearm	Pronation	Tissue stretch (soft)
	Supination	Tissue stretch (soft)
Wrist	Flexion	Tissue stretch (soft)
	Extension	Tissue stretch (soft)
	Radial Deviation	Tissue stretch (firm)
	Ulnar Deviation	Tissue stretch (firm)
Thumb (CMC)	Flexion	Tissue stretch (soft)
	Extension	Tissue stretch (soft)
	Abduction	Tissue stretch (soft)
	Adduction	Tissue stretch (soft)
Thumb (MCP)	Flexion	Tissue stretch (soft)
	Extension	Tissue stretch (soft)
	Abduction	Tissue stretch (soft)
	Adduction	Tissue stretch (soft)
Thumb (IP)	Flexion	Tissue stretch (firm)
	Extension	Tissue stretch (firm)
Finger (MCP)	Flexion	Tissue stretch (firm)
	Extension	Tissue stretch (soft)
	Abduction	Tissue stretch (soft)
	Adduction	Tissue stretch (soft)
Finger (PIP & DIP)	Flexion	Tissue stretch (soft)
	Extension	Tissue stretch (firm)

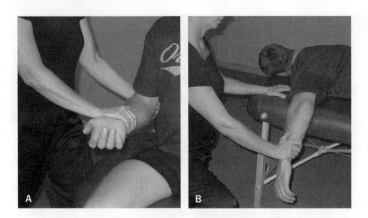

Figure 11.9 Resisted elbow flexion (A) and extension (B).

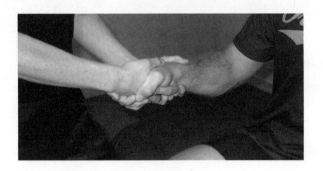

Figure 11.10 Resisted forearm pronation or supination.

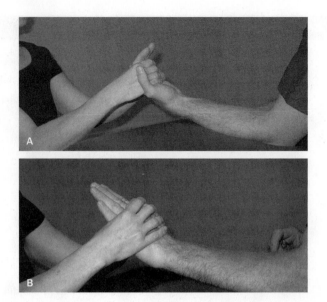

Figure 11.11 Resisted wrist flexion (A) and extension (B).

table with the humerus abducted to 90⁰ and supported by the table and the elbow at the table's edge. The client's arm is brought into full or partial extension. The practitioner places a hand on the client's distal forearm and the client holds this position while the practitioner attempts to push the client's arm into flexion (Figure 11.9).

Forearm
RESISTED PRONATION AND SUPINATION
The client is standing or seated. The practitioner grasps the client's hand as if shaking hands. The practitioner's other hand stabilizes the client's forearm. The client holds the position as the practitioner attempts to either supinate (to test pronation) or pronate (to test supination) the client's forearm (Figure 11.10).

Wrist
RESISTED FLEXION AND EXTENSION
The client is seated with the forearm supinated or pronated and supported by the treatment table with the wrist at the table's edge. The practitioner grasps the client's hand with one or both hands. (The other hand can stabilize the client's forearm on the table if desired). To test flexion, the client's forearm is supinated and the client holds the hand stationary while the practitioner attempts to pull the wrist into extension (Figure 11.11). To test extension, the forearm is pronated and the practitioner attempts to move the wrist into flexion (Figure 11.11).

RESISTED RADIAL AND ULNAR DEVIATION
The client is seated with the forearm in neutral and supported by the treatment table with the wrist at the table's edge. The practitioner grasps the client's hand with one or both hands. (The other hand can stabilize the forearm if desired). The client holds the wrist stationary while the practitioner attempts to pull the wrist into ulnar deviation (to test radial deviation) or into radial deviation (to test ulnar deviation) (Figure 11.12).

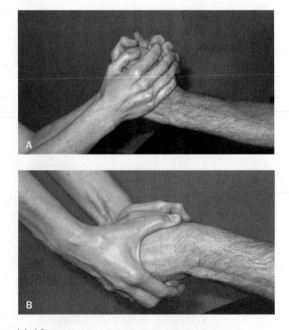

Figure 11.12 Resisted radial (A) and ulnar deviation (B).

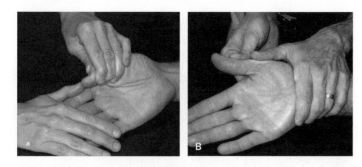

Figure 11.13 Resisted thumb flexion (A) and extension (B).

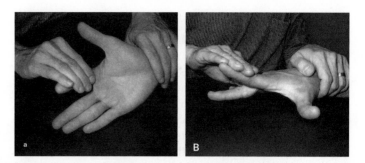

Figure 11.15 Resisted finger flexion (A) and extension (B).

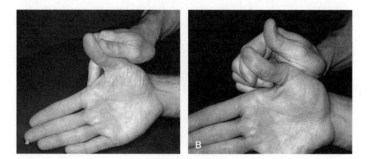

Figure 11.14 Resisted thumb abduction (A) and adduction (B).

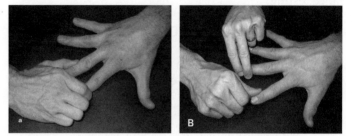

Figure 11.16 Resisted finger abduction (A) and adduction (B).

Thumb

RESISTED FLEXION AND EXTENSION

The client is seated with the forearm and hand supported by the treatment table. The practitioner uses one hand to stabilize the client's hand while the other hand offers resistance to the client's thumb movement. The client is instructed to pull the thumb medially across the palm to test flexion or to pull the thumb away from the palm to test extension (Figure 11.13).

RESISTED ABDUCTION AND ADDUCTION

The client is seated with the forearm and hand supported by the treatment table. The forearm is supinated so the hand rests on the treatment table. The practitioner uses one hand to stabilize the client's hand, while the other hand offers resistance to the client's thumb movement. To test abduction, the client attempts to pull the thumb upwards, away from the table, as the practitioner pushes against the thumb. To test adduction, the practitioner positions the client's thumb in abduction and the client pulls the thumb toward the table as the practitioner resists the movement (Figure 11.14).

Fingers

RESISTED FLEXION AND EXTENSION

The client is seated with the forearm and hand supported by the treatment table. The practitioner uses one hand to stabilize the client's hand while the other controls the motion of the finger. To test flexion, the forearm is supinated and the practitioner brings the client's finger into partial flexion at the MCP joint. The client holds this position as the practitioner attempts to push the finger into

extension (Figure 11.15).

To test extension, the forearm is pronated. The client starts with the finger in a partially extended position and holds it stationary as the practitioner attempts to push the finger into flexion (Figure 11.15).

RESISTED ABDUCTION AND ADDUCTION

The client is seated with the forearm and hand supported by the treatment table and the forearm in a pronated or supinated position. The practitioner uses one hand to stabilize the client's wrist and the other hand to control the finger motion. The client holds their fingers apart. To test abduction, the practitioner attempts to push the fingers back together as the client resists (Figure 11.16). To test adduction, the client attempts to pull the fingers back together while the practitioner resists (Figure 11.16)

BOX 11.7 CLINICAL NOTES

Evaluating finger motions

Because the fingers have multiple joints it is possible to evaluate manual resistance at each specific joint-- MCP, PIP, and DIP. However, due to the difficulty in isolating motions, flexion and extension are usually evaluated with the entire finger instead of at each joint.

Structural and Postural Deviations

The following section covers common structural or postural deviations unique to the elbow, forearm, wrist, and hand. Under each condition there is a brief description of its characteristics followed by likely HOPRS findings. If applicable, orthopedic tests are included in the special tests section. If no special orthopedic test is listed for that condition, evaluation should focus on other portions of the assessment process, such as range-of-motion or resistance testing.

EXCESSIVE CUBITAL VALGUS

Excessive cubital valgus is a structural deviation involving the *carrying angle* at the elbow that can lead to upper extremity disorders.

Characteristics

In anatomical position there is a natural angulation of the forearm called the **cubital valgus** or carrying angle, which allows the forearm to swing away from the body during the normal walking stride (Figure 11.17). A *valgus angulation* is a lateral deviation of the distal end of a bony segment. The carrying angle prevents objects carried in the hand from hitting the body and is normally 5^0–15^0. **A carrying angle that exceeds 15^0 is considered excessive.** Although excessive cubital valgus has no specific symptoms, it can lead to various conditions such as *cubital tunnel syndrome, medial epicondylitis, apophysitis,* and *myofascial trigger points.*

Excessive cubital valgus usually results from genetics, but could be caused by an injury such as a fracture. Epiphyseal injuries or fractures can cause a related condition where the carrying angle has a varus angulation, called *cubital varus* or *gunstock deformity.*

History

Ask the client about pain or symptoms being experienced and any history of injuries or fractures. Also ask whether the client is aware of the deviation. If the condition results from an injury, the nature of the injury and damage to adjacent structures should be identified.

Observation

A significant valgus angulation of the forearm will be apparent when the client stands in anatomical position; compare the angulations of each side to determine similarity and differences. To determine if the angle is excessive, measure it with a goniometer.

Palpation

Palpation produces no specific findings. Irritation to the ulnar nerve or attachment sites of the flexor muscles may cause tenderness in those areas. An injury may produce residual tenderness in the elbow region.

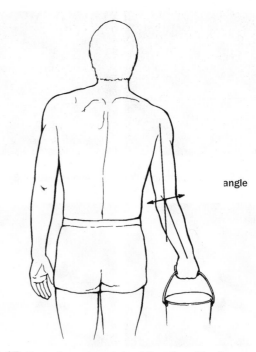

Figure 11.17 Normal carrying angle at the elbow. The forearm angles more in a lateral direction in excessive cubital valgus. (Mediclip image copyright, 1998 Williams & Wilkins. All rights reserved).

Range-of-Motion and Resistance Testing

AROM: Active range of motion is not impaired unless the excessive cubital valgus results from traumatic injury that otherwise limits motion. If the postural distortion is considerable, pain or irritation might develop near the end of full elbow flexion as the ulnar nerve and flexor tendons are pulled taut.
PROM: The same principles apply as for active motion.
MRT: No unusual findings with manual resistive tests.

Suggestions for Treatment

No treatment is generally recommended for excessive cubital valgus, but resulting soft-tissue disorders may need treatment. If there is nerve impairment or recurrent nerve pain, the client should be referred to a physician. If nerve irritation is severe or impedes function, surgery can be performed that repositions the ulnar nerve.

DUPUYTREN'S CONTRACTURE

Dupuytren's contracture is a condition that produces fibrous restriction in both the palmar fascia and the flexor tendons of the fingers.

Characteristics

Dupuytren's contracture is a **fibrosis of the palmar fascia that affects the tendons of the fingers,** causing *flexion contractures* that force the fingers to curl into flexion at the MCP, PIP, or DIP joints (Figure 11.18). It usually affects both hands, but the hands can have different degrees of severity. Shaffer[6] describes three stages of fibrous thicken-

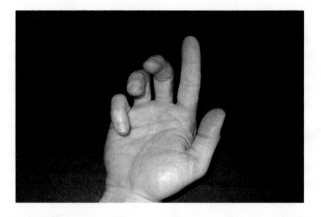

Figure 11.18 Common hand distortion involving flexion deformity seen in Dupuytren's contracture.

ing in Dupuytren's contracture: in the *proliferative phase*, myofibroblasts develop; in the *involutional phase*, the myofibroblasts align along tension lines; and in the *residual phase*, tissue becomes acellular and leaves thick bands of collagen. The condition begins with a loss of range of motion in the fingers and progresses as the flexion contractures develop, leading to loss of finger extension. In time, the fingers are held in a constant, but varied, degree of flexion. The condition is more pronounced in the 4th and 5th digits.

The causes for the condition are not well understood, but there are factors that increase the risk of its development. Studies show a greater incidence in people who have diabetes, seizure disorders, smoke, or drink alcohol excessively.[7-9] There is some indication that the increased incidence in patients with seizure disorders is related to use of phenobarbital for seizure treatment.[6] Some people have a genetic predisposition to developing the condition, with a greater incidence occurring in descendants of Scandinavian cultures.[10] The condition is more likely to affect men than women.[11, 12]

History
Symptoms will depend on the development stage, but include thickening sensations just under the skin on the palm, pain, or tightness and loss of motion in the fingers. In more advanced stages, the fingers will be permanently flexed.

Ask whether the client has discussed the condition with a physician. Identify any history of seizures or diabetes and types of medications used. Ask about patterns of alcohol or nicotine use that are greater than average. Explore the occurrence of this or other similar conditions in family members and if the client descends from a northern European culture. There could be multiple precipitating factors.

Observation
Thickening of the palmar fascia may be observable. Fibrosis gathers around the flexor tendons causing them

to look somewhat cord-like. Flexion deformities occur typically at the 4th and 5th digits (Figure 11.18). Pitting and loss of mobility in the skin of the palm is evident during some hand movements.

Palpation
Palpable fibrous nodules may be present in the palm or joints of the fingers. These nodules can develop into cord-like structures that are palpable under the skin. The skin feels firm or tight throughout the palm and fingers.

Range-of-Motion and Resistance Testing
AROM: Active finger flexion and extension is impaired.
PROM: There is typically crepitus or stiffness in the tissues with passive motion. Passive flexion can be limited; extension is limited due to the contractures.
MRT: Weakness with resisted flexion and extension and reduced grip strength is likely. Resisted flexion may cause pain.

Differential Evaluation
Stenosing tenosynovitis, nerve compression pathologies, rheumatoid arthritis, synovial ganglions, tumors, or fibrositic processes in the hand.

Suggestions for Treatment
A number of treatments are used, including splinting, ultrasound, stretching and flexibility exercises, as well as injection therapy.[6] When these conservative measures fail, surgery is sometimes used. Although there is no available literature on using massage for treating Dupuytren's contracture, empirical reports indicate that stripping and myofascial techniques are helpful in reducing the fibrosis and increasing range of motion.

RHEUMATOID ARTHRITIS

Rheumatoid arthritis (RA) **is a systemic autoimmune disorder that is** *polyarticular* (affecting multiple joints), with the hands and feet affected more frequently than other joints. In more advanced stages it affects tissues other than joints. The cause of RA is not known, although there is speculation that viruses, bacteria, or fungi are involved.[13] Other research suggests genetic or environmental factors.[14] An antibody called *rheumatoid factor* is usually present in RA and the client is tested for this by a physician. It is particularly helpful if RA is treated in its early stages.

Characteristics
In RA, the body's **immune system erroneously attacks the lining of the synovial membrane** surrounding the joints through an enzymatic reaction that causes *articular degeneration*.[15] The condition is progressive. Initially there is inflammation and proliferation of fibrous tissue, causing swelling, heat, puffiness, and fibrin deposits that cause movement pain.[16] Range of motion is decreased

due to stiffness and pain, which is generally worse in the morning due to accumulation of fluid in the synovial tissues during the night. Symptoms are common in the distal extremities, particularly in the hands. Other regions of the body may also be affected, and fever, fatigue, and anemia may be present.

Many symptoms of RA are intermittent because the disease can flare up and then go into remission. During flare-up, the joints of the body become stiff and sore. Because it is a systemic autoimmune disorder, both sides of the body are typically affected simultaneously. The condition often begins in the hands and wrists and spreads to other joints such as the knees, ankles, feet, and cervical spine.[16] One of the main characteristics that distinguishes RA from *osteoarthritis* is the degree of swelling and deformity in the hands, which is more pronounced in RA. This condition can produce *stenosing tenosynovitis* (trigger finger) as a result of inflammation in the synovial sheaths of the flexor tendons.

As the condition progresses there is continued thickening of the synovial membrane, which can lead to a destructive phase involving tendon adhesions and ruptures, loosening of the joint capsules, subluxations, and permanent joint deformities.[17] Temporary or permanent joint deformities occur at the **MCP finger joints**. Due to the mobility in both the sagittal and frontal planes of the MCP joints, there is a greater degree of distortion possible in these joints than in the IP joints of the fingers.[17] The fingers are sometimes held in a flexion deformity or forced laterally or medially. Due to joint mechanics, it is rare for the deformity to fix the fingers in extension at the MCP joint. In the frontal plane, the fingers can be forced medially into what is called an *ulnar drift*, where the fingers deviate toward the ulnar side of the hand. Other common deviations include the *swan-neck* and *boutonniere deformities* (Figure 11.19).[4,18]

The condition occurs more in older individuals and women are affected 2–3 times more than men.[15, 19] Oral contraceptives and pregnancy are associated with a decreased risk of developing the condition, while there is higher risk in the postpartum period.[13] Other factors increase an individual's risk for the condition, including cigarette smoking, obesity, or blood transfusions.[13, 20, 21] Certain environmental conditions may play a role in the

condition, although exact causes are not established.[14, 22]

The incidence of RA is very low in African and Southeast Asian cultures and higher in American Indian and Alaska Native populations. Research is ongoing about whether this increased incidence is a genetic factor or related to lifestyle and environmental issues.

History
The client complains of swelling and pain in various joints, particularly the hands and feet. Pain is normally symmetrical between both sides of the body, but can be unilateral. Pain is felt while at rest and magnified during movement of the affected joint. Joint stiffness and limited range of motion is pronounced in the morning and ordinarily dissipates over the course of several hours. Clients with advanced stages of the condition frequently have deformities in their hands and complain of pain or movement limitations. Fatigue and periodic fever might be reported as well. Ask the client if he or she has seen a physician, as a referral is warranted.

Observation
Joints affected by RA characteristically become enlarged with visible nodules. The skin may appear puffy, red, or shiny during the initial inflammatory reaction.[16] Look for characteristic hand and finger distortions such as ulnar drift and the swan-neck and boutonniere deformities described above.

Palpation
The practitioner is likely to feel heat, swelling, or nodules at the affected joints. The tissues surrounding the joints are often painful when palpated. If there is fibrosity and disuse, the practitioner will feel stiffness in the muscles and other soft tissues of the hand.

Range-of-Motion and Resistance Testing
AROM: Any active motion that involves the affected joint(s) is usually painful. Motion is not always painful when the condition is not flared up. If the condition is advanced, active motion is limited in various directions due to pain and/or fibrosity within the joint.
PROM: Because the pathology involves inflammation of synovial tissue, the tissues are irritated during passive as well as active motion. Any motion at the affected joint(s) could be painful. As with active motion there is greater tenderness if the RA is flared up.
MRT: It is more common to see muscle weakness than pain with an MRT. Weakness can be due to neurological inhibition and to fibrositic changes in the muscle-tendon unit. MRTs that engage muscles acting on the affected joints may produce pain.

Differential Evaluation
Stenosing tenosynovitis, Dupuytren's contracture, osteoarthritis, degenerative joint disease, gout, peripheral nerve compression, tendinosis, tenosynovitis.

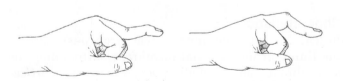

Figure 11.19 Swan-neck (A) and boutonniere deformity (B). (image courtesy of Primal Pictures Ltd. www.primalpictures.com.)

Suggestions for Treatment

There is no known cure for rheumatoid arthritis. If RA is suspected, practitioners should refer the client to a physician and get clearance before providing palliative care. Some clients find relaxation massage beneficial, but caution is advised. Massage is helpful in certain stages, but is also considered a contraindication in the more acute stages as it may increase inflammatory activity.[19, 25] The primary goals of treatment are to manage symptoms, prevent further inflammation, and reduce the risk of permanent joint damage. In some cases, NSAIDS and corticosteroids are used to address the inflammation. Heat is used to relieve joint pain and stiffness, while cold is used during acute bouts of inflammation. Some studies show dietary treatment with omega-3 fatty acids to be beneficial.[26]

Common Injury Conditions

LATERAL EPICONDYLITIS (TENNIS ELBOW)

Lateral epicondylitis (LE) is a common overuse syndrome of the elbow, affecting 1–3% of the population.[27,28] This increased incidence is due to several factors such as repetitive motion activities and poor conditioning. Although LE occurs among tennis players, this group only accounts for a small percentage of the population that suffers from the condition.[29, 30] LE is more prevalent in the occupational sector.

Characteristics

Recent studies indicate that in the majority of cases lateral epicondylitis is not an inflammatory condition, but **chronic *collagen degeneration* in the extensor tendons and *enthesopathy* (irritation of the attachment site) at the lateral epicondyle of the humerus** (Figure 11.20).[31-35] Tendon degeneration is more accurately called *tendinosis*. Some research shows inflammation during early onset that could lead to chronic degeneration if not immediately resolved.[27]

Repeated tensile stress on the tendons leads to *collagen degeneration* and *enthesopathy*. The **extensor carpi radialis brevis (ECRB)** is the most affected due to its anatomical arrangement and line of pull.[36] However, the tendon fibers from all the wrist extensor muscles blend near the attachment site at the lateral epicondyle and may also be involved in the condition.[37]

Pain is aggravated by actions that engage the extensor muscles in a contraction (concentric, isometric, or eccentric). Motions requiring wrist flexion produce pain due to the extensor tendons being stretched. In a few acute cases, pain results from fiber tearing in the tendon or periosteal tears at the attachment site of the ECRB tendon.[38]

Any activities that stress the tendons can produce LE. Sports, occupations, or hobbies that require the repetitive grasping of objects, such as tennis rackets, tools, or a computer mouse, can lead to the condition. Repetitive

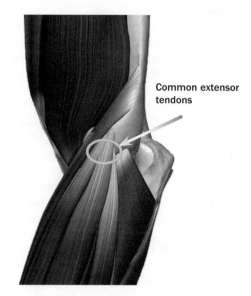

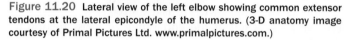

Figure 11.20 Lateral view of the left elbow showing common extensor tendons at the lateral epicondyle of the humerus. (3-D anatomy image courtesy of Primal Pictures Ltd. www.primalpictures.com.)

supination or pronation may also cause LE.[41] Symptoms are generally unilateral, but could be bilateral if symmetrical upper extremity forearm activities are performed. The condition is seen most frequently in occupational activities, for example massage therapy, computer work, or construction, where chronic stress comes from holding static positions.[39, 40] Using a mouse or holding a hammer requires the wrist and hand extensors to be under constant isometric contraction, sufficient to cause tendon degeneration.

It is not unusual for other conditions to co-exist with lateral epicondylitis or be related to its onset. For example, *myofascial trigger points* that cause the extensor muscles to be hypertonic create an excess tensile load on the tendons and can lead to the epicondylitis.[42]

History

The client reports pain in the lateral elbow region that radiates into the forearm. Discomfort is typically a generalized aching, although if highly aggravated the client describes the pain as sharp. Acute onset is rare, but inquire about whether onset was gradual or sudden. Ask about activities requiring repetitive gripping or static contractions of the forearms and wrist. The extensors are used to stabilize the wrist in many activities and the client may report difficulty grasping or lifting a smaller item, such as a glass or book.

Observation

There are rarely visible indicators of LE as it is not an inflammatory condition. Even when there is inflammation at the insertion site, such as a periosteal tear or enthesitis, the inflammatory reaction is rarely visible.

Palpation

Tenderness and pain are likely where the extensor tendons attach at the lateral epicondyle of the humerus. The wrist extensors characteristically feel hypertonic as well. Pain is increased if the wrist is put in flexion and the muscles or tendons are palpated. A fibrotic or ropy feel to the extensor tendons and the extensor muscles in the forearm can be present. Palpate the path of the extensor carpi radialis brevis muscle and tendon as it is often affected.

Pain referrals from myofascial trigger points may be evident near the elbow or forearm when forearm muscles are palpated. Entrapment of the posterior interosseous nerve near the attachment of the extensor tendons could produce pain down the forearm with palpation.[43]

Range-of-Motion and Resistance Testing

AROM: Pain may or may not be present with active wrist extension, as only a minor contraction is required in wrist extension. Pain occurs at the end range of active wrist flexion as the extensor tendons are stretched.

PROM: Pain is felt at the end range of wrist flexion as the affected tendons are stretched. Pain or discomfort is uncommon with passive wrist extension as the muscles and tendons are not stressed.

MRT: Pain is present with resisted wrist extension. Reflex muscular inhibition characteristically produces weakness. Weakness can result not only from LE, but from posterior interosseous nerve compression in the radial tunnel near the lateral humeral epicondyle (see Radial Tunnel Syndrome).

Special Test

Tennis Elbow Test

The client is standing or seated. The practitioner wraps one hand around the client's elbow so the thumb is pressing on the extensor tendons just distal to the lateral epicondyle of the humerus. Be careful not to press on the ulnar nerve on the posterior side of the elbow while holding the elbow. The practitioner's other hand grasps the client's hand and uses it to resist the client's wrist extension. Only offer resistance to wrist extension and do not push the client's arm toward the floor, as this recruits other muscles that may confuse the test. This test is simply a manual resistive test for wrist extension with pressure being placed simultaneously on the affected tendons (Figure 11.21).

Explanation: Contracting the wrist extensors causes pain as the affected tendons are pulled near the attachment site. By pressing on the tendons while in contraction, stress to the damaged tissues is exaggerated, making the test more sensitive than a manual resistive test alone.

Differential Evaluation

Radial tunnel syndrome, myofascial trigger point activity, ligament damage near the elbow, radial neuropathy, cervical radiculopathy, joint pathology of the elbow joints, medial epicondylitis.

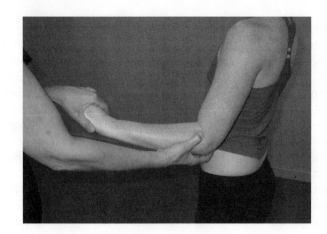

Figure 11.21 Tennis elbow test.

Suggestions for Treatment

This condition is treated conservatively. Ultrasound, stretching, range-of-motion exercises, and electrical stimulation are common physical therapy modalities used for treatment. Anti-inflammatory medications are sometimes used with beneficial results in the early stages of treatment.[27] Many individuals use various elastic bands for support although the therapeutic benefits of these is questioned due to their impact on circulation and function.[44]

Lateral epicondylitis responds well to massage. Deep friction is applied directly on the affected tendons in order to stimulate collagen production in the damaged tendon fibers.[45] Deep longitudinal stripping, myofascial approaches, and massage with active engagement are all beneficial to restore optimum function to the wrist extensors. Although beneficial in the long run, many of these treatments can be uncomfortable when administered, so exercise caution when applying them. Teaching the client how to perform self massage is advantageous for regular stimulation of collagen production during what is ordinarily a slow healing process.

MEDIAL EPICONDYLITIS (GOLFER'S ELBOW)

Medial epicondylitis (ME) occurs in the golfing population, but also exists in other populations who engage in repetitive activities.[46, 47] The populations at risk for lateral epicondylitis are also susceptible to medial epicondylitis.

Characteristics

ME is similar to *lateral epicondylitis* except the tendons affected are the **wrist flexors where they attach to the medial epicondyle of the humerus** instead of the extensors at the lateral epicondyle (Figure 11.22). ME is not inflammatory. **Excessive tensile stress on the flexor tendons causes chronic collagen degeneration (*tendinosis*) and *enthesopathy* at the attachment site.**[41, 48] The condition develops from repetitive or prolonged contractions

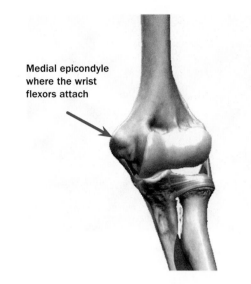

Medial epicondyle where the wrist flexors attach

Figure 11.22 Anterior view of the left elbow showing attachment site of the wrist flexors. (3-D anatomy image courtesy of Primal Pictures Ltd. www.primalpictures.com.)

of the wrist flexor group.[49] Because the wrist and finger flexors are responsible for grasping and holding objects, the condition frequently develops in the occupational sector due to the manipulation of tools and equipment with the hands. The actions involved in throwing also make ME a common sports injury.[50]

Problems may derive from repetitive supination and pronation of the forearm because of the stress placed on the **pronator teres muscle**.[41] While the pronator teres is not a flexor of the wrist, the proximity of its attachment site at the medial epicondyle and its coordinated effort with the wrist flexors cause it to be involved in ME in some cases.[41]

Actions that engage the flexor muscles in a contraction (concentric, isometric, or eccentric) aggravate pain. Pain might also occur in motions requiring wrist extension where the flexor tendons are being stretched. Pain is felt during activity and generally subsides shortly after activity has ceased. Poor conditioning is a cause of ME and should be identified in the history.[50]

It is possible for ME to be a result of an injury, eventually leading to chronic tendon irritation. For example, hitting the ground hard during a golf swing can be the initial stressor that leads to ME at a later date. Similar to lateral epicondylitis, there may be some initial inflammation with minor tendon fiber tearing that is a precursor to the more chronic tendon degeneration usually associated with the condition.[38]

Other conditions are seen regularly along with ME or are related to its onset. Workers with ME have a higher prevalence of other work-related musculoskeletal disorders, such as *carpal tunnel syndrome*.[51] When the flexor tendons are overused, it can lead to *tenosynovitis* in the carpal tunnel causing compression of the median nerve.[43]

The client might also complain of neurological sensations in the 4th and 5th digits, suggesting *ulnar nerve pathology*. Ulnar nerve involvement could arise from compression in the cubital tunnel by the **flexor carpi ulnaris** muscle (see Cubital Tunnel Syndrome). Part of the flexor carpi ulnaris attaches to the medial epicondyle so tightness could result in both medial epicondylitis and ulnar nerve compression.[47]

History

The client reports pain on the medial side of the elbow that radiates into the forearm. Pain is typically generalized aching, although if highly aggravated the client describes it as sharp. Similar to LE, normal onset is gradual rather than acute. Ask about activities requiring repetitive gripping or static contractions of the forearm and wrist. If the client developed the condition through work, try to identify ergonomic factors that overuse the flexor muscles. Inquire about sudden changes in activity level that could be related to poor conditioning.

The client may report pain when shaking hands as this action engages the affected muscles. Inquire about symptoms related to nerve pathologies, such as cubital or carpal tunnel syndromes, or pronator teres syndrome. The client's symptoms provide important clues for distinguishing tendinosis from these other nerve compression problems.

Observation

There are rarely visible indicators of medial epicondylitis as it is not an inflammatory condition. Even when there is inflammation at the insertion site, such as enthesitis, the inflammatory reaction is not visible. Some structural problems such as excessive cubital valgus are visible and may contribute to ME, but a structural problem is not necessarily a symptom of epicondylitis.

Range-of-Motion and Resistance Testing

AROM: Pain is possible in active wrist flexion, but only if the condition is severe. Without additional resistance there are not enough muscle fibers recruited to put adequate tension on the tendon and its attachment site. As the condition worsens less force is required to cause pain. There is pain at the end range of active extension as the affected tendons are stretched. Pain may also be felt at the end range of supination because the pronator teres is stretched.

PROM: Pain is felt at the end range of wrist hyperextension as the affected tendons are stretched and could occur at the end range of supination if the pronator teres is involved. Pain with passive wrist flexion or pronation is uncommon since these motions relieve the tensile load on the affected tendons.

MRT: Resisted wrist flexion produces pain. If the pronator teres is involved, pain is felt during resisted pronation. Weakness in either action is possible and results from reflex muscular inhibition.

Special Test

Golfer's Elbow Test

The client is standing or seated. The practitioner grasps the client's elbow so that the thumb is pressing on the flexor tendons just distal to their attachment site at the medial epicondyle. Be careful not to press on the ulnar nerve on the posterior side of the elbow. The practitioner's other hand is used to offer resistance to the client's wrist flexion. Only offer resistance to wrist flexion. Do not push the client's forearm arm toward the floor as this recruits other muscles that may confuse the test. This test is simply a manual resistive test for wrist flexion with pressure being placed simultaneously on the affected tendons (Figure 11.23).

Explanation: Engaging the wrist flexors in a contraction causes the pain of medial epicondylitis as there is tensile force on the affected tendons. Pressing on the tendons simultaneously, stresses the damaged tissue making the test more sensitive than a manual resistive test alone.

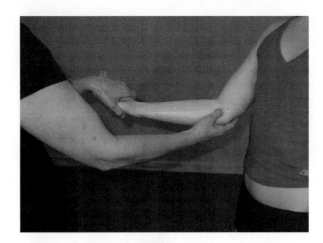

Figure 11.23 Golfer's elbow test.

Differential Evaluation

Arthritis, pronator teres strain, cubital tunnel syndrome, cervical radiculopathy, pronator teres syndrome, median nerve compression near the elbow, thoracic outlet syndrome, ulnar collateral ligament injury, osteochondritis dissecans, epicondylar apophysitis (little league elbow), stress fractures, ulnar nerve pathology, flexor muscle strain.

Suggestions for Treatment

Treatment suggestions for this condition are the same as for lateral epicondylitis except for the region where the treatment is applied. The primary tendons to be targeted are those of the wrist flexors on the medial forearm just distal to the medial epicondyle of the humerus. When performing massage treatment, attention should focus on the wrist flexors and pronator teres muscles.

OLECRANON BURSITIS

The pain that is experienced when one strikes the elbow on something comes from the direct impact on the olecranon process of the ulna. The bursa that lies superficial to the olecranon process is highly susceptible to compression trauma and the subsequent inflammatory reaction of *olecranon bursitis* that sometimes results.

Characteristics

The **olecranon bursa** sits directly superficial to the **olecranon process of the ulna** to protect it and reduce friction between the bony prominence and the overlying skin (Figure 11.24). The primary cause of olecranon bursitis is **compression of the bursa, which is followed by inflammation**. The compressive force may result from an acute injury or from chronic compressive loads over time. Acute bursitis occurs from a direct blow to the elbow. Chronic bursitis can develop from repeated compression, such as leaning on the elbows each day at work.

Other causes of olecranon bursitis include *infection, systemic disorders,* or *medical procedures* such as kidney dialysis.[52-55] In some cases, especially those involving systemic disorders, the bursa becomes infected and medical treatment is required.[56] Unlike systemic causes of bursitis, compressive bursitis is not serious, causes relatively minor movement restrictions, and is easily treated.

History

The client reports pain with various movements. If the condition is an acute injury, the client should be able to identify a traumatic event. If the condition appeared gradually, identify factors in the client's daily activities that might involve chronic compression of the elbow.

If there is no history of acute injury or chronic compression of the elbow, consider the possibility of a systemic disorder. In this case, if the client does not already have such a diagnosis they should be referred to a physician for further evaluation. Subsequent research into the client's history could show a relationship between the onset of a systemic disorder and that of the bursitis.

Observation

The clearest visual indicator of olecranon bursitis is a large lump on the posterior side of the elbow. In severe cases, this lump approaches the size of a golf ball or larger. Redness due to the inflammatory reaction may be visible. If present, redness and inflammation appear the same regardless of whether the condition is acute, chronic, or caused by a systemic disorder.

Palpation

The posterior elbow is tender to touch and even mild pressure produces pain. The amount of pain does not always coincide with the degree of inflammation in the bursa. Excess fluid around the posterior elbow is palpable. The area could feel warm due to inflammation. There is less likelihood of increased heat or redness with chronic bursitis.[56] In some cases where there is a systemic infection,

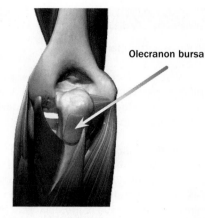

Figure 11.24 Posterior view of the left elbow showing the olecranon bursa which provides protection and reduces friction. (3-D anatomy image courtesy of Primal Pictures Ltd. www.primalpictures.com.)

heat may be felt in other areas due to fever.

Contrary to some anatomy illustrations, a normal bursa is only a few cell layers thick and therefore difficult, if not impossible, to palpate when not enlarged.[56] When the bursa is aggravated from either compression or systemic irritation, the cells multiply and the bursa begins to fill with excess fluid making it more palpable.[57]

Range-of-Motion and Resistance Testing
AROM: Active elbow flexion or extension may be painful, although pain at the end range of flexion is more common. In elbow flexion, the skin is pulled taut over the posterior elbow and increases pressure on the inflamed bursa. In extension the posterior structures of the elbow become crowded and, depending on fluid levels, could increase pain.
PROM: The same principles apply as for active motion.
MRT: Increase in pain from MRT is not likely. In certain positions, pain results from the skin and superficial fascia being pulled taut. Tensile stress on the muscle-tendon units around the elbow should not increase pain or cause weakness.

Differential Evaluation
Rheumatoid arthritis, olecranon process fracture, ligament sprain of the elbow, synovial cyst, ulnar nerve compression.

Suggestions for Treatment
In either acute or chronic bursitis, the principles of PRICE (protection, rest, ice, compression, and elevation) generally apply, but compression should be avoided in treatment, because the problem originated from pressure on the bursa. Anti-inflammatory medication is often prescribed. Bursitis that results from infection (septic bursitis), or another systemic disorder, is treated with anti-inflammatory medications such as NSAIDS or antibiotics.[56] There is no benefit to direct massage of the affected bursa and should be avoided until inflammation has subsided.

CUBITAL TUNNEL SYNDROME

Nerve compression problems frequently cause pain and dysfunction in the upper extremity. Those who work in the occupational environment are particularly at risk. Although not as present in the popular literature as carpal tunnel syndrome, *cubital tunnel syndrome* is the second most common peripheral compression neuropathy in the upper extremity.[58]

Characteristics
The **cubital tunnel** is located where the **ulnar nerve** passes between the two heads of the **flexi carpi ulnaris (FCU)** (Figure 11.25).[43] One head of the FCU blends with the **flexor tendon** attachments at the medial epicondyle of the humerus; the other head originates on the medial aspect of the **olecranon process**. The cubital tunnel is spanned by an aponeurotic band connecting the two heads of the FCU.[43] **Cubital tunnel syndrome occurs when the ulnar nerve is compressed between the two heads of the FCU or by the aponeurotic band**.[59] Space within the tunnel decreases as much as 55% during elbow flexion, making nerve compression possible.[58] During flexion the ulnar nerve is increasingly pulled taut, which may aggravate symptoms.[60, 61] Subluxation (shifting position) of the ulnar nerve as the elbow moves into flexion could produce symptoms as well.[62]

Cubital tunnel syndrome develops from either acute or chronic compression at the elbow. Biomechanical or structural factors could also play a role. For example, *excessive cubital valgus* decreases space within the cubital tunnel and can compress the ulnar nerve. The condition could also be produced by *bone spurs, synovial ganglions, fibrous bands* within the muscle, or *mechanical compression* of the nerve during elbow flexion.[58, 61] *Hypertonicity* of the FCU is one of the familiar causes. The ulnar nerve is increasingly sensitive to compression if there are more proximal nerve compression pathologies (see the *double crush phenomenon* in Chapter 2).[63]

Cubital tunnel syndrome usually produces a variety of sensory symptoms including pain, burning, tingling, and paresthesia. It is often a chronic condition. More men than woman are affected, although it is unclear as to why.[61] Motor symptoms, such as weakness or atrophy, are likely and ordinarily affect the intrinsic muscles of the hand. The symptom pattern of cubital tunnel syndrome is due to the arrangement of the sensory and motor fibers in the ulnar nerve at the cubital tunnel. Near the elbow, the ulnar nerve's sensory and motor fibers to the intrinsic hand muscles are superficial (located on the periphery of the nerve) and are affected by compression of the nerve. The fibers deep within the nerve are primarily those to the FCU and the flexor digitorum profundus (FDP). Compression pathologies in the cubital tunnel cause sensory symptoms as well as weakness or atrophy to the intrinsic hand muscles, but rarely to the FCU and FDP muscles unless the compression is severe.[61]

History

The client typically reports pain, aching, burning sensations, or paresthesia in the ulnar nerve distribution of the hand (Figure 11.45).[64, 65] Weakness, clumsiness in the hand, or difficulty performing precise movements with the thumb and fingers may also be reported. Identify actions that require repetitive or static flexion of the elbow. Night symptoms might be reported if the client sleeps with the elbow in a flexed position.

Observation

Cubital tunnel syndrome has no specific visual indicators, unless excessive cubital valgus is involved. There may be muscle atrophy in the intrinsic muscles of the hand, which could be caused by ulnar nerve compression anywhere along the length of the nerve. For example, nerve compression in Guyon's canal in the wrist could produce muscular atrophy identical to that which might occur with cubital tunnel syndrome (see Guyon's Canal Syndrome). Other conditions may cause atrophy of intrinsic hand muscles (see General Neuromuscular Pathologies near end of chapter).

The primary intrinsic hand muscle to evaluate is the adductor pollicis. Muscle atrophy is apparent with a decrease in size of the muscle mass or webbing between the thumb and fingers compared to the unaffected side. Other intrinsic hand muscles innervated by the ulnar nerve are those of the hypothenar eminence (the fleshy bundle of muscles near the base of the hand on the ulnar side) and muscle wasting might occur in that group.

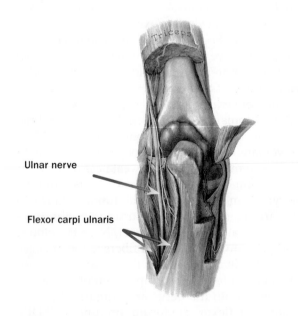

Ulnar nerve

Flexor carpi ulnaris

Figure 11.25 Posterior view of the right elbow where the ulnar nerve enters the space between the two heads of the flexor carpi ulnaris muscle, the cubital tunnel. (Mediclip image copyright, 1998 Williams & Wilkins. All rights reserved).

Ulnar nerve entrapment

There are several locations in the upper extremity where the ulnar nerve can become entrapped. Unfortunately they can produce identical symptoms, making identification of the injury site challenging.

For a clear estimation of what is happening, it is best to cross reference the various methods of evaluating ulnar nerve dysfunction. Look for indicators of sensory as well as motor dysfunction, but keep in mind that impaired motor function is more likely in the hand than in the forearm, even though muscles in both areas are innervated by the ulnar nerve.

Palpation

Pressing on the cubital tunnel elicits the client's symptoms. Palpate the region when the elbow is in neutral, as well as full flexion. Cubital tunnel syndrome may be implicated if the symptoms are exaggerated during flexion. Some anatomic obstructions in the cubital tunnel are palpable, such as bone spurs or synovial masses. Tenderness or hypertonicity may be evident throughout the FCU muscle.

Range-of-Motion and Resistance Testing

AROM: Symptoms are likely to increase during elbow flexion and decrease during extension. Symptoms may not be felt when the elbow is brought rapidly into full flexion and immediately returned to neutral. However, if the elbow is held in flexion for longer than a minute, symptoms are usually felt. The longer the nerve is compressed, the more likely it is to produce pathological symptoms.

PROM: The same principles apply as for active motion.

MRT: Pain is not expected in resisted movements. Palpating the cubital tunnel during resisted wrist flexion, typically exacerbates symptoms. Symptoms ordinarily occur if resisted wrist flexion is performed while the elbow is flexed. Weakness is possible in resisted adduction or flexion of the thumb, because these are primary motions of the adductor pollicis muscle. Weakness of this muscle is more specifically tested with the Froment's sign discussed in the section on *Guyon's canal syndrome*.

Special Tests
Elbow Flexion Test

The client is standing or seated and brings both elbows into full flexion with the forearms supinated and the wrists hyperextended (Figure 11.26). The client should adopt the position on both sides at the same time so a comparison with the unaffected side can be made. If symptoms are reproduced within about 60 seconds, compression of the ulnar nerve in the cubital tunnel is likely.[66, 67]

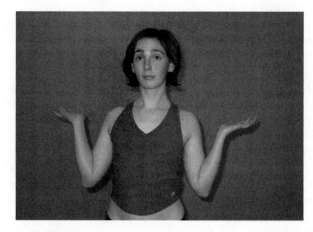

Figure 11.26 Elbow flexion test.

Explanation: The position puts tensile stress on the ulnar nerve while decreasing space within the cubital tunnel. If the condition is present, these actions aggravate the client's symptoms. Note the similarity of this test position to the upper limb neurodynamic test #4. The variation of adding shoulder abduction makes this test more sensitive.

Froment's sign
See Guyon's Canal Syndrome.

Upper limb neurodynamic test #4
See General Neuromuscular Pathologies near the end of the chapter.

Differential Evaluation
Guyon's canal syndrome, thoracic outlet syndrome, carpal tunnel syndrome, other regions of ulnar nerve compression or tension, systemic disease, space-occupying lesions in the elbow, ligament damage in the elbow, cervical radiculopathy, myofascial trigger point referral, diabetic neuropathy, osteophytes in the elbow region.

Suggestions for Treatment
Relieving compression on the affected nerve is the primary goal of treatment. Encourage the client to eliminate activities that keep the elbow flexed for long periods or apply pressure to the cubital tunnel (leaning on the elbows, for example). Splints that keep the elbows in extension are helpful for people who sleep with the elbows in flexion. Even low levels of compression, if left on the nerve for long periods, can require a lengthy period of rehabilitation to restore normal function. If conservative measures are not successful, surgery is sometimes performed. A common surgical procedure involves moving the ulnar nerve to a different location so it is not compressed within the tunnel.

Massage is helpful for cubital tunnel syndrome because a primary cause is muscular hypertonicity in the flexor carpi ulnaris (FCU). Techniques such as deep stripping or massage with active engagement help reduce overall tension in the muscles and decrease compression on the ulnar nerve. Particular caution should be observed in applying pressure to the flexor carpi ulnaris near the region of ulnar nerve entrapment so as not to aggravate the pathology.

PRONATOR TERES SYNDROME

The symptoms of *pronator teres syndrome (PTS)* and *carpal tunnel syndrome* can be identical because they are both peripheral median nerve compression syndromes. Some authors suggest that PTS is under-diagnosed due to the increased attention given carpal tunnel syndrome.[43]

Characteristics
PTS develops from **compression of the median nerve by the pronator teres muscle,** sometimes referred to as *pronator syndrome*. According to Wertsch, the term *pronator syndrome* also includes median nerve compression by other structures in the elbow such as the **ligament of Struthers** or the **bicipital aponeurosis (lacertus fibrosus).**[68]

As the median nerve passes the elbow it runs between the two heads of the **pronator teres muscle,** where the nerve may be compressed (Figure 11.27). Compression can be due to muscle *hypertonicity* or *fibrous bands* within the muscle pressing on the nerve.[69,70] In some cases pressure is placed on the nerve by **anatomical anomalies,** such as the nerve traveling deep to both heads of the pronator teres.[71] In this situation, the nerve may be compressed against the ulna by the pronator teres muscle itself.

PTS results from repetitive motions that cause *hypertonicity* in the pronator teres. Occupational activities such as hammering, cleaning fish, or performing any activity that requires continual manipulation of tools can cause overuse of the pronator teres.[72] The hypertonicity then causes nerve compression and the symptoms are felt in the **anterior forearm** and the **median nerve distribution in the hand** (Figure 11.45). Women are affected more than men, but the reason for this is not clear.

Most symptoms of nerve compression radiate distal to the site of compression. Aching forearm pain and paresthesia along with pain in the median nerve distribution in the hand is likely to be PTS and should not be assumed to indicate carpal tunnel syndrome.[73] In some cases, nerve compression pain can radiate proximal to the site of compression. All potential sites of compression should be considered in the differential evaluation process.[74]

While PTS and carpal tunnel syndrome both affect the median nerve and have similar symptoms, there are distinct differences. PTS pain is exacerbated by repetitive elbow flexion and symptoms arise in the forearm as well as the hand. Carpal tunnel syndrome is aggravated by wrist movements and pain is not experienced as much in the forearm. In both cases, atrophy is possible in the

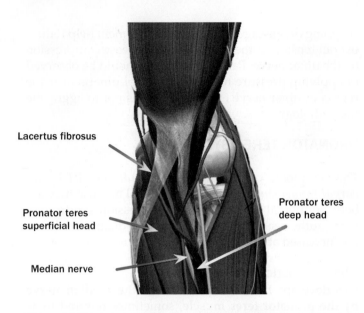

Lacertus fibrosus

Pronator teres
superficial head

Median nerve

Pronator teres
deep head

Figure 11.27 Anterior view of the left elbow showing the two heads of the pronator teres muscle. The median nerve runs between the two heads and is compressed in this region in pronator teres syndrome. (3-D anatomy image courtesy of Primal Pictures Ltd. www.primalpictures.com.)

thenar muscles of the hand, which are innervated by branches from the median nerve. The median nerve can be compressed in more than one location. There could be carpal tunnel compression and pronator teres compression simultaneously (see *double or multiple crush phenomenon* in Chapter 2).

Another cause of median nerve compression near the pronator teres involves a fibrous band from the **biceps brachii muscle**. This band connects the distal portion of the biceps brachii to the ulna on the forearm and is called the **lacertus fibrosus or bicipital aponeurosis.** The median nerve runs under the lacertus fibrosus and may be compressed by it, particularly during strong repetitive contractions of the biceps brachii.[43]

In some cases, pronator teres compression pathologies affect the **anterior interosseous nerve (AIN)** and not the median nerve. The AIN branches off the median nerve as it passes between the two heads of the pronator teres. Some authors consider AIN compression part of pronator teres syndrome, but AIN involvement is also called *anterior interosseous nerve syndrome*.[75] AIN syndrome rarely produces sensory symptoms because the nerve is almost exclusively composed of motor fibers.[43] If the AIN is compressed it shows up clinically as motor weakness in the index finger and thumb, making it difficult to form a pinch grip with those two digits (see description of the Pinch Grip Test below).[76]

History

The client reports aching, shooting, or sharp, electrical-type pain, as well as paresthesia in the median nerve distribution of the hand. These symptoms might be felt in the anterior forearm as well. Pain is aggravated when performing activities that use the pronator teres muscle against resistance, such as using a screwdriver or hand-held power tool.[72, 77] Ask about repetitive elbow movements that aggravate symptoms.

Clients with carpal tunnel syndrome frequently report night pain, while individuals with PTS generally do not.[43] Prolonged wrist flexion during sleep aggravates carpal tunnel syndrome because it decreases the space in the carpal tunnel and presses on the median nerve. Because wrist flexion does not affect the pronator teres muscle, this wrist position does not increase nerve compression symptoms in PTS.

Observation

There are no prominent visual indicators of pronator teres syndrome. Nerve compression may cause atrophy of the forearm and hand muscles supplied by the median nerve (see General Neuromuscular Pathologies near the end of the chapter for muscles supplied by the median nerve). If only one hand is symptomatic, it should be compared with the opposite side to determine differences in muscle size. The muscles of the thenar eminence (fleshy bundle of muscles on the thumb side of the hand) are likely to show signs of atrophy when compared to the unaffected side.

Palpation

Tenderness and hypertonicity are common in the forearm flexor muscles and the pronator teres muscle. Symptoms are aggravated when palpating the pronator teres, because the palpation increases pressure in the region of nerve compression.

Range-of-Motion and Resistance Testing

AROM: Active motion without resistance rarely causes discomfort in any direction unless the condition is advanced. There may be slight discomfort at the end of active supination if the wrist is hyperextended and the supination is performed with the elbow extended. Pain or discomfort with this maneuver is due to simultaneous stretching of the pronator teres and the median nerve, which pulls the nerve taut against the dense muscular fibers. Symptoms present if active motions are performed against resistance (holding a heavy implement in the hand during motion, for example).

PROM: Passive supination produces pain if the wrist is hyperextended and the elbow is extended, due to simultaneous stretching of the pronator teres and median nerve.

MRT: Pain might be felt during resisted forearm pronation and possibly during resisted elbow flexion. Weakness may be evident in the flexors of the hand or fingers, due to impairment of motor signals from the median nerve.

Special Tests
Pronator Teres Test
The client is standing with the elbow in 90⁰ of flexion. The practitioner places one hand on the client's elbow for

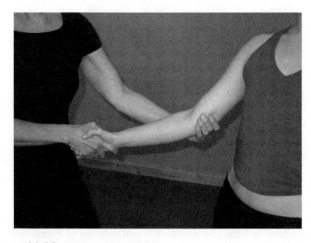

Figure 11.28 Pronator teres test.

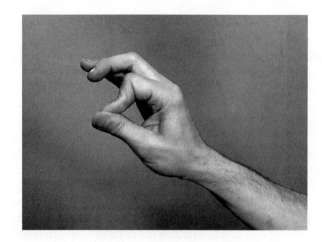

Figure 11.29 Pinch grip test. Image shows inability to prevent the index finger DIP joint from extending during pinch grip.

stabilization and the other hand grasps the client's hand in a handshake position. The client holds this position as the practitioner attempts to supinate the client's forearm (forcing the client to contract the pronator muscles). While holding the resistance against pronation, the practitioner extends the client's elbow (Figure 11.28). If the client's pain or discomfort is reproduced there is a good chance of median nerve compression by the pronator teres. The client should keep the elbow relaxed during the test, because holding the elbow firmly in flexion will not allow elbow extension.

Explanation: The pronator teres is engaged in an isometric contraction, which increases compression of the median nerve. Once the pronator teres is contracted and the elbow is extended, the contracted muscle is forcefully lengthened, producing greater potential nerve compression.

Pinch Grip Test
This test is specific to anterior interosseous nerve syndrome. The client firmly pinches the tips of the thumb and index finger together (Figure 11.29). If the client is unable to do this without hyperextending the DIP joint of the index finger, anterior interosseous nerve motor signals could be impaired due to proximal compression of the nerve near the elbow. This test is similar to Froment's sign (see Guyon's Canal Syndrome in this chapter), although motor signals in different nerves are tested.

Explanation: The anterior interosseous nerve innervates the flexor digitorum profundus muscle that flexes the DIP joint of the index finger. This muscle is also necessary to hold the finger in a normal pinch grip without hyperextending the DIP joint. If the nerve is compressed, impaired motor signals cause muscle weakness and the individual is unable to prevent DIP hyperextension.

Differential Evaluation
Carpal tunnel syndrome, other median nerve entrapment sites, cervical radiculopathy, thoracic outlet syndrome, tumors or space-occupying lesions of the anterior elbow,

medial epicondylitis, medial apophysitis (little league elbow), myofascial trigger point referrals, diabetic neuropathy.

Suggestions for Treatment
The primary focus of treatment is reducing compression on the median nerve. If the primary pathology is hypertonicity of the pronator teres, the condition is easier to address than if there are other anatomical considerations. Massage is helpful, as it can be directly applied to the pronator teres muscle. Static compression methods are used to treat myofascial trigger point activity aggravating the pronator teres and surrounding muscles. Deep stripping or pin-and-stretch methods are also helpful.

Traditional treatment includes splints or braces that are used to change elbow biomechanics and reduce compression on the affected nerve. Stretching methods are valuable to decrease nerve compression by improving flexibility in the pronator teres.

RADIAL TUNNEL SYNDROME

Chronic pain around the lateral elbow region is often ascribed to *lateral epicondylitis* (tennis elbow), but could result from nerve compression. *Radial tunnel syndrome (RTS)* is sometimes called *resistant tennis elbow* because it causes pain in the same region as tennis elbow, but does not improve with standard epicondylitis treatments.[78, 79]

Characteristics
The primary problem in RTS is compression of a branch of the radial nerve that travels through several fibro-osseous tunnels in the elbow region. The elbow region is one of only a few locations where the radial nerve is susceptible to compression. RTS affects the terminal motor branch of the radial nerve called the **posterior interosseous nerve (PIN)**. Compression pathologies affecting this nerve usually cause symptoms of **weakness or atrophy**, because the PIN is comprised almost completely of **motor fibers**.

Pain or paresthesia is felt in the forearm due to the few **sensory fibers** that supply the extensor muscles. Pain can also come from the sensory receptors within the PIN. This symptom variation leads some authors to classify the problem as two conditions—*posterior interosseous nerve syndrome* as the motor problem and RTS as the sensory variation. Other authors consider the variations as part of a single condition involving motor and/or sensory symptoms from the radial nerve or its branches.[43] In this text both are considered part of RTS.

RTS is caused by the anatomical relationship between the posterior interosseous nerve and the supinator muscle.[80] The **supinator muscle** is composed of two heads. The superficial head, which is more proximal, arises from the **lateral epicondyle of the humerus** and has fibers that also originate from the **radial collateral** and **annular ligaments**. The deep head originates on the **supinator crest** and the **fossa of the ulna** (Figure 11.30).

The path of the PIN runs between the two divisions of the supinator muscle. The passage under the edge of the supinator is called the **arcade of Frohse** (Figure 11.31). In about 30% of the population, the PIN passes under a firm tendinous band at the arcade of Frohse which may become the entrapment site in RTS.[43] Although the superficial sensory branch of the radial nerve does not pass under the arcade of Frohse, the PIN remains susceptible to compression and could produce motor or sensory symptoms. In some cases, *fibrous bands* or *hypertonicity* from myofascial trigger point pain referral in the supinator muscle produce compression of the PIN. Nerve compression from **cysts** or **other soft-tissue masses** is also possible.[81]

The pain sensations of RTS develop mostly near the lateral epicondyle of the humerus, but periodically radiate into the anterior and lateral forearm as well. RTS is frequently mistaken for lateral epicondylitis because the pain sites are similar.[78]

History

The client reports pain, paresthesia, or numbness near the lateral epicondyle of the humerus. Pain is described as an aching sensation and commonly extends distally into the anterior or lateral forearm. Pain may also radiate proximally into the arm, although not often. Ask about activities involving prolonged isometric contractions of the forearm muscles, such as handwriting or tool use in recreation or occupation. The client may also report weakness when gripping or holding objects.

Observation

There are no distinguishing visual characteristics of radial tunnel syndrome. Resultant motor impairment is observed during some movements or positions. The client may be able to extend the wrist, but find it difficult or impossible to fully hyperextend the fingers at the MCP joint or the finger joints becuase of muscle weakness (Figure 11.32).

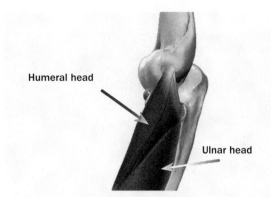

Humeral head

Ulnar head

Figure 11.30 Lateral view of the left elbow showing the two heads of the supinator muscle. (3-D anatomy image courtesy of Primal Pictures Ltd. www.primalpictures.com.)

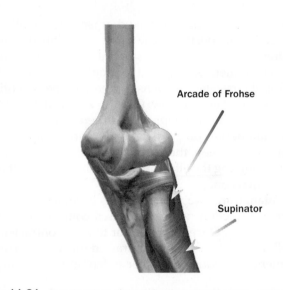

Arcade of Frohse

Supinator

Figure 11.31 Anterior view of the left elbow showing the supinator muscle and the arcade of Frohse where the posterior interosseous nerve is entrapped. (3-D anatomy image courtesy of Primal Pictures Ltd. www. primalpictures.com.)

Palpation

When the practitioner presses directly on the supinator muscle just distal to the lateral epicondyle of the humerus, pain is reproduced. Palpation in this area is one way to distinguish RTS from lateral epicondylitis, where pain is more exaggerated at the extensor attachment on the lateral epicondyle of the humerus.

Range-of-Motion and Resistance Testing

AROM: Active motion performed without resistance is unlikely to be painful. Pain might occur at the end of full pronation when the supinator is pulled taut against the underlying nerve.

PROM: The same principles apply as for active motion.

MRT: If supinator muscle fibers are compressing the posterior interosseous nerve, resisted supination of the forearm can aggravate the symptoms and pain is

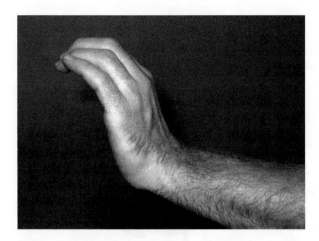

Figure 11.32 Hand impairment pattern in radial tunnel syndrome. The individual can hyperextend the wrist, but has difficulty extending the fingers.

increased. This test should be performed with the elbow extended in order to decrease the contribution of the biceps brachii to the supination effort.[43] RTS is more likely to produce weakness with this resisted action, whereas lateral epicondylitis is painful with resisted wrist extension. Weakness in response to MRT is possible in all muscles innervated by the posterior interosseous nerve (see General Neuromuscular Pathologies near the end of the chapter for muscles innervated by the PIN).

Special Test
Upper Limb Neurodynamic Test #3
Although not specifically designed for radial tunnel syndrome, this test is helpful for identifying various compression or tension pathologies that affect the radial nerve. The test is valuable when considered in conjunction with other evaluation procedures (see General Neuromuscular Pathologies at the end of the chapter for a description of ULNT #3).

Differential Evaluation
Lateral epicondylitis, tumors or synovial masses in the elbow region, ligament sprains in the elbow joint, cervical radiculopathy, thoracic outlet syndrome, myofascial trigger point referrals, other proximal radial nerve lesions, diabetic or other systemic neuropathies.

Suggestions for Treatment
Massage and soft-tissue therapy play a beneficial role in treating RTS. Addressing all the areas of potential radial nerve entrapment is important to determine if there are multiple nerve crush or neural tension problems. Pay attention to the wrist and finger extensors in the forearm, as well as the supinator muscle. Deep longitudinal stripping techniques on these muscles will help free neural restrictions in the distal region of the radial nerve and

decrease tension. Deep broadening techniques for the wrist extensors are also helpful.

Techniques that reduce nerve compression at the interface between the PIN and the arcade of Frohse are beneficial, such as pin-and-stretch methods for the supinator. The practitioner should be careful not to aggravate symptoms by putting additional pressure on the compressed nerve.

CARPAL TUNNEL SYNDROME

Of all the upper extremity entrapment neuropathies, *carpal tunnel syndrome (CTS)* has received the most attention. Due to the substantial amount of research on the condition, CTS is well defined.[43,82,83] The research focus on CTS has led to the condition becoming a popular diagnosis. The condition's familiarity could lead a healthcare professional to assume CTS is involved rather than pursuing less known conditions, leading to misdiagnosis. Other upper extremity nerve entrapment problems with similar symptoms, such as *pronator teres syndrome* or *thoracic outlet syndrome,* have symptoms sometimes misinterpreted as CTS.

Characteristics
The **carpal tunnel** is located at the base of the hand with the dorsal aspect created by the **carpal bones** and the palmar border by the **transverse carpal ligament**. The transverse carpal ligament attaches to the **pisiform** and **hamate** on the medial side and spans the tunnel to connect to the **trapezium** and **scaphoid** on the lateral side (Figure 11.33, 34). The tunnel contains the median nerve and nine tendons: four from the flexor digitorum superficialis group, four flexor digitorum profundus tendons, and one from the flexor pollicis longus. The tendons are enclosed in a common synovial sheath.

CTS involves compression of the median nerve under the transverse carpal ligament (also called the **flexor retinaculum**). The condition develops when space decreases within the tunnel and the nerve is compressed against the transverse carpal ligament. The median nerve is the most superficial structure in the tunnel, which is why it is at risk of compression against this ligament (Figure 11.34).[68]

Tenosynovitis of the flexor tendons is a frequent cause of CTS.[43] An inflammatory reaction between the tendon and its sheath results from overuse, and the subsequent edema causes additional pressure on the median nerve. If the compression is perpetuated, fibrosis and tendon thickening eventually occurs. **Fibrous proliferation** in the area may also tether the median nerve to adjacent structures, such as the transverse carpal ligament, thereby exacerbating symptoms.

CTS is a widespread occupational disorder among those who use tools, computers, or machines that require repetitive flexion and extension of the wrist. Women develop CTS more than men, however it is unclear why.[84]

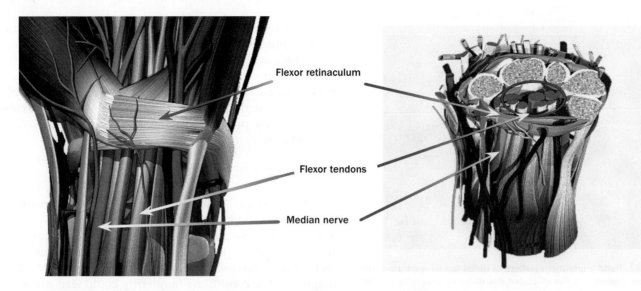

Figure 11.33 Anterior view of the left wrist showing nine flexor tendons and the median nerve that travel underneath the flexor retinaculum in the carpal tunnel. (3-D anatomy image courtesy of Primal Pictures Ltd. www. primalpictures.com.)

Figure 11.34 Anterior view of a left wrist cross-section showing the carpal tunnel. (3-D anatomy image courtesy of Primal Pictures Ltd. www. primalpictures.com.)

It is possible that women are more highly represented in jobs that are at a high risk for CTS such as data entry, food processing, packaging, and cleaning jobs.[85]

CTS can result from an **acute injury** that causes direct crushing trauma to the median nerve. An acute injury can cause a secondary reaction in the tissues that leads to CTS. An example is *Volkmann's contracture,* where CTS often results from an acute injury that causes edema and produces increased pressure within the compartments of the forearm.[43] Structural changes that affect the size of the carpal tunnel are fluid retention during pregnancy, *osteophytes, structural anomalies, tumors in the wrist,* or *obesity.* Some people are predisposed to CTS by nature of their anatomy. The **structure of the wrist** that makes it more square reduces the space in the tunnel.

While the majority of causes are mechanical compression from overuse, other systemic factors could play a role in the condition. Systemic conditions that contribute to CTS include *gout, nerve ischemia, diabetes, alcoholism, rheumatoid arthritis, vitamin B6 deficiency, and kidney failure.*[84, 86–90] Restriction in blood flow (ischemia) could cause the nerve to be hypersensitive and produce CTS symptoms.

It is not unusual for CTS to exist at the same time as other upper extremity overuse problems, such as *medial epicondylitis.* The *double crush phenomenon* (described in Chapter 2) also makes the median nerve more susceptible to compression in the carpal tunnel.

As with other nerve compression syndromes, the pressure causes varying stages of *demyelination* of the median nerve (*neurapraxia, axonotmesis,* or *neurotmesis*). Sensory symptoms are felt in the hand within the region of cutaneous innervation of the median nerve (Figures 11.45). The longer the duration of the condition and severity of the compression, the more recovery time

is needed for healing (see Chapter 2 for a discussion of the stages of nerve compression).

There is no single assessment procedure for CTS. Successful evaluation of the condition requires a comprehensive process including all phases of the HOPRS procedure.[91] In some cases, electrodiagnostic studies and an MRI provide more information. However, nerve conduction tests have not proved sufficiently more reliable than a thorough clinical evaluation.[92, 93] There are also concerns about the accuracy of some special tests.[92, 94] Using a comprehensive HOPRS procedure is the best approach to evaluating CTS.[95, 96]

History

Ask the client about repetitive wrist or hand activities, such as occupational or recreational requirements. Common symptoms are paresthesia, numbness, or pain in the median nerve distribution of the hand and fingers. Symptoms either appear gradually or suddenly and are more often sensory than motor. The preponderance of sensory symptoms occurs because the median nerve at the wrist is composed of over 90% sensory fibers and less than 10% motor.[97] If motor symptoms are present, it is usually an indication of a more advanced problem. As the condition progresses, the client reports a decrease in tactile sensitivity in the fingertips, clumsiness, loss of dexterity, and weakened grip strength because most of the wrist and finger flexors are innervated by the median nerve.

In the absence of repetitive motion, symptoms appear gradually if the condition is chronic and caused by a systemic disorder or obstruction within the carpal tunnel. Ask the client about recent injuries to the wrist. Inquire about symptoms of nerve involvement in the more proximal regions of the upper extremity. Night symptoms result from the client sleeping with the wrist flexed, which increases compression of the nerve.

Observation

Some CTS symptoms are visible during physical examination. The thenar muscles in the hand, which are innervated by the median nerve, may be atrophied and reduced in size compared to the unaffected hand. When atrophied, the thenar eminence sometimes appears to have an indentation instead of a smooth, rounded surface.

A ratio of measurement can be performed that indicates whether the wrist has more of an oval or square shape. For accuracy, these measurements should be done with a caliper. If the height of the wrist (anterior to posterior measurement) is divided by the width of the wrist (medial to lateral measurement) and the result is greater than .70, the individual is said to have a **square-shaped wrist** and be more prone to CTS symptoms.[94] In the absence of measurements a visual estimation is possible, although this method is less accurate.

Palpation

Tenderness and reproduction of sensory symptoms are likely when the region over the carpal tunnel (at the base of the hand) is palpated. Pressure applied directly to the median nerve in this region is sometimes called the median nerve compression test or the carpal compression test.[98] In this procedure, pressure is applied to the carpal tunnel and held for about 30 seconds. This test is not reliable on its own and is not a definitive indicator of CTS without validation from other portions of the assessment.

Hypertonicity in the wrist and finger flexors is a common finding in CTS, particularly when other overuse conditions such as medial epicondylitis are involved. The wrist and finger flexors should also be evaluated for myofascial trigger points that contribute to overall tightness or refer pain and other symptoms. Fluid retention could be palpable in the wrist. Atrophy of the thenar muscles might be apparent when compared to the unaffected side.

Range-of-Motion and Resistance Testing

AROM: Active motion reproduces symptoms near the end range of either wrist flexion or extension and may reduce the available range. Space within the carpal tunnel is decreased more in flexion than extension. In extension the median nerve is stretched, so an increase in symptoms is expected.

PROM: The same principles apply as for active motion.

MRT: Pain or weakness may be apparent in resisted wrist flexion, finger flexion, or thumb abduction. Pain is often absent when the wrist is in a neutral position during the test, but results if the wrist position stretches or compresses the nerve.

Special Tests
Phalen's Test

Phalen's test is a common evaluation for carpal tunnel syndrome. Its accuracy is increased when performed in conjunction with other procedures, such as the carpal compression test (see Palpation above).[99] The client presses the back of the hands together so the wrists are flexed close to 90° (Figure 11.35). If the sensory symptoms of pain, paresthesia, or numbness in the median nerve distribution are reproduced within about 60 seconds, the test is considered positive.

This test can also be performed passively, with the practitioner placing the client's hands in the position. In a variation called the reverse Phalen's test, the wrists are placed in full hyperextension and held for 60 seconds. The reverse Phalen's test is best used as an adjunct to, rather than a replacement, for the standard Phalen's test.[100]

Explanation: When the wrists are in full flexion, space is decreased within the carpal tunnel and pressure is applied to the median nerve causing symptoms. The

---

Box 11.9 Clinical Notes

Median nerve compression in the wrist

CTS is just one of several nerve entrapment syndromes that can produce symptoms in the hand. Other conditions refer pain to the hand as well. Hasty assumptions about the presence of CTS can lead to inadeqate treatment and exacerbated symptoms, and create an environment for a slow and painful healing process.

Careful evaluation of sensory symptoms in the hand along with a thorough assessment of signs and symptoms allows the practitioner to arrive at an accurate picture of the condition, which may not involve the median nerve at all.

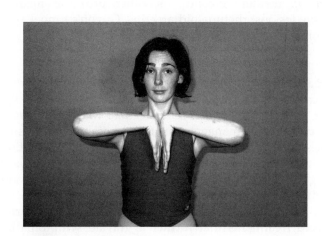

Figure 11.35 Phalen's test.

Phalen's test compresses the nerve and impairs blood flow within the nerve as well. The rate at which symptoms appear indicates the degree of pathology. If symptoms are perceived immediately, the problem is more advanced than if it takes a full minute for presentation.

Tinel's Sign

The practitioner lightly taps on the carpal tunnel at the base of the hand. If neurological symptoms are reproduced with each tap, it is an indication of CTS (Figure 11.36). While Tinel's sign is in widespread use, it is not one of the more accurate ways of identifying CTS.[101] The test's value lies in its ability to provide additional information when performed in conjunction with other testing procedures.

Explanation: Tapping directly on the carpal tunnel places sudden compressive force on the affected nerve, producing sensory symptoms in the hand.

Tethered Median Nerve Stress Test

The wrist is held in extension and supination. While in this position the index finger is pulled into hyperextension as far as motion allows (Figure 11.37). The finger movement can be performed by the practitioner or by the client. The final position is held for about 60 seconds. As with several CTS special tests, this test is not considered highly accurate if used alone, but it is a valuable component of a comprehensive clinical examination.[102]

Explanation: Space within the carpal tunnel is decreased when the wrist is held in extension. By pulling the index finger into hyperextension, the median nerve is pulled taut. If there is pressure on the median nerve from structures within the tunnel, pressure on the nerve is increased. This test may also be positive when there are adhesions between the median nerve and the transverse carpal ligament that prevent the nerve from sliding adjacent to the ligament.[87]

Differential Evaluation

Cervical radiculopathy, thoracic outlet syndrome, myofascial trigger point referrals, pronator teres syndrome, medial epicondylitis, other proximal median nerve lesions, rheumatoid arthritis, Guyon's tunnel syndrome, diabetic neuropathy, Volkmann's contracture.

Suggestions for Treatment

Treatment for CTS focuses on conservative approaches such as wrist splints, stretching, and in some cases the use of anti-inflammatory medication. Massage plays a valuable role in management of CTS, because it addresses the soft tissues that compress the median nerve. Attention should focus on reducing hypertonicity in the wrist and finger flexor muscles. Deep longitudinal stripping and active engagement methods are particularly beneficial applied to the wrist and finger flexors in the forearm. Avoid treatments that further aggravate symptoms by compressing the affected nerve directly over the tunnel.

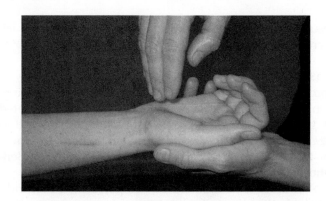

Figure 11.36 Tinel's sign at the carpal tunnel.

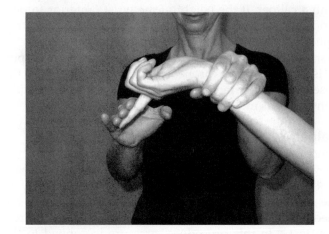

Figure 11.37 Tethered median nerve stress test.

Myofascial methods may be beneficial for stretching the fascial tissues lying over the carpal tunnel, which could help reduce symptoms.[103]

GANGLION CYST

Ganglion cysts are the most common tumors of the hand and wrist.[104] Exactly how and why they form is poorly understood, making treatment challenging. Despite the similarity in name, a ganglion cyst is different from the *ganglion* that is a collection of nerve cells.

Characteristics

The ganglion cyst is **a fibrous swelling that occurs near joints** and is located near and often attached to the joint capsule or tendon sheaths. The cysts could be growths on the tendon retinacula, knots of dysfunctional tissue, or herniations of the synovial sheath of an associated joint.[105] The cyst contains a clear mucinous fluid that is different from the synovial fluid contained within joint capsules. What causes the cysts is not established, but there are various hypotheses proposed. One idea is that they result from mucoid degeneration of collagen and connective tissues. Additional causes include ligament stress, subluxation of local joints, or other lesions.[105]

The majority of ganglions, 60–70%, are dorsal wrist ganglions and develop as a **herniation or extension of the joint capsule or tendon sheath**.[104] Dorsal wrist ganglions are often **connected to the scapholunate ligament with a fibrous stalk**.[106] About 20% of ganglions occur on the volar surface of the wrist, while the remaining percentage develop in other regions of the body.[105] Ganglions take place with more frequency in women than in men. Hand dominance does not appear to be responsible for ganglion development .[107]

The size of the cystic mass can become pronounced and cause concern about the severity of the problem, for example cancer is often feared. While it is important to evaluate these other possibilities, the majority of wrist ganglions are benign cystic tumors. In many cases the ganglion is not painful, but may cause pain due to its location. Ganglions can interfere with hand activities because of pain.

Ganglion cysts complicate *nerve compression* conditions, as either a sole cause of the problem or a contributing factor.[81, 108] Ganglions can cause compression of the ulnar nerve in Guyon's canal or the median nerve in the carpal tunnel. A ganglion might be overlooked as a cause of nerve entrapment in favor of a familiar explanation.

History

The client reports weakness, paresthesia, or dull, aching pain in the region of the cyst. The client frequently experiences pain when the cyst is struck or compressed. Pain occurs with flexion or extension as the cyst is pulled or compressed, but generally not felt when the wrist is held in a neutral position. Symptoms are intermittent and directly related to motions of the wrist that stretch or compress the cyst. The client may note that the cyst changes in size or appearance. Ask about wrist trauma as cysts can appear after an acute injury, although no confirming evidence supports this cause.

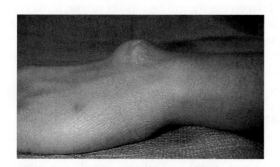

Figure 11.38 A dorsal ganglion cyst on the left wrist.

Observation

The obvious visible characteristic of a ganglion cyst is a bump that appears near the wrist (Figure 11.38). Ganglion cysts are typically only a few centimeters wide, but range from a small rise under the skin to a pronounced bump. In some cases the cysts are not visible; these are called *occult ganglions*. These cysts develop more often on the dorsal surface of the wrist where they are associated with the tendon sheaths of the wrist and finger extensors. Occult cysts on the volar surface of the wrist are frequently associated with nerve compression.[81, 108, 109]

Palpation

The ganglion cyst is characteristically tender to palpation. Tenderness is out of proportion to the amount of pressure used. If the client can tolerate pressure on the cyst it may feel soft, as if filled with a gel-like substance. In advanced cases the ganglion feels firmer due to thickening of fibrous tissue within the cyst.

Range-of-Motion and Resistance Testing

AROM: Active motion may cause pain when the wrist is moved, depending on the location of the cyst. Pain is most likely when the movement further compresses the cyst. For example, the dorsal cyst is usually painful at the end of wrist extension. Pain can arise as tissues attached to the cyst are stretched in flexion.

PROM: The same principles apply as for active motion.

MRT: Manual resistance does not aggravate the cyst unless the test position compresses or pulls on the cyst. For example, a dorsal wrist ganglion could be painful during resisted extension if the wrist is fully hyperextended during the MRT. Pain does not occur during resisted flexion as there is no tension or compression on the dorsal ganglion. This pattern would be opposite for volar ganglions.

Differential Evaluation

Distal nerve compression pathologies, tenosynovitis, tendinosis, localized infection, carpal fracture if it is acute, carpal ligament sprain.

Suggestions for Treatment

There are only a couple of options for treating ganglion cysts. Ironically, some physicians still advocate using a striking force to put pressure directly on the ganglion. This treatment approach does not effectively eliminate the cyst and causes further problems. It is best to refer the client to a physician for further evaluation. Massage is not a beneficial treatment for ganglion cysts, but may temporarily relieve overall achy pain associated with the condition. Ganglions can be aspirated to remove excess fluid, although the cyst often returns. In some cases the cyst may be surgically removed, but recurrence is still possible. Some people find alternative approaches helpful, such as altering wrist activities, changing the diet, or experimenting with supplements.

GUYON'S CANAL SYNDROME

While *carpal tunnel syndrome* is a familiar nerve compression pathology of the wrist, there is another tunnel in the wrist where nerve compression is possible. *Guyon's canal syndrome (GCS)* **develops when the ulnar nerve is compressed in Guyon's canal,** or tunnel, on the medial side of the wrist. This condition is also called *ulnar tunnel syndrome.*

Characteristics

The **flexor retinaculum,** also called the **transverse carpal ligament,** splits into two bands toward the middle of the wrist (Figure 11.39). On the ulnar side, the flexor retinaculum attaches to the **pisiform** and **hamate;** on the radial side, it attaches to the **scaphoid** and **trapezium.** The space between the broad, deeper band and the shorter, superficial band of the flexor retinaculum is called **Guyon's canal** or the tunnel of Guyon (Figure 11.39). The ulnar nerve and artery pass through Guyon's canal.

Generally, **GCS occurs from external pressure on the palm,** such as holding something tightly or an impact on the palm. **Internal compression** can also derive from structures such as ganglion cysts, but this is not as common.[108] Unlike carpal tunnel syndrome, tenosynovitis is not a cause of nerve compression as there are no tendons that run through Guyon's canal.

There are three variations of ulnar nerve compression identified at the Guyon canal and symptoms vary based on the location of the compression.[43] **Type I** compression occurs proximal to Guyon's canal and involves both the superficial (sensory) and deep (motor) branches of the ulnar nerve causing mixed sensory and motor symptoms. Motor symptoms include weakness and atrophy in the hypothenar muscles, as well as the adductor pollicis.

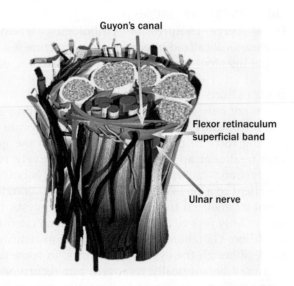

Guyon's canal

Flexor retinaculum superficial band

Ulnar nerve

Figure 11.39 Anterior view of a left wrist cross-section showing Guyon's canal.(3-D anatomy image courtesy of Primal Pictures Ltd. www.primal-pictures.com.)

Sensory symptoms include paresthesia and numbness in the ulnar nerve distribution (Figures 11.45). **Type II** compression is most common and are within the canal, involving the **deep branch of the ulnar nerve** and producing strictly motor deficits, such as atrophy and weakness. Compression of the superficial branch of the ulnar nerve by the **palmaris brevis muscle** produces **Type III** pathologies and generates exclusively sensory symptoms.

Because GCS mainly develops from **external compression,** occupational disorders are a primary cause. A tight grip on tools, such as screwdrivers or handles, can cause compression of the nerve as the grip forces the hard object into the palm. If the symptoms arise as a result of an acute injury, like falling on an outstretched hand, *carpal fractures* or *dislocations* may cause the nerve compression. Long distance cyclists frequently experience this condition. The position of the hands on the handlebars places pressure directly over the Guyon's canal; thus the condition's alternate name of *handlebar palsy.*[110, 111] People who use walking canes develop the condition as well.

History

The client is likely to report pain and paresthesia in the ulnar nerve distribution of the hand (Figures 11.45). Symptoms can be felt proximally in the forearm, although this is not common. The client's pain worsens with certain motions and is exacerbated with additional pressure on the base of the hand. There may also be reports of weakness in grip strength as the adductor pollicis muscle is an important component of thumb gripping and it is innervated by the ulnar nerve.

Ask if the client experienced any sudden force to the base of the hand, such as using the base of the palm to strike something. If there is a space-occupying lesion or cyst within the canal, there may be simultaneous compression of the ulnar artery or vein. Reported symptoms would then include cold intolerance, swelling, fullness, puffiness, or coldness in the hand and fingers.

Observation

The prominent visible indicator of GCS is atrophy of the muscles innervated by the ulnar nerve, particularly the wasting of the hypothenar eminence (the fleshy base of the hand on the ulnar side). Atrophy of the adductor pollicis would be evident by a decrease in size of the webbing between the thumb and index finger. If the condition is unilateral it is helpful to compare it with the hand on the unaffected side. If a cyst or other mass is pressing on the ulnar nerve near Guyon's canal, it might be visible on the volar aspect of the medial wrist near the base of the hand.

Palpation

Palpation directly over Guyon's canal can be painful and reproduce symptoms. Pressure on the ulnar nerve, both proximal and distal to Guyon's canal, can increase the symptoms.

Range-of-Motion and Resistance Testing

AROM: Active wrist extension is likely to be painful or reproduce neurological symptoms at the end range of motion as the ulnar nerve is stretched through the tunnel. There may also be pain or neurological sensations at the end of wrist flexion as the ulnar nerve is compressed.

PROM: The same principles apply as for active motion.

MRT: Because no tendons run through Guyon's tunnel, pain is unlikely to increase with manual resistance. There may be weakness in muscles innervated by the ulnar nerve distal to the canal, particularly the adductor pollicis which is a primary flexor and adductor of the thumb.

Special Test
Froment's Sign

The client holds a piece of paper between the thumb and base of the index finger, as if holding a key. The practitioner attempts to pull the paper out of the client's grip (Figure 11.40). If the client is able to hold the paper firmly and the practitioner has difficulty pulling it from the client's grasp, there is no perceivable weakness in the adductor pollicis muscle. The test is positive if the practitioner is able to easily pull the paper from the client's grasp. This test is similar to the pinch grip test for anterior interosseous nerve pathology (see Pronator Teres Syndrome), but the position of the thumb pinch is different.

Explanation: The adductor pollicis contributes greatly to thumb flexion, which is the motion performed while attempting to grip the paper. The adductor pollicis is innervated by the deep branch of the ulnar nerve and its compression can cause muscle weakness.

Upper Limb Neurodynamic Test #4

See General Neuromuscular Pathologies near the end of the chapter.

Differential Evaluation

Carpal tunnel syndrome, cubital tunnel syndrome, synovial ganglion cysts, carpal ligament damage, other regions of ulnar nerve pathology, thoracic outlet syndrome, cervical radiculopathy, myofascial trigger point pain referrals, diabetic neuropathy.

Suggestions for Treatment

Treatment for GCS requires removing external compressive forces so the nerve can begin healing. Wrist splints may decrease symptoms by holding the wrist in a neutral position. If the nerve is compressed for a long time, healing is slower. If conservative treatments are not successful, surgery can be performed to make more space for the ulnar nerve and its branches within the tunnel.

Massage affords some symptomatic relief in the area, especially if there is neural tension in other regions of the ulnar nerve. Massage techniques that directly compress the Guyon's canal are not recommended, as they aggravate the condition.

DE QUERVAIN'S TENOSYNOVITIS

Tenosynovitis is an inflammatory irritation between a tendon and its synovial sheath. Synovial sheaths are common in the distal extremities. *De Quervain's tenosynovitis* affects two tendons and their sheath in an area called the **anatomical snuff box** in the wrist. This condition is a repetitive stress injury, affecting people who use their thumbs or hands extensively.

Characteristics

The **abductor pollicis longus (APL)** and **extensor pollicis brevis (EPB)** tendons are surrounded by a synovial sheath as they course under the **extensor retinaculum** on the radial side of the wrist. This region is often called the *anatomical snuff box* (Figure 11.41). Repetitive or overuse activities involving the thumb can lead to **tendon irritation and the subsequent inflammation can cause thickening and adhesions between the tendons and their synovial sheath** (see Chapter 4 for a discussion of tenosynovitis).[112]

Tenosynovitis in these tendons can also result from anatomical anomalies. Surgical research shows the presence of a **septum** or **fascial wall** between the **APL** and **EPB tendons** in a large percentage of the population. One study reported septum presence in 77% of the cadaver specimens dissected.[113] The septum decreases the space around the tendons, increasing the risk of friction and

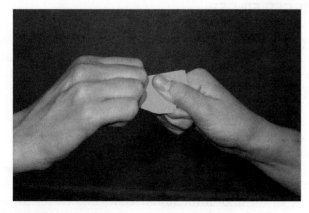

Figure 11.40 Froment's sign.

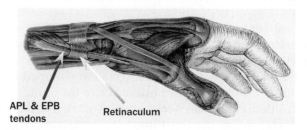

APL & EPB tendons   Retinaculum

irritation.[114] The septum is not identifiable with physical examination.

De Quervain's tenosynovitis occurs in occupations where the hands are used extensively, particularly when tools are held or manipulated. Extensive use of the thumb, such as in massage therapy, is also likely to lead to the problem. If local inflammation presses on the nearby radial nerve, paresthesia may be felt along the thumb, dorsum of the hand, or index finger.[97]

History

The client reports localized pain in the distal radial forearm near the wrist, which sometimes refers to nearby areas. Pain is expected during activities where something is pinched between the thumb and fingers, as the tendons used stabilize the base of the thumb.[112] Pain could also cause reflex muscular inhibition and subsequent muscle weakness in the thumb or hand. The client usually describes a repetitive motion activity engaging the thumb or wrist that preceded a gradual onset of symptoms.

Observation

Although there is inflammatory activity, there are no significant visible factors in de Quervain's tenosynovitis.

Palpation

Direct palpation of the anatomical snuff box reveals tenderness. The areas proximal and distal to the snuff box may also be tender. If the tendons are irritated from overuse, pain could present in the proximal attachment sites of the APL and EPB muscles on the radius due to enthesopathy. In severe cases, palpable edema is possible around the retinaculum near the styloid process of the radius. If the condition has progressed, fibrous thickening of the tendons is palpable.

Range-of-Motion and Resistance Testing

AROM: Active motion is painful at the end of thumb extension as the tendons are pulled against the binding retinaculum. Pain or discomfort may also occur at the end of ulnar deviation of the wrist or flexion of the thumb as the affected tendons are stretched.

PROM: The same principles apply as for active motion.

MRT: Pain and/or weakness resulting from reflex muscular inhibition may be apparent in thumb gripping and resisted extension or abduction of the thumb.

Special Test

Finkelstein Test

The client pulls the thumb into full flexion across the anterior face of the palm. The fingers are wrapped over the thumb to hold it in this position. Once the thumb is in this position, either the client (actively) or the practitioner (passively) moves the wrist into ulnar deviation (Figure 11.42). De Quervain's tenosynovitis is likely if pain is reproduced near the styloid process of the radius at the end range of motion.

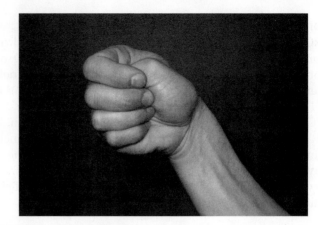

Figure 11.42 Finklestein test.

Explanation: Bringing the thumb across the anterior surface of the palm stretches the affected tendons. Positioning the wrist into ulnar deviation extends that stretch. Stretching the tendons and their synovial sheaths in the presence of inflammation or adhesions reproduces the pain of de Quervain's tenosynovitis.

Differential Evaluation

Carpal tunnel syndrome, rheumatoid arthritis, distal radial nerve entrapments, myofascial trigger point referrals, tendinitis, osteoarthritis, enthesitis of affected tendons, carpal bone or ligamentous injury, distal radial styloid injury.

Suggestions for Treatment

Fibrous adhesion between the tendon and its sheath can be addressed with deep friction massage performed transverse to the fiber direction of the affected tendons. Massage will mobilize the tendons within their sheaths and improve overall mobility. Attention should also focus on reducing tension in the affected muscles (abductor pollicis longus and extensor pollicis brevis) with deep longitudinal stripping methods as well as active engagement techniques.

TRIGGER FINGER

Trigger finger develops when tendon thickening prevents free movement of the tendon within its synovial sheath. It is not a serious problem, but can cause pain and be a hindrance to normal function of the hand.

Characteristics

Tendons in the hand and fingers must bend around numerous joints while maintaining smooth, gliding movement. Sometimes tendons become thickened and their ability to easily glide past other structures is limited. The tendons of the **flexor digitorum superficialis** and **flexor digitorum profundus** are surrounded by synovial sheaths to enhance mechanical function during finger flexion. There are thickened sections of the tendon sheath, called **pulleys**, close to the joints. The pulley located closest to the MCP joint is the **A1 pulley** (Figure 11.43). A frequent location for a fibrous nodule binding on the tendon is at the A1 pulley.[115, 116] During flexion and extension, the tendon slides back and forth under the pulley. Trigger finger develops when **a fibrous nodule or thickening develops on the surface of the tendon and prevents smooth gliding action**.

As the finger is extended, the fibrous nodule gets caught proximal to the pulley and prevents the finger from completing the motion until it snaps under the pulley (like a trigger). In some cases, the nodule can also be caught distal to the pulley as the individual attempts finger flexion producing a snapping sensation as the finger is finally allowed to flex.

Trigger finger is sometimes called *stenosing tenosynovitis,* although the term is being abandoned because there is rarely inflammation or other characteristics of true tenosynovitis in the affected tissues.[117] It is not clear what causes the tendon thickening of trigger finger; it is sometimes attributed to systemic diseases such as *diabetes, hypothyroidism, gout, or rheumatoid arthritis.*[118] In many cases, there is no systemic pathology and it is unclear why the condition developed. The condition affects women more often than men and mainly affects those 45–60 years-old. There does not appear to be an association with repetitive activity or overuse.

History

The client reports locking or catching sensations in the finger during flexion or extension, which may be painful. Pain, if present, is felt in the palm or the affected digit. Trigger finger generally occurs in only one finger, but can affect multiple digits in some systemic disorders such as *rheumatoid arthritis* or *diabetes.*[119] The condition's onset is usually gradual.

Observation

The nodule on the affected tendon may be visible, especially during flexion or extension of the finger. In some cases, movement into extension is so impaired that the finger is held in flexion, causing a flexion deformity. Visible indicators of systemic conditions, such as rheumatoid arthritis, which affect the joints are cause for concern and a correlation exists between trigger finger and these disorders.[118]

Palpation

The tendinous nodule is likely to be palpable and can be at any of the flexor pulleys, but usually the A1 pulley. It is also frequently tender to the touch. Crepitus during flexion and extension may be felt by the client or practitioner if the finger is lightly palpated during motion. A fibrous feeling to the fascia of the palm or fingers is possible.

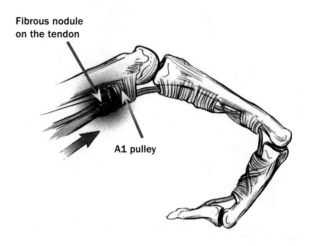

Fibrous nodule on the tendon

A1 pulley

Figure 11.43 A fibrous nodule catching on the A1 pulley at the MCP joint making it difficult to perform extension in trigger finger. (3-D anatomy image courtesy of Primal Pictures Ltd. www.primalpictures.com.)

Range-of-Motion and Resistance Testing

AROM: Active motion is painful and limited in finger flexion or extension depending on where the fibrous nodule is catching on the pulley. Pain with extension is more common because the nodule often occurs proximal to the pulley.[119] The catching and snapping of the digit takes place during either flexion or extension.

PROM: The same principles apply as for AROM. In serious cases there is greater PROM than active.

MRT: Resisted finger flexion or extension may be painful if the tendinous nodule is pulled against the edge of the pulley during contraction. Weakness can develop as pain causes reflex muscular inhibition.

Differential Evaluation

Carpal tunnel syndrome, other median nerve entrapments, gout, rheumatoid arthritis, Dupuytren's contracture, diabetes mellitus, ganglion cysts.

Suggestions for Treatment

Although inflammation is usually not present, traditional treatment commonly consists of corticosteroid injections and anti-inflammatory medications. Physical therapy may be used to encourage movement. When other conservative treatments fail, surgical release of the A1 pulley is performed with a simple office procedure. No evidence supports the use of massage or other soft-tissue manipulation for trigger finger. Practitioners should consult the client's physician prior to engaging in massage treatments of this condition.

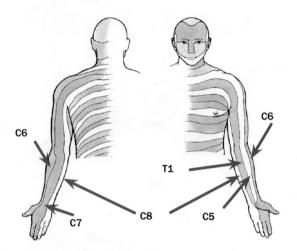

Figure 11.44 Dermatomes of the upper extremity (Mediclip image copyright, 1998 Williams & Wilkins. All rights reserved).

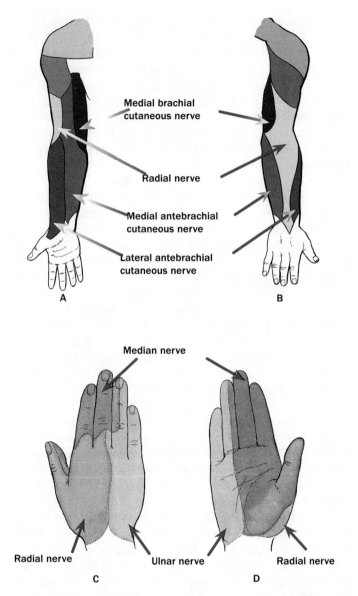

Figure 11.45 Cutaneous innervation of the upper extremity in the anterior arm (A) posterior arm (B) dorsal hand (C) and palmar hand (D). (Mediclip image copyright, 1998 Williams & Wilkins. All rights reserved).

General Neuromuscular Disorders

In many cases, soft-tissue dysfunctions are not given a specific name. Adequate assessment is required to determine the tissues most likely involved and to take into account pathologies that may or may not have specific titles. Chapter 4 provides a discussion of the pathological processes of hypertonicity, myofascial trigger points, muscle strains, nerve compression and tension, tendinosis, tenosynovitis, ligament sprains, and osteoarthritis in any region of the body. Chapter 4 also includes the history, observation, palpation, relevant tests, and treatment suggestions sections for these conditions. The principles are the same for these conditions wherever they occur in the body. Included in this section are specific tables and graphics for the distal upper extremity, including dermatomes, cutaneous innervation, trigger point referral patterns, and findings for MRTs.

Nerve compression or tension pathologies produce symptoms in the elbow, forearm, wrist, or hand from either a cervical radiculopathy (spinal nerve root compression) or a peripheral neuropathy (peripheral upper extremity nerve injury). There are numerous locations in the distal upper extremity where peripheral neuropathies could occur; many are discussed as discrete conditions earlier in the chapter. Other common regions where nerve compression might develop in the elbow, forearm, wrist, and hand are listed in Box 11.10.

Sensory symptoms from a radiculopathy may also be felt in the distal upper extremity and are experienced within the dermatome associated with that nerve root (Figure 11.44). Sensory symptoms of peripheral neuropathy are felt in the region of cutaneous innervation for the nerve affected (Figure 11.45). Radiculopathies or peripheral neuropathies may cause motor dysfunction and produce weakness in the muscles innervated by the affected nerve (Box 11.11). Special tests for nerve compression or tension pathology are provided below. A list

---

Box 11.10 Regions of Possible Nerve Entrapment

Radial and Posterior Interosseous Nerves
   Spiral groove on the posterior aspect of the humerus
   Under the supinator muscle in the radial tunnel

Median and Anterior Interosseous Nerves
   Under the bicipital aponeurosis (lacertus fibrosus)
   Beneath the Ligament of Struthers
   Between the two heads of pronator teres muscle
   Carpal tunnel

Ulnar Nerve
   Cubital tunnel
   Guyon's tunnel

BOX 11.11 INNERVATION OF DISTAL UPPER EXTREMITY MUSCLES

Radial Nerve
Main Trunk
  Brachialis
  Triceps brachii
  Anconeus
  Brachioradialis
  Extensor carpi radialis longus

Posterior Interosseous Branch
  Supinator
  Extensor carpi radialis brevis
  Extensor digiti minimi
  Extensor carpi ulnaris
  Extensor digitorum
  Extensor indicis
  Abductor pollicis longus
  Extensor pollicis brevis
  Extensor pollicis longus

Median Nerve
Main Trunk
  Flexor carpi radialis
  Pronator teres
  Palmaris longus
  Flexor digitorum superficialis
  Abductor pollicis brevis
  Opponens pollicis
  Flexor pollicis brevis (superficial head)
  Lumbricales (1st & 2nd)

Anterior Interosseous Branch
  Flexor pollicis longus
  Flexor digitorum profundus (lateral part)
  Pronator quadratus

Ulnar Nerve
  Adductor pollicis
  Abductor digiti minimi
  Opponens digiti minimi
  Flexor digiti minimi brevis
  Flexor digitorum profundus (medial part)
  Flexor carpi ulnaris
  Lumbricales (3rd & 4th)
  Palmaris brevis
  Palmar interossei
  Dorsal interossei
  Flexor pollicis brevis (deep head)

---

of primary upper extremity motor nerves and the muscles they innervate is provided in Box 11.11. Table 1 provides a chart of muscles, their resisted actions, and potentially affected nerves or nerve roots.

Muscular hypertonicity occurs in the distal upper extremity as a result of chronic overload or repetitive motion stress. Myofascial trigger points can refer pain or characteristic neurological sensations to various regions of the elbow, forearm, wrist, and hand. Trigger points in muscles outside of the upper extremity can also refer pain to this region (see Chapters 9 and 10). Common myofascial trigger point referral patterns for the major muscles in this region are shown in Figure 11.50–51.

Special Tests

Upper limb neurodynamic tests (ULNTs) evaluate symptoms in neural tension or compression pathologies, such as carpal tunnel syndrome, cubital tunnel syndrome, and ulnar nerve entrapment. They are also helpful assessing less specific nerve pathologies, such as scar tissue binding the median nerve close to the elbow. In many cases there are problems in more than one location along a nerve's path and the ULNTs are valuable for identifying multiple sites of dysfunction.

Each neurodynamic test includes a series of steps that progressively add more tension to the nerve, testing its mobility. When tension is increased on the nerve, symptoms from nerve pathologies become evident. The tests can be performed actively or passively, but are usually performed passively so that muscular involvement is minimized. The order of steps can be varied to focus attention on a particular region of nerve pathology. For example, if a problem is suspected in the distal median nerve, the practitioner could begin ULNT #1 with wrist and finger extension and then eventually add movements at the elbow and the shoulder. If pain is felt initially

before elbow and shoulder movements are added, there is a greater chance of distal nerve pathology.

There are four common ULNTs: the first two test the median nerve, the radial is tested by the third, and the fourth tests the ulnar. The numbering of these tests is not consistent in medical texts; in this text they are numbered ULNT 1–4. To avoid confusion in treatment notes, identify the ULNT used by the nerve being stressed during the test. For example, treatment notes might state, "ULNT #2 with median nerve bias."

General instructions: The practitioner performs a series of movements that gradually increase tension on the nerve. Symptoms, if present, will increase as movements are added. Movements are performed in the order listed with each test. During testing, ask the client about changes in symptoms after each movement. Once the client experiences symptoms, it is not necessary to complete the remainder of the movements, especially if the symptoms are strong.

Upper Limb Neurodynamic Test #1 (Median nerve bias)

The client is in a supine position. The practitioner stands facing the client's head on the testing side. The client's elbow is flexed to 90⁰ at the beginning of the test. The final position of the shoulder in ULNT #1 is contraindicated if shoulder instability is present (Figure 11.46)

Test Movements
1. Shoulder is brought into depression.
2. Arm is abducted to about 110⁰.
3. Forearm is supinated.
4. Wrist and fingers are hyperextended.
5. Shoulder is laterally rotated.
6. Elbow is extended.
7. Neck is contralaterally flexed.

Explanation: The positions used in ULNT #1 gradually increase tension on the median nerve. The final position provides maximal stretch on the nerve. Pathological tension is created when the nerve is tethered or bound along its length. Compression pathologies are symptomatic because they create new tension points for the nerve and greater tensile force is thus applied along the nerve's length during movement. Each progressive step places more tension on the nerve, exacerbating symptoms.

Upper Limb Neurodynamic Test #2 (Median nerve bias)

The client is supine and slightly diagonal on the treatment table so the shoulder of the test side is off the table edge. The practitioner stands near the client's head, facing the feet. The practitioner places a thigh on the superior aspect of the client's shoulder to hold the it in depression. Shoulder is held in slight abduction in test (Figure 11.47).

Test Movements
1. Elbow is extended.
2. Shoulder is laterally rotated, forearm is supinated.
3. Wrist and fingers are hyperextended.
4. Neck is contralaterally flexed.

Explanation: As with ULNT #1, tension is progressively added to the median nerve through each successive movement. ULNT #2 is not as sensitive as ULNT #1 because the shoulder is not abducted very far during the test. This is a good alternative test if the client has a history of shoulder instability.

Upper Limb Neurodynamic Test #3 (Radial nerve bias)

The client is supine and slightly diagonal on the table with the test side shoulder off the table edge. The practitioner stands near the client's head, facing the feet. The practitioner places a thigh on the superior aspect of the client's shoulder to hold the shoulder in depression. The shoulder is held in slight abduction during the entire test. Same starting position as ULNT #2 (Figure 11.48).

Test Movements
1. Elbow is extended.
2. Shoulder is medially rotated, forearm pronated.
3. Wrist and fingers are flexed.
4. Neck is contralaterally flexed.

Explanation: Tension is progressively added to the radial nerve through each successive movement. Since the radial nerve lies along the lateral and posterior aspect of the forearm, it is most fully stretched when the forearm is pronated and the wrist and fingers are flexed.

Upper Limb Neurodynamic Test #4 (Ulnar nerve bias)

The client is in a supine position. The practitioner is standing facing toward the client's head on the same side of the treatment table as the side being tested. The client's elbow is in extension at the beginning of this test (Figure 11.49).

Test Movements
1. Shoulder is depressed.
2. Wrist and fingers are hyperextended.
3. Forearm is pronated, shoulder laterally rotated.
4. Elbow is flexed.
5. Shoulder is abducted.
6. Neck is contralaterally flexed.

Explanation: Tension is progressively added to the ulnar nerve through each successive movement. Because the ulnar nerve lies along the posterior elbow and the anterior wrist through Guyon's canal, the nerve is most stretched when the elbow is flexed and the wrist and fingers are hyperextended. This test requires shoulder abduction, as in ULNT #1, and provides more tension on the ulnar nerve. The test may be contraindicated for a client with shoulder instability.

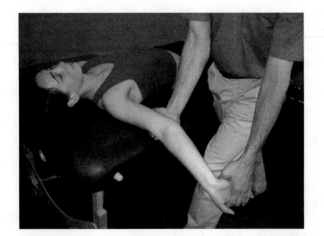

Figure 11.46 Final position for ULNT #1, median nerve bias.

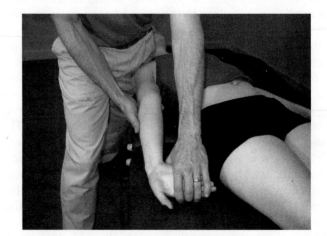

Figure 11.47 Final position for ULNT #2, median nerve bias.

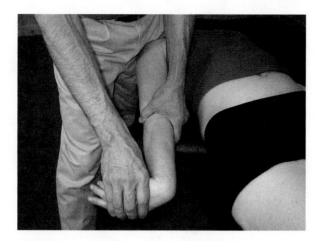

Figure 11.48 Final position for ULNT #3, radial nerve bias.

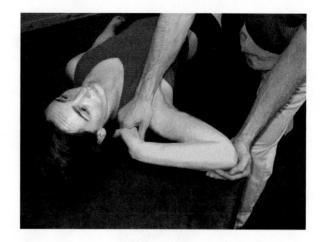

Figure 11.49 Final position for ULNT #4, ulnar nerve bias.

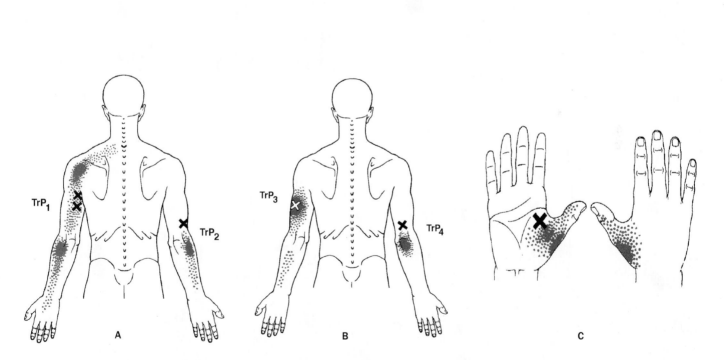

Figure 11.50 Myofascial trigger point referral patterns: Triceps brachii (A, B), Adductor pollicis (C). (Images courtesy of Mediclip, copyright 1998 Williams & Wilkins. All rights reserved).

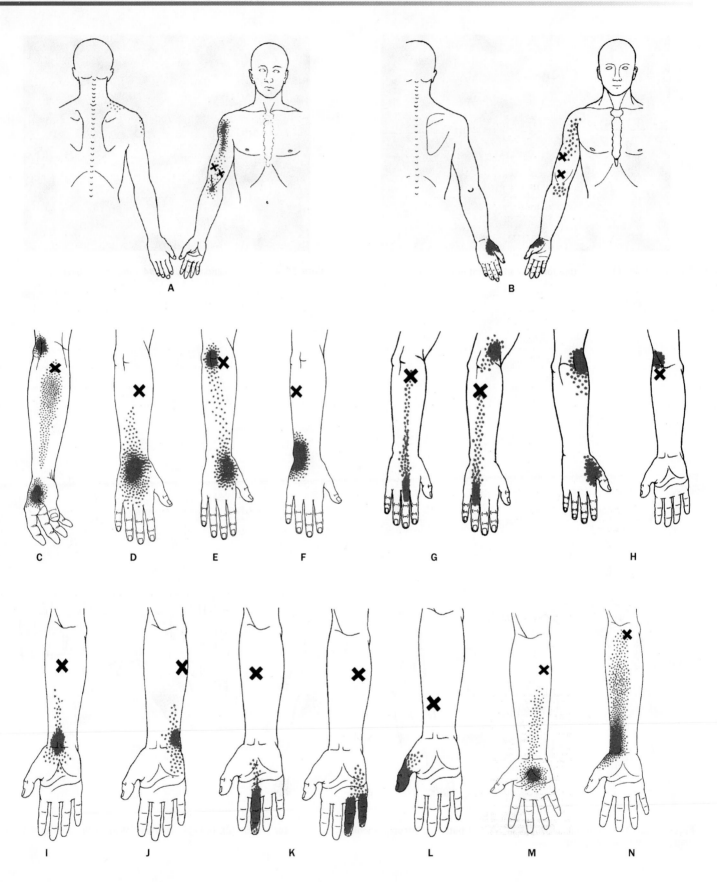

Figure 11.51 Myofascial trigger point referral patterns: Biceps brachii (A), Brachialis (B), Brachioradialis (C), Extensor carpi radialis brevis (D), Extensor carpi radialis longus (E), Extensor carpi ulnaris (F), Extensor digitorum (G), Supinator (H), Flexor carpi radialis (I), Flexor carpi ulnaris (J), Flexor digitorum profundus & superficialis (K), Flexor pollicis longus (L), Palmaris longus (M), Pronator teres (N). (Images courtesy of Mediclip, copyright 1998 Williams & Wilkins. All rights reserved).

TABLE 1 WEAKNESS WITH MANUAL RESISTIVE TEST AND POSSIBLE NERVE INVOLVEMENT

Muscle	Resisted Action	Possible nerve involvement if action weak
Abductor pollicis brevis	Thumb abduction	Median (C7-C8)
Abductor pollicis longus	Thumb abduction	Radial (C7-C8)
Adductor pollicis	Thumb adduction	Ulnar (C8-T1)
Anconeus	Elbow extension	Radial (C6-C8)
Biceps brachii	Elbow flexion	Musculocutaneous (C5-C6)
Brachialis	Elbow flexion	Musculocutaneous (C5-C6)
Brachioradialis	Elbow flexion	Radial (C5-C6)
Extensor carpi radialis brevis	Wrist extension	Radial (C7-C8)
Extensor carpi radialis longus	Wrist extension	Radial (C6-C7)
Extensor carpi ulnaris	Wrist extension	Radial (C7-C8)
Extensor digitorum	Finger extension (MCP joint)	Radial (C7-C8)
Extensor pollicis brevis	Thumb extension	Radial (C7-C8)
Extensor pollicis longus	Thumb extension	Radial (C7-C8)
Flexor carpi radialis	Wrist flexion	Median (C6-C7)
Flexor carpi ulnaris	Wrist flexion	Ulnar (C7-T1)
Flexor digitorum profundus	Finger flexion (DIP joint)	Median (C8-T1)
Flexor digitorum superficialis	Finger flexion (PIP joint)	Median (C8-T1)
Flexor pollicis longus	Thumb flexion	Median (C7-C8)
Palmaris longus	Wrist flexion	Median (C7-C8)
Pronator quadratus	Forearm pronation	Median (C7-C8)
Pronator teres	Forearm pronation	Median (C7-C8)
Supinator	Forearm supination	Radial (C6-C7)
Triceps brachii	Elbow extension	Radial (C6-C8)

TABLE 2 JOINTS, ASSOCIATED MOTIONS, PLANES OF MOTION IN ANATOMICAL POSITION, AXIS OF ROTATION, AND AVERAGE ROM				
Joint	Motion	Plane of Motion	Axis of Rotation	Avg. ROM (degrees)
Elbow	Flexion	Sagittal	Medial-lateral	150
	Extension	Sagittal	Medial-lateral	*
Forearm	Pronation	Transverse	Vertical	80
	Supination	Transverse	Vertical	80
Wrist	Flexion	Sagittal	Medial-lateral	80
	Extension	Sagittal	Medial-lateral	70
	Radial Deviation	Frontal	Anterior-posterior	20
	Ulnar Deviation	Frontal	Anterior-posterior	30
Thumb (CMC)	Flexion	Frontal	Anterior-posterior	15 (CMC & MCP)
	Extension	Frontal	Anterior-posterior	20 (CMC & MCP)
	Abduction	Sagittal	Medial-lateral	70 (CMC & MCP)
	Adduction	Sagittal	Medial-lateral	*
Thumb (MCP)	Flexion	Frontal	Anterior-posterior	15 (CMC & MCP)
	Extension	Frontal	Anterior-posterior	20 (CMC & MCP)
	Abduction	Sagittal	Medial-lateral	70 (CMC & MCP)
	Adduction	Sagittal	Medial-lateral	*
Thumb (IP)	Flexion	Frontal	Anterior-posterior	80
	Extension	Frontal	Anterior-posterior	*
Finger (MCP)	Flexion	Sagittal	Medial-lateral	90
	Extension	Sagittal	Medial-lateral	30
	Abduction	Frontal	Anterior-posterior	*
	Adduction	Frontal	Anterior-posterior	*
Finger (PIP)	Flexion	Sagittal	Medial-lateral	100
	Extension	Sagittal	Medial-lateral	*
Finger (DIP)	Flexion	Sagittal	Medial-lateral	85-90
	Extension	Sagittal	Medial-lateral	*

*Average range-of-motion values are either 0 or not usually calculated

References

1. Cyriax J. Textbook of Orthopaedic Medicine Volume One: Diagnosis of Soft Tissue Lesions. Vol 1. 8th ed. London: Bailliere Tindall; 1982.
2. Hislop H, Montgomery J. Daniels and Worthingham's Muscle Testing. Philadelphia: W.B. Saunders; 2002.
3. Berryman Reese N, Bandy WD. Joint Range of Motion and Muscle Length Testing. Philadelphia: W.B. Saunders Co.; 2002.
4. Neumann DA. Kinesiology of the Musculoskeletal System. St. Louis: Mosby; 2002.
5. Kendall F, Kendall-McCreary E, Geise-Provance P. Muscles: Testing and Function. 4th ed. Baltimore: Williams & Wilkins; 1993.
6. Shaffer K, Shaffer J. Dupuytren Contracture.

eMedicine [web page]. 4-28-04. Available at: www.emedicine.com. Accessed February 7, 2005.
7. Ravid M, Dinai Y, Sohar E. Dupuytren's disease in diabetes mellitus. Acta Diabetol Lat. May-Aug 1977;14(3-4):170-174.
8. Attali P, Ink O, Pelletier G, et al. Dupuytren's contracture, alcohol consumption, and chronic liver disease. Arch Intern Med. Jun 1987;147(6):1065-1067.
9. Burge P, Hoy G, Regan P, Milne R. Smoking, alcohol and the risk of Dupuytren's contracture. J Bone Joint Surg Br. Mar 1997;79(2):206-210.
10. Benson LS, Williams CS, Kahle M. Dupuytren's contracture. J Am Acad Orthop Surg. Jan-Feb 1998;6(1):24-35.
11. McFarlane RM. On the origin and spread

Reference Table for Condition Assessment

This table lists a number of pathological conditions along the left-hand column. The top of the table lists common evaluation procedures. A ◆ in the box associated with a pathological condition and an evaluation procedure indicates the procedure is commonly used to identify that pathology. A ● in the box associated with the condition and a range-of-motion or resistance test, indicates pain is likely with that test for that pathology. Conditions are listed alphabetically.

TABLE 3 REFERENCE TABLE FOR CONDITION ASSESSMENT

	AROM	PROM	MRT	Elbow flexion test	Finklestein test	Froment's sign	Golfer's elbow test	Phalen's test	Pinch grip test	Pronator teres test	Tennis elbow test	Tethered median nerve stress test	Tinel's sign	ULNT #1	ULNT #2	ULNT #3	ULNT #4
Carpal Tunnel Syndrome	●	●						◆	◆			◆	◆	◆	◆		
Cubital Tunnel Syndrome	●	●		◆		◆							◆				◆
De Quervain's Tenosynovitis	●	●	●		◆												
Ganglion Cyst	●	●	●														
Guyon's Canal Syndrome	●	●				◆							◆				◆
Lateral Epicondylitis	●	●	●								◆						
Medial Epicondylitis	●	●	●				◆										
Muscle Strains	●	●	●				◆				◆						
Muscular Hypertonicity	●	●															
Nerve Compression & Tension	●	●		◆		◆		◆	◆	◆		◆	◆	◆	◆	◆	◆
Olecranon Bursitis	●	●															
Pronator Teres Syndrome	●	●						◆	◆				◆	◆	◆		
Radial Tunnel Syndrome	●	●														◆	
Trigger Finger	●	●	●														

of Dupuytren's disease. J Hand Surg [Am]. 2002;27(3):385-390.

12. Zerajic D, Finsen V. Dupuytren's disease in Bosnia and Herzegovina. An epidemiological study. BMC Musculoskelet Disord. Mar 29 2004;5(1):10.

13. Silman AJ, Pearson JE. Epidemiology and genetics of rheumatoid arthritis. Arthritis Res. 2002;4 Suppl 3:S265-272.

14. Gabriel SE, Crowson CS, O'Fallon WM. The epidemiology of rheumatoid arthritis in Rochester, Minnesota, 1955-1985. Arthritis Rheum. Mar 1999;42(3):415-420.

15. Lee DM, Weinblatt ME. Rheumatoid arthritis. Lancet. Sep 15 2001;358(9285):903-911.

16. Rattray F, Ludwig L. Clinical Massage Therapy: Understanding, Assessing and Treating over 70 Conditions. Toronto: Talus Incorporated; 2000.

17. Neumeister M, Nguyen M. Rheumatoid Hand. eMedicine [web page]. 11-17-2004. Available at: www.emedicine.com. Accessed February 7, 2005.

18. Jacobs JL. Hand and Wrist. In: Richardson J, Iglarsh ZA, eds. Clinical Orthopaedic Physical Therapy. Philadelphia: W.B. Saunders; 1994.

19. King R. Rheumatoid Arthritis. eMedicine [web page]. 12-28-2004. Available at: www.emedicine.com. Accessed February 7, 2005.

20. Symmons DP, Bankhead CR, Harrison BJ, et al. Blood transfusion, smoking, and obesity as risk factors for the development of rheumatoid arthritis: results from a primary care-based incident case-control study in Norfolk, England. Arthritis Rheum. Nov 1997;40(11):1955-1961.

21. Uhlig T, Hagen KB, Kvien TK. Current tobacco smoking, formal education, and the risk of

rheumatoid arthritis. J Rheumatol. Jan 1999;26(1):47-54.

22. Shichikawa K, Inoue K, Hirota S, et al. Changes in the incidence and prevalence of rheumatoid arthritis in Kamitonda, Wakayama, Japan, 1965-1996. Ann Rheum Dis. Dec 1999;58(12):751-756.

23. Ferucci ED, Templin DW, Lanier AP. Rheumatoid arthritis in American Indians and Alaska Natives: A review of the literature. Semin Arthritis Rheum. Feb 2005;34(4):662-667.

24. Templin DW, Boyer GS, Lanier AP, et al. Rheumatoid arthritis in Tlingit Indians: clinical characterization and HLA associations. J Rheumatol. Jul 1994;21(7):1238-1244.

25. Werner R, Benjamin B. A Massage Therapist's Guide to Pathology. Baltimore: Williams & Wilkins; 1998.

26. Ariza-Ariza R, Mestanza-Peralta M, Cardiel MH. Omega-3 fatty acids in rheumatoid arthritis: an overview. Semin Arthritis Rheum. Jun 1998;27(6):366-370.

27. Disabella VN. Lateral Epicondylitis. eMedicine. 10-26-2004. Available at: www.emedicine.com. Accessed January 30, 2005.

28. Hong QN, Durand MJ, Loisel P. Treatment of lateral epicondylitis: where is the evidence? Joint Bone Spine. Sep 2004;71(5):369-373.

29. Jobe FW, Ciccotti MG. Lateral and Medial Epicondylitis of the Elbow. J Am Acad Orthop Surg. 1994;2(1):1-8.

30. Noteboom T, Cruver R, Keller J, Kellogg B, Nitz AJ. Tennis elbow: a review. J Orthop Sports Phys Ther. 1994;19(6):357-366.

31. Kraushaar BS, Nirschl RP. Tendinosis of the elbow (tennis elbow). Clinical features and findings of histological, immunohistochemical, and electron microscopy studies. J Bone Joint Surg Am. 1999;81(2):259-278.

32. Nirschl RP. Elbow tendinosis/tennis elbow. Clin Sports Med. 1992;11(4):851-870.

33. Khan KM, Cook JL, Maffulli N, Kannus P. Where is the pain coming from in tendinopathy? It may be biochemical, not only structural, in origin. Br J Sports Med. 2000;34(2):81-83.

34. Goguin JP, Rush, Fr. Lateral epicondylitis. What is it really? Current Orthopedics. 2003;17:386-389.

35. Boyer MI, Hastings H, 2nd. Lateral tennis elbow: "Is there any science out there?" J Shoulder Elbow Surg. Sep-Oct 1999;8(5):481-491.

36. Leach RE, Miller JK. Lateral and medial epicondylitis of the elbow. Clin Sports Med. Apr 1987;6(2):259-272.

37. Greenbaum B, Itamura J, Vangsness CT, Tibone J, Atkinson R. Extensor carpi radialis brevis. An anatomical analysis of its origin. J Bone Joint Surg Br. 1999;81(5):926-929.

38. Kumar VS, Shetty AA, Ravikumar KJ, Fordyce MJ. Tennis elbow-outcome following the Garden procedure: A retrospective study. J Orthop Surg (Hong Kong). Dec 2004;12(2):226-229.

39. Haahr JP, Andersen JH. Physical and psychosocial risk factors for lateral epicondylitis: a population based case-referent study. Occup Environ Med. May 2003;60(5):322-329.

40. Ono Y, Nakamura R, Shimaoka M, et al. Epicondylitis among cooks in nursery schools. Occup Environ Med. Mar 1998;55(3):172-179.

41. Stockard AR. Elbow injuries in golf. J Am Osteopath Assoc. Sep 2001;101(9):509-516.

42. Simons DG. Review of enigmatic MTrPs as a common cause of enigmatic musculoskeletal pain and dysfunction. J Electromyogr Kinesiol. 2004;14(1):95-107.

43. Dawson D, Hallett M, Wilbourn A. Entrapment Neuropathies. 3rd ed. Philadelphia: Lippincott-Raven; 1999.

44. Knebel PT, Avery DW, Gebhardt TL, et al. Effects of the forearm support band on wrist extensor muscle fatigue. J Orthop Sports Phys Ther. 1999;29(11):677-685.

45. Gehlsen GM, Ganion LR, Helfst R. Fibroblast responses to variation in soft tissue mobilization pressure. Med Sci Sport Exercise. 1999;31(4):531-535.

46. Plancher KD, Halbrecht J, Lourie GM. Medial and lateral epicondylitis in the athlete. Clin Sports Med. Apr 1996;15(2):283-305.

47. Grana W. Medial epicondylitis and cubital tunnel syndrome in the throwing athlete. Clin Sports Med. 2001;20(3):541-548.

48. Almekinders LC, Temple JD. Etiology, Diagnosis, and Treatment of Tendinitis - An Analysis of the Literature. Med Sci Sport Exercise. 1998;30(8):1183-1190.

49. Ciccotti MC, Schwartz MA, Ciccotti MG. Diagnosis and treatment of medial epicondylitis of the elbow. Clin Sports Med. Oct 2004;23(4):693-705, xi.

50. Chen FS, Rokito AS, Jobe FW. Medial elbow problems in the overhead-throwing athlete. J Am Acad Orthop Surg. 2001;9(2):99-113.

51. Descatha A, Leclerc A, Chastang JF, Roquelaure Y. Medial epicondylitis in occupational settings: prevalence, incidence and associated risk factors. J Occup Environ Med. Sep 2003;45(9):993-1001.

52. Salzman KL, Lillegard WA, Butcher JD. Upper extremity bursitis. Am Fam Physician. 1997;56(7):1797-1806, 1811-1792.

53. Ho G, Jr., Tice AD, Kaplan SR. Septic bursitis in the prepatellar and olecranon bursae: an analysis of 25 cases. Ann Intern Med. Jul 1978;89(1):21-27.

54. Senecal L, Leblanc M. Olecranon bursitis in chronic haemodialysis patients. Nephrol Dial Transplant. Sep 2001;16(9):1956-1957.

55. Zimmermann B, 3rd, Mikolich DJ, Ho G, Jr. Septic bursitis. Semin Arthritis Rheum. Jun 1995;24(6):391-410.

56. McFarland EG, P. M, Queale WS, Cosgarea AJ. Olecranon and prepatellar bursitis. Physician Sportsmed. 2000;28(3).

57. Reilly JP, Nicholas JA. The chronically inflamed bursa. Clin Sports Med. Apr 1987;6(2):345-370.

58. Bozentka DJ. Cubital tunnel syndrome pathophysiology. Clin Orthop. 1998(351):90-94.

59. Miller RG. The cubital tunnel syndrome: diagnosis and precise localization. Ann Neurol. 1979;6(1):56-59.

60. Butler D. Mobilisation of the Nervous System. London: Churchill Livingstone; 1991.

61. Verheyden JR, Palmer AK. Cubital Tunnel Syndrome. eMedicine. December 18, 2002. Available at: www.emedicine.com. Accessed January 30, 2005.

62. Childress HM. Recurrent ulnar-nerve dislocation at the elbow. Clin Orthop. May 1975(108):168-173.

63. Upton AR, McComas AJ. The double crush in nerve entrapment syndromes. Lancet. Aug 18 1973;2(7825):359-362.

64. Wadsworth TG. The external compression syndrome of the ulnar nerve at the cubital tunnel. Clin Orthop. 1977(124):189-204.

65. Clark CB. Cubital tunnel syndrome. Jama. 1979;241(8):801-802.

66. Buehler MJ, Thayer DT. The elbow flexion test. A clinical test for the cubital tunnel syndrome. Clin Orthop. 1988(233):213-216.

67. Novak CB, Lee GW, Mackinnon SE, Lay L. Provocative testing for cubital tunnel syndrome. J Hand Surg [Am]. 1994;19(5):817-820.

68. Wertsch JJ, Melvin J. Median nerve anatomy and entrapment syndromes: a review. Arch Phys Med Rehabil. Dec 1982;63(12):623-627.

69. Fuss FK, Wurzl GH. Median nerve entrapment. Pronator teres syndrome. Surgical anatomy and correlation with symptom patterns. Surg Radiol Anat. 1990;12(4):267-271.

70. Tulwa N, Limb D, Brown RF. Median nerve compression within the humeral head of pronator teres. J Hand Surg [Br]. 1994;19(6):709-710.

71. Nebot-Cegarra J, Perez-Berruezo J, Reina de la Torre F. Variations of the pronator teres muscle: predispositional role to median nerve entrapment. Arch Anat Histol Embryol. 1991;74:35-45.

72. Stal M, Hagert CG, Moritz U. Upper extremity nerve involvement in Swedish female machine milkers. Am J Ind Med. 1998;33(6):551-559.

73. Gessini L, Jandolo B, Pietrangeli A. The pronator teres syndrome. Clinical and electrophysiological features in six surgically verified cases. J Neurosurg Sci. 1987;31(1):1-5.

74. Olehnik WK, Manske PR, Szerzinski J. Median nerve compression in the proximal forearm. J Hand Surg [Am]. 1994;19(1):121-126.

75. Hill NA, Howard FM, Huffer BR. The incomplete anterior interosseous nerve syndrome. J Hand Surg [Am]. Jan 1985;10(1):4-16.

76. Mysiew WJ, Colachis SC, 3rd. The pronator syndrome. An evaluation of dynamic maneuvers for improving electrodiagnostic sensitivity. Am J Phys Med Rehabil. 1991;70(5):274-277.

77. Hartz CR, Linscheid RL, Gramse RR, Daube JR. The pronator teres syndrome: compressive neuropathy of the median nerve. J Bone Joint Surg Am. 1981;63(6):885-890.

78. Rosenbaum R. Disputed radial tunnel syndrome. Muscle Nerve. 1999;22(7):960-967.

79. Younge DH, Moise P. The radial tunnel syndrome. Int Orthop. Oct 1994;18(5):268-270.

80. Erak S, Day R, Wang A. The role of supinator in the pathogenesis of chronic lateral elbow pain: a biomechanical study. J Hand Surg [Br]. Oct 2004;29(5):461-464.

81. Mileti J, Largacha M, O'Driscoll SW. Radial tunnel syndrome caused by ganglion cyst: treatment by arthroscopic cyst decompression. Arthroscopy. May 2004;20(5):e39-44.

82. Slater R. Carpal tunnel syndrome: current concepts. Journal of Southern Orthopedic Association. 1999;8(3).

83. Preston DC. Distal median neuropathies. Neurol Clin. 1999;17(3):407-424, v.

84. Becker J, Nora DB, Gomes I, et al. An evaluation of gender, obesity, age and diabetes mellitus as risk factors for carpal tunnel syndrome. Clin Neurophysiol. Sep 2002;113(9):1429-1434.

85. McDiarmid M, Oliver M, Ruser J, Gucer P. Male and female rate differences in carpal tunnel syndrome injuries: personal attributes or job tasks? Environ Res. 2000;83(1):23-32.

86. Hirano M, Kuroda K, Kunimoto M, Tanohata K, Inoue K. [A case of carpal tunnel syndrome caused by a ganglion cyst--diagnosis and follow-up study with magnetic resonance imaging]. Rinsho Shinkeigaku. Jan 1995;35(1):80-82.

87. LaBan MM, Friedman NA, Zemenick GA. "Tethered" median nerve stress test in chronic carpal tunnel syndrome. Arch Phys Med Rehabil. 1986;67(11):803-804.

88. LaBan MM, MacKenzie JR, Zemenick GA. Anatomic observations in carpal tunnel syndrome as they relate to the tethered median nerve stress test. Arch Phys Med Rehabil. 1989;70(1):44-46.

89. Franzblau A, Rock CL, Werner RA, Albers JW, Kelly MP, Johnston EC. The relationship of vitamin B6 status to median nerve function and carpal tunnel syndrome among active industrial workers. J Occup Environ Med. May 1996;38(5):485-491.

90. Keniston RC, Nathan PA, Leklem JE, Lockwood RS. Vitamin B6, vitamin C, and carpal tunnel syndrome. A cross-sectional study of 441 adults. J Occup Environ Med. Oct 1997;39(10):949-959.

91. D'Arcy CA, McGee S. The rational clinical

examination. Does this patient have carpal tunnel syndrome? Jama. 2000;283(23):3110-3117.

92. Szabo RM, Slater RR, Jr., Farver TB, Stanton DB, Sharman WK. The value of diagnostic testing in carpal tunnel syndrome. J Hand Surg [Am]. 1999;24(4):704-714.

93. Redmond MD, Rivner MH. False positive electrodiagnostic tests in carpal tunnel syndrome. Muscle Nerve. 1988;11(5):511-518.

94. Kuhlman KA, Hennessey WJ. Sensitivity and specificity of carpal tunnel syndrome signs. Am J Phys Med Rehabil. 1997;76(6):451-457.

95. Gerr F, Letz R. The sensitivity and specificity of tests for carpal tunnel syndrome vary with the comparison subjects. J Hand Surg [Br]. 1998;23(2):151-155.

96. Gunnarsson LG, Amilon A, Hellstrand P, Leissner P, Philipson L. The diagnosis of carpal tunnel syndrome. Sensitivity and specificity of some clinical and electrophysiological tests. J Hand Surg [Br]. 1997;22(1):34-37.

97. Verdon ME. Overuse syndromes of the hand and wrist. Prim Care. 1996;23(2):305-319.

98. Fertl E, Wober C, Zeitlhofer J. The serial use of two provocative tests in the clinical diagnosis of carpal tunel syndrome. Acta Neurol Scand. 1998;98(5):328-332.

99. Edwards A. Phalen's test with carpal compression: testing in diabetics for the diagnosis of carpal tunnel syndrome. Orthopedics. May 2002;25(5):519-520.

100. Werner RA, Bir C, Armstrong TJ. Reverse Phalen's maneuver as an aid in diagnosing carpal tunnel syndrome. Arch Phys Med Rehabil. Jul 1994;75(7):783-786.

101. Kuschner SH, Ebramzadeh E, Johnson D, Brien WW, Sherman R. Tinel's sign and Phalen's test in carpal tunnel syndrome. Orthopedics. Nov 1992;15(11):1297-1302.

102. Raudino F. Tethered median nerve stress test in the diagnosis of carpal tunnel syndrome. Electromyogr Clin Neurophysiol. 2000;40(1):57-60.

103. Sucher BM. Myofascial release of carpal tunnel syndrome. J Am Osteopath Assoc. 1993;93(1):92-94, 100-101.

104. Nahra ME, Bucchieri JS. Ganglion cysts and other tumor related conditions of the hand and wrist. Hand Clin. Aug 2004;20(3):249-260, v.

105. Kouris G, Derman G. Ganglion Cyst. eMedicine.

April 30, 2004. Available at: www.emedicine.com. Accessed October 14, 2004.

106. Schena A, Terrill RQ. Ganglions. eMedicine. 7-23-2004. Available at: www.emedicine.com. Accessed Jaunary 30, 2005.

107. Dodge LD, Brown RL, Niebauer JJ, McCarroll HR, Jr. The treatment of mucous cysts: long-term follow-up in sixty-two cases. J Hand Surg [Am]. Nov 1984;9(6):901-904.

108. Elias DA, Lax MJ, Anastakis DJ. Musculoskeletal images. Ganglion cyst of Guyon's canal causing ulnar nerve compression. Can J Surg. Oct 2001;44(5):331-332.

109. Shu N, Uchio Y, Ryoke K, Yamamoto S, Oae K, Ochi M. Atypical compression of the deep branch of the ulnar nerve in Guyon's canal by a ganglion. Case report. Scand J Plast Reconstr Surg Hand Surg. Jun 2000;34(2):181-183.

110. Capitani D, Beer S. Handlebar palsy--a compression syndrome of the deep terminal (motor) branch of the ulnar nerve in biking. J Neurol. Oct 2002;249(10):1441-1445.

111. Noth J, Dietz V, Mauritz KH. Cyclist's palsy: Neurological and EMG study in 4 cases with distal ulnar lesions. J Neurol Sci. Jul 1980;47(1):111-116.

112. Corrigan B, Maitland GD. Musculoskeletal and Sports Injuries. Oxford: Butterworth Heinemann; 1994.

113. Mahakkanukrauh P, Mahakkanukrauh C. Incidence of a septum in the first dorsal compartment and its effects on therapy of de Quervain's disease. Clin Anat. 2000;13(3):195-198.

114. Nagaoka M, Matsuzaki H, Suzuki T. Ultrasonographic examination of de Quervain's disease. J Orthop Sci. 2000;5(2):96-99.

115. Sampson SP, Badalamente MA, Hurst LC, Seidman J. Pathobiology of the human A1 pulley in trigger finger. J Hand Surg [Am]. Jul 1991;16(4):714-721.

116. Moore JS. Flexor tendon entrapment of the digits (trigger finger and trigger thumb). J Occup Environ Med. May 2000;42(5):526-545.

117. Rayan GM. Distal stenosing tenosynovitis. J Hand Surg [Am]. Nov 1990;15(6):973-975.

118. Saldana MJ. Trigger digits: diagnosis and treatment. J Am Acad Orthop Surg. Jul-Aug 2001;9(4):246-252.

119. Foye PM, Stitik TP. Trigger Finger. eMedicine. 6-14-2004. Available at: www.emedicine.com. Accessed February 14, 2005.

Glossary

Accessory Motion— motion that is within the anatomical limits of the joint's range, but is achieved by passive movement of the joint past the point where active motion stops

Apprehension sign—visible guarding or resistance to motion or position, demonstrated by facial expression or limited movement.

Avulsion— tearing of an attachment (usually a tendon) away from the bone.

Axial load— a force applied along the long axis of a bone, group of bones, or other rigid structure.

Axis of rotation— the imaginary line around which any object or bone segment rotates. The axis of rotation is perpendicular to the plane in which movement occurs.

Biomechanics— the branch of science that studies the application of principles of mechanical physics to living systems.

Bucket-handle tear— tear in cartilage tissue (usually meniscus or labrum) where the outer rim is torn away from the reminder of the structure creating a shape that looks like the handle of a bucket.

Congenital— a condition that is present at birth or related to heredity.

Contracture— permanent or semi-permanent muscle contraction due to spasm or paralysis.

Cutaneous innervation— region of skin that is supplied by a single peripheral nerve.

Dermatome— region of skin innervated by fibers from a single nerve root.

Dislocation— displacement of a bone or other body part from its normal position.

Double crush— pressure on a nerve in more than one location.

Dysesthesia— impairment of the sensation of touch.

Ecchymosis— movement of blood from ruptured blood vessels into the subcutaneous tissues. A synonym for bruising.

Enthesitis— irritation or inflammation of the attachment site of a tissue (usually ligament or tendon) into bone.

Exostosis— calcium build up at the site of mechanical stress on a bone. Also called a bone spur.

Fibrosis— formation of excess fibrous connection of adjacent tissues.

Foramen— opening or orifice, usually in a bone.

Ground reaction force— force that is equal in magnitude and opposite in direction to the force that the body exerts on a supporting surface.

Hyperesthesia— exaggerated sensitivity to touch.

Laxity— excess mobility, usually associated with joint disorders.

Lesion— localized pathological change in body tissue.

Nociceptors— neurological receptors sensitive to pain sensations.

Orthotic— artificial support or brace, for example shoe inserts that correct faulty biomechanics.

Osteophytes— small, abnormal bony growth.

Paresthesia— sensations of pins and needles resulting from neurological pathology.

Proprioception— sensations of movement or spatial

orientation resulting from sensory information generated within the body.

Reciprocal inhibition— a principle suggesting that a muscle is neurologically prevented from achieving its full contraction stimulus while its antagonist is in a degree of contraction.

Reflex muscular inhibition— neurologically mediated reduction in muscle contraction strength or function as a direct result of pain.

Subcutaneous— located beneath the skin.

Subluxation— partial or incomplete joint dislocation.

Sulcus— indentation or groove in the contour of a body region.

Torque— the tendency of a force to produce rotation about an axis. The magnitude of torque is related to the distance that the force is applied from the axis of rotation. The greater is the distance from the axis of rotation, the greater is the torque force.

Valgus— lateral deviation of the distal end of a bony segment.

Varus— medial deviation of the distal end of a bony segment.

Index

calcaneus, 54, 64, 75-76
capsule, 98, 224
cervical, 157-158, 186-187, 192, 196
compartment, 73, 75, 80-81, 84, 86, 118
cruciate ligament, 93, 101, 103, 126
drawer test, 93, 104-105, 125
drop of the tibia, 105
edge of the band, 112
femoral cutaneous nerve, 87, 122-123, 140, 147
fibers of the ITB, 111
innominate rotation test, 135-136
interosseous nerve, 15, 40, 260, 267-269
longitudinal ligament, 168-169, 193-194, 198-199, 201
pelvic rotation, 163, 166
sacroiliac ligaments, 142
shin splints, 55, 82-84, 89
talofibular ligament, 63
tibial
    artery, 73
    nerve, 73
tibiofibular ligaments, 66-67
tibiotalar, 65
vertebral structures, 134, 162, 164, 166-167, 191, 193
Postural
adaptation, 6, 169
alterations, 195
chain, 138
compensation, 97, 157, 185
dysfunctions, 98
evaluation, 9, 22
grid chart, 22, 157, 160, 185-186
muscles, 161-162, 186
overload, 37
re-education, 162
reference grid, 162
retraining, 100, 136, 158, 191, 215-216,
Prepatellar
bursa, 16, 117
bursitis, 286, 93, 117, 125, 127
Prescription medication, 197
Previous
injury, 22, 38, 68
medical history, 21
medications, 80
surgeries, 155
PRICE, 64, 67, 263
Primary
action, , 39, 121, 141, 222, 225
anti-gravity muscles, 9
frozen shoulder, 218
impingement, 224
osteoarthritis, 45, 47
weight-bearing structure, 161
Prior injury, 233
Progressive degeneration, 223
Prolapse/extrusion, 168
Proliferation of fibrous tissue, 257
Proliferative phase, 257
Pronation, 39, 49-51, 55-57, 70, 247-248, 250-251, 253-254, 259, 261, 266-268, 283-284
Pronator
quadratus, 251, 279, 283
syndrome, 265, 287

teres
    syndrome, 247, 261-262, 265-266, 269, 272, 275, 285, 287
    test, 247, 266-267, 285
Prone knee bend test, 153, 171-172, 177
Proper shock absorption, 54, 162
Proprioception, 42, 98
Proprioceptors, 235
Protective spasm, 103
Protruding disc, 199
Proximal
musculotendinous junction, 121
nerve compression, 74, 140, 263
neuropathy, 82, 84-85
vascular entrapment, 82
Proximity of sensitive neurological structures, 168
Pulmonary embolism, 118
Pulposus, 6, 14, 153, 162-163, 165, 167-168, 170, 174, 177, 181, 185, 192, 198, 201, 206
Pump bump, 76
Push-off, 68, 70

Q
Quadratus femoris, 132, 149-150
Quadriceps
atrophy, 109, 116
femoris, 115, 126
retinaculum, 108-110
rupture, 118
strains, 121
tendon, 108, 115
Quality of pain, 21, 116
Quebec Task Force, 193, 207

R
Radial
collateral, 268
nerve, 15, 190, 238-239, 267-269, 276, 278-281
neuropathy, 260
pulse, 189-190
Tunnel Syndrome, 247, 260, 267-269, 285, 287
Radial, 15, 190, 238-239, 267-269, 276, 278-281,
Radiculopathies, 69, 71, 85, 122, 147, 238, 278
Radiographic evaluation, 245
Raynaud's syndrome, 191
Recent medications, 78
Reciprocal inhibition, 161, 186-187, 215
Rectus
abdominis, 155, 176-177
capitis posterior minor, 183, 205
femoris, 9, 96, 121-125, 132, 134-136, 149-150
Recurrent
hamstring strains, 120
nerve pain, 256
Redness, 22, 38, 76, 117, 195, 221, 234, 262
Referral
pattern, 8-9, 203
zones, 215
Reflex muscular inhibition, 30, 52, 64, 66-67, 78, 95, 102, 104, 109-110, 114, 116, 132, 146, 155, 167, 184, 196, 213, 219, 222-223, 225, 227, 229, 237, 252, 260-261, 276-277,
Region of
cutaneous innervation, 40, 85, 122, 147, 238, 270, 278

analysis, 22, 78, 135, 158

indicators, 22, 83, 143, 264, 266

VMO, 109, 111

Volar ganglions, 273

W

WAD, 192-197, 202, 207

Wall chart grid, 22

Wallerian degeneration, 14

Wear pattern, 54, 56-57, 83

Wearing

high-heeled shoes, 68, 76, 161

narrow toe-box shoes, 68

of a heavy knapsack, 189

orthotics, 58

Weight-bearing phase, 56, 111

Whiplash-Associated Disorders, 193, 207

Width of the wrist, 271

Windlass mechanism, 70-71, 91

Work-related musculoskeletal disorders, 261

Wright Abduction Test, 181, 189-190, 200

Wrist

pain, 35

splints, 272, 275

Wry neck, 197

X

X-ray

procedures, 31

viewing, 32

Y

Yes-no questions, 21

Z

Zygapophysial, 158, 164, 178, 186, 191, 206-207